Research and Development in
Clinical Nursing Practice

Research and Development in Clinical Nursing Practice

Edited by

Brenda Roe

Honorary Senior Research Fellow, Institute of Human Ageing,
University of Liverpool

and

Christine Webb

Professor of Health Studies, University of Plymouth

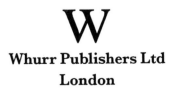

Whurr Publishers Ltd
London

© 1998 Whurr Publishers Ltd
First published 1998 by
Whurr Publishers Ltd
19b Compton Terrace, London N1 2UN, England

Reprinted 1999 and 2000

British Library Cataloguing in Publication Data
A catalogue record for this book is available from the
British Library.

ISBN 1 86156 057 5

Printed and bound in the UK by Athenaeum Press Ltd,
Gateshead, Tyne & Wear

Contents

Contributors

Francine M. Cheater MA (Hons), PhD, RGN. Senior Lecturer in Clinical Audit, Eli Lilly National Clinical Audit Centre, Department of General Practice and Primary Health Care, University of Leicester.

S. José Closs BSc (Hons), MPhil, PhD, RGN. Senior Lecturer in Nursing Research, School of Health, University of Hull.

Nicola J. Crichton BSc (Hons), MSc, PhD. Lecturer in Statistics and Research, Royal College of Nursing Institute, London.

Kathryn Getliffe BSc (Hons), MSc, PhD, DN Cert. Senior Lecturer, European Institute of Health and Medical Sciences, University of Surrey.

Crispin Jenkinson DPhil. Deputy Director, Health Services Research Unit, Department of Public Health and Primary Care, University of Oxford.

Ann McMahon BSc, MSc, RGN, RMN. RCN Research and Development Adviser, School of Nursing, Midwifery and Health Visiting, University of Manchester.

Carl May PhD. Senior Research Fellow, Department of General Practice, University of Manchester.

Anne Mulhall BSc, MSc, PhD. Independent Research and Training Consultant, West Cottage, Hook Hill Lane, Woking, Surrey GU22 OPT.

David Pontin BSc, MSc, RN, RSCN. Health Visiting Student, University of the West of England.

Sheila Rodgers BSc, MSc, RGN. Lecturer, Department of Nursing Studies, University of Edinburgh.

Brenda Roe BSc (Hons), MSc, PhD, RN. Honorary Senior Research Fellow, Institute of Human Ageing, University of Liverpool.

Kate Seers BSc (Hons), PhD, RGN. Senior Research Fellow, Royal College of Nursing Institute, Oxford.

Fahera Sindhu BSc, DPhil. Research Methodologist, National Audit Office, 157–197 Buckingham Palace Rd, Victoria, London SW1W 9SP.

David R. Thompson BSc, MA, PhD, RN, FRCN, AFBPsS. Professor of Nursing, School of Health, University of Hull.

Pat Turton PhD, RN, DN Tut Cert. 51 Great Clarendon St, Oxford OX2 6AX.

Heather Waterman Bsc (Hons), PhD, RGN, OND, DipN. Lecturer, School of Nursing, Midwifery and Health Visiting, University of Manchester.

Christine Webb PhD, RN, RNT. Professor of Health Studies, University of Plymouth.

Anne Williams PhD, RGN. Professor of Nursing, Department of Nursing, Midwifery and Health Care, University of Wales, Swansea.

Foreword

This book is unique. It is more than simply a research textbook. Rather than covering the range of research approaches and methods, it links research and development policy with the day-to-day practice of nursing. Up-to-date topics not previously found in research texts for nurses include evidence-based practice, systematic reviews and meta-analysis. The contributors include a wide variety of nurses and other researchers who provide a practical guide on how to conduct research using state-of-the-art techniques.

Previously this new material was only available in widely scattered sources such as journals and conference presentations. By synthesising the information in one readily available place, the authors have made accessible a wealth of detail so that practising nurses can readily use and benefit from its lessons.

Research, which was once a topic confined to academic circles, has now become part of nurses' everyday worlds and is vital to improving nursing practice. The Royal College of Nursing has always been at the forefront in promoting developments such as clinical audit, clinical guidelines and evidence-based nursing. Therefore I am delighted to recommend this book to nurses at a time when it has never been more vital to demonstrate that a rigorous research approach underlies nursing practice and that patient care benefits from nursing involvement in the research approaches and techniques featured in this book.

Christine Hancock
General Secretary
Royal College of Nursing

Preface

The topic of research and development (R and D) in clinical nursing practice is unique to this book. Many others have focused on research methods and their application for nurses, but none has yet specifically made links between state-of-the-art thinking in R and D policy for health services, nursing practice at the 'grassroots', and research methods. Slogans such as 'nursing must be a research-based profession' have been around for a long time, and more recently initiatives such as nursing development units (NDUs), quality assurance and evidence-based practice have moved to the forefront. These have placed nursing in a leadership position amongst health professions in taking seriously the promotion of rational care based on critical appraisal of past practices and the evaluation of innovations in care.

This book brings together key authors with a track record in R and D in clinical nursing practice or health services research and who are pioneers in taking forward R and D. The emphasis throughout the book is on reader-friendliness, by using accessible language and a wealth of illustrative examples drawn from clinical practice.

As the title states, the primary readership will be undergraduate and postgraduate nurses in all clinical specialties, along with purchasers and providers responsible for clinical development, evidence-based health care and clinical effectiveness. However, students and practitioners in other health care related professions such as physiotherapy, occupational therapy and social work will find a great deal to interest them and to relate to their own practice development and evaluation.

The book is divided into three sections. The first 'Background' section gives an overview of research in the context of nursing. The second section, 'Research Methods', is a detailed examination of a whole range of methods appropriate to health care research. Finally, the third section focuses on the 'Development of Clinical Practice'. Each chapter looks at theoretical matters, including definitions, strengths and weaknesses of its chosen topic or method, and illustrates its arguments with nursing-related examples. Rather than have a separate chapter or section on ethical issues, these run throughout the book as an interwoven theme. The aim in all chapters is to show how the topics discussed relate to everyday health care practice.

In Chapter 1 Brenda Roe gives an overview of R and D in clinical nursing practice, looking at its history both in the UK and USA. She notes the increasing emphasis on teaching research in nurse education programmes on both sides of the Atlantic, and most recently in Project 2000 courses in the UK. She links developments within nursing with policy development at the national level and the NHS R and D strategy. Thus the NDU 'movement' in the UK, the Conduct and Utilization of Research in Nursing project in the US, and the growth of approaches such as clinical guidelines are seen as ways of trying to overcome the barriers to considering research and its implementation in practice which have been so well documented. The most up-to-date concern is with evidence-based practice (EBP), and this is a theme that recurs many times throughout the book.

In Chapter 2 David Thompson considers whether it is 'art' or 'science' that predominates in nursing R and D. He asks questions about 'what is science' and believes that there has been a polarisation between art and science that mirrors a polarisation of quantitative and qualitative research methods. His conclusion is that everyone in health care needs to work together, both so that multi-disciplinary care becomes the norm but also so that research methods are chosen appropriately rather than on a polemical basis. Research is a moral activity requiring a balance between rigour and creativity in research practice.

Starting off the section on Research Methods, Anne Williams in Chapter 3 discusses qualitative research designs. Heather Waterman in Chapter 4 and Carl May in Chapter 5 continue the discussion of qualitative methods by writing very practically about methods of data collection and data analysis. Heather focuses on interviews and participant observation, using her own research experience to give essential down-to-earth guidance on mundane but essential matters such as equipment, planning the data collection session (including making sure you know how to get there!), and carrying out the method. She discusses the need for reflexivity in monitoring the data collection process, as well as considering emotional issues both for researchers and participants. She illustrates her chapter with examples from her research in ophthalmic nursing. Carl takes a similarly practical approach to qualitative data analysis, at the same time emphasising the importance of the creative aspect. He questions the use of automated techniques such as computer software and suggests that lists and grids may be better for organising data. He reminds readers that analysis begins in the planning stages and carries on through data collection, right to the presentation stage: in order to keep track of processes and thinking, a journal should be kept to provide a decision trail. He suggests a threefold approach to the 'serious business of analysis', using 'structure', 'agency' and 'discourse' as a framework and taking account of 'deviant' cases as well as sources of agreement among participants. In presenting research conclusions, he draws attention to the need to discuss ethical issues such as confidentiality and privacy, as well as the typicality of quoted examples and the research context. His emphasis on getting and staying organised throughout the research applies not only to qualitative but also quantitative research.

In Chapter 6 Fahera Sindhu looks at systematic reviews of the literature and meta-analyses. She distinguishes between different types of reviews, before focusing in depth on meta-analysis – its definition, evolution, uses and criticisms. A very clear flowchart gives step-by-step details of how to go about meta-analysis, including pitfalls that may be encountered.

With Chapter 7 by Kathy Getliffe on quantitative research designs, the book moves on to various aspects of quantitative research. Kathy explores the aims and purposes of quantitative research designs and the general principles, before considering different types of experimental and non-experimental designs. She emphasises that selection of an appropriate design is crucial and depends on whether the aim of the research is descriptive, explanatory, predictive or interventional.

In Chapter 8 Anne Mulhall continues the quantitative focus, with a discussion of methods of data collection. She sets the scene for the chapter by considering definitions of terms that are often confused, including paradigms, methodology and methods, and believes that, far from being boring, research methods are actually exciting! The methods considered in detail are observation, asking questions via questionnaires and interviews, and taking measurements, with each illustrated by clinical examples. Validity and reliability are also given attention, and ethical aspects of these methods are highlighted.

Health status measures and outcomes are the concern of Crispin Jenkinson in Chapter 9. He notes that one of the reasons for the recent concern with health status measures and outcomes is increasing recognition of the importance of patient perceptions in developing and evaluating health care. This type of measure is also increasingly being used in audit, cost-containment and prioritisation work. He gives an in-depth consideration of rigour in relation to outcome measures, illustrating this with varied examples and their benefits and limitations. He ends with the caution that more research is needed on the appropriateness, sensitivity and validity of these instruments with different categories of patients.

Statistical considerations and analysis are the focus taken by Nicola Crichton in Chapter 10. It can be very difficult to write about statistics in a way that both promotes understanding and holds the reader's attention, but Nicola's approach succeeds extremely well. She writes directly to readers and illustrates what she is saying with vivid examples from existing clinical nursing research. Using this approach, she explains about sampling, size and power calculation, graphical presentation of data and choice of statistical tests. Her section on confidence intervals and estimation of the size of effects is exemplary in its clarity. She ends with a call for larger studies in nursing research to strengthen the conclusions that can be drawn on the basis of statistical analysis.

Section 3 on the Development of Clinical Practice begins with Chapter 11, in which Ann McMahon discusses developing practice through research. She traces the influence of many government policy statements on research and development and links these with the nursing development 'movement' sponsored, among others, by the King's Fund and Department of Health. Other key influences in clinical practice development featured in the chapter are the Foundation of Nursing Studies and the broad range of initiatives and activities based on the Royal College of Nursing's Dynamic Quality Improvement Network (DQI) programme. Strategies to enable practice development through research are discussed, including journal clubs and action research. Ann concludes that nurses are professionally accountable for the development of their practice and for justifying this with research evidence. However, appropriate structures and resources are needed so that research-based practice developments can be spread throughout the service.

This development theme is continued by Sheila Rodgers in Chapter 12, writing about dissemination and utilisation of research findings. She describes the increasing importance of dissemination and utilisation questions in health service policies, and the growing concern with effectiveness, efficiency and evidence-based practice. Within nursing, she sees these as an important means for realising accountability. The chapter includes information on sources of information for research dissemination and utilisation, as well as discussion of the barriers to and influences on these. Sheila concludes that education and reading are crucial for nurses, as well as a sense of ownership and authority when introducing new practices. Ultimately, however, she believes that a culture shift is needed towards new ways of thinking and working towards evidence-based practice so that this becomes a way of life in nursing as well as other fields of health care work.

Chapter 13 on clinical guidelines and their role in the development of practice is written by Kate Seers. The chapter includes discussion on the research and other bases for guidelines development, how to evaluate guidelines, and why they may not always be adopted by practitioners. After describing various initiatives in guideline development, she concludes that it is essential that the implementation of guidelines is itself subject to evaluation both by practitioners and those for whom they care.

Developments in action research are the theme of Chapter 14 by Christine Webb, Pat Turton and David Pontin. After discussing different definitions and types of action research and its use in nursing, controversial issues emerging from growing experience of its use are examined. These include securing access and collaboration, questions of power and control in research, and ethical issues to do with informed consent and anonymity. The theme of rigour, which appears in many other chapters, is picked up again here. David Pontin's project evaluating nursing developments in an acute hospital and Pat Turton's work developing community nursing services for gay men with symptomatic HIV are given as examples of action research in very different nursing contexts. The chapter ends by claiming that action research is a flexible approach that can and should be adapted to develop practice in different health care settings.

Brenda Roe in Chapter 15 writes about evaluation research for developing health care and health services. She differentiates between evaluation and evaluation research, the criteria for the latter being pre-specification of goals or objectives and measurement of success in achieving these. She illustrates the importance of outcome measurement in nursing with two examples – a single case study and a randomised controlled trial. Evaluation is important at the level of health care for individuals and of overall health services, and Brenda shows how this can be done through a presentation of the examples of continence care – one of her own areas of specialist research and practice – as well as other topics. She concludes with a reminder that evaluation research uses systematic empirical approaches, and research designs and questions that measure outcomes of specific goals or objectives, and her examples show how this can be done.

Clinical audit and research, their similarities and differences, are the focus of Chapter 16 by Francine Cheater and José Closs. They define audit as aiming to ask 'Are we doing what we should?' whereas research asks 'What should we be doing?' In other words audit is concerned with the present and what is, while research deals with the future and what ought to be. Nevertheless there are links between the two and these are brought out in the detailed discussion in the chapter. Audit may also be part of wider quality initiatives such as total quality management (TQM). Indeed both research and audit are essential to achieving the highest standards in health.

Chapter 17, by Brenda Roe and Christine Webb, draws the themes of the book together and makes suggestions for the way forward for research and development in clinical nursing practice.

PART ONE: BACKGROUND

Chapter 1
Research and development in clinical nursing practice: an overview

Brenda Roe

Introduction

Research has been a key feature of the expansion and professionalisation of nursing within this century. The development and improvement of clinical nursing practice by either undertaking or using research has only featured since the Second World War. This chapter sets research and development (R and D) within clinical nursing practice in context and looks at the history of research in nursing within the UK and the USA by way of comparison. It goes on to look at key NHS research and development policies and their relationship to nursing. Recent recognition of the importance of development in health services and health care is covered and set in the context of development work within nursing, such as nursing development units and attempts to change nursing practice within clinical settings. Strengths and limitations of the early development work are explored and the need for rigorous evaluation examined. Finally research and development within clinical nursing practice are viewed in the present day and the scene is set for the chapters that follow.

Brief history of nursing research in the UK

Florence Nightingale systematically collected data in the clinical setting to inform the organisation and delivery of nursing care, and

3

was recognised as one of the first nurses to undertake and apply research. Following her death there was an absence of research in nursing practice for nearly a quarter of a century (1910–35) (Abdellah and Levine, 1965). Early research work in nursing in the United Kingdom was funded mainly by charitable organisations and attempted to investigate manpower planning and other resource issues, such as numbers of nursing staff required within hospitals following the end of the Second World War and the establishment of the NHS. Analysis of nursing work and the related tasks provides early examples of this research (Goddard, 1953; Menzies, 1959). A number of small-scale research studies in nursing were funded in 1968 by the Department of Health and Social Security. These studies had a clinical emphasis, examined the quality of nursing care and were published in a research series by the Royal College of Nursing (Department of Health, 1993a: 6). Since this time the Department has been the principal source of 'ring fenced' or protected funding for research into all aspects of nursing, midwifery and health visiting. The Department went on to fund two research units (the Nursing Education Research Unit, University of London and the Nursing Practice Research Unit, formerly at Northwick Park Hospital, Harrow, and latterly at the University of Surrey) along with directly commissioned research programmes and individual projects on nursing as well as research training studentships and fellowships specifically for nurses (Department of Health, 1993a: 6).

During the last two decades educational curricula have also been developed and now include teaching on research methods as well as the research evidence underpinning clinical practice (UKCC, 1986; Macleod Clark and Hockey, 1989: 6). Research has formed such a basic tenet in undergraduate and postgraduate education that nursing departments have been included in all three research assessment exercises undertaken by the Higher Education Funding Council for England (Times Higher Education Supplement, 1996).

Comparison with research in nursing in the United States

The development of research in nursing within the United States has followed a similar path to that within the United Kingdom but appeared to start in an organised way earlier, from 1900. Some of the early research work from 1900 to 1940 looked at education, partly due to the fact that nursing leaders undertook graduate and postgraduate studies in this subject rather than in clinical nursing practice (Abdellah and Levine, 1965; Polit and Hungler, 1987). An increase in hospital admissions following the Second World War also led to studies that looked at manpower planning and staffing. An interest in research in nursing accelerated from the 1950s onward, with the establishment of a government-funded nursing research centre to look specifically at nursing practice, the Walter Reed Army Institute of Research, and an increased amount of money available from government and private foundations for funding research projects, in particular on subjects related to clinical nursing practice. The first journal, *Nursing Research,* was also published and there were more nurses registering for undergraduate courses. The 1960s saw development in the conceptual and theoretical aspects of nursing, although research into clinical practice continued to be a priority for further investigation. These developments in education, management, theoretical concepts and clinical practice have continued throughout the 1970s to the present day (Polit and Hungler, 1987). Nursing research in the United States, although commencing earlier, has shown parallel developments to that in the United Kingdom, initially focusing on education, then on resources and moving on to clinical nursing practice and conceptual models.

Relationship to NHS research and development policy

In 1991 a strategy for developing a framework for the direction and management of research and development (R and D) within the NHS was published in 1991 (Department of Health, 1991). It formed a comprehensive approach to developing a national research and development infrastructure for health services and health care. The strategy has included medicine, nursing and the professions allied to medicine, without specific reference to any one health profession, its objective being

> to ensure that the content and delivery of care in the NHS is based on high quality research relevant to improving the health of the nation. (Department of Health, 1991: 2)

The Department of Health (DH) research and development programme comprises a DH centrally managed programme (including public health) and an NHS R and D programme managed by the regional executive offices. The NHS R and D programme is based on priority areas identified by the Central Research and Development Committee (CRDC).

An aim of the wider strategy was to form links between the DH and NHS research programmes, the research councils, universities, charities and industry to foster close alliances, avoid duplication and to adopt a more strategic and managed approach to research and development. The idea was that these links would benefit those involved in health care and health services research, whether as researchers, funders or users of research findings. Within the strategy, consideration was also given to resourcing the national and regional programmes, including locally organised research schemes. It also considered the education and training requirements of personnel and the importance of an information strategy for sharing details of research so as to avoid duplication of effort and to make findings readily accessible to those delivering and managing health care.

The strategy was reviewed in 1993 to summarise progress and to chart its future direction in relation to the identified priorities and health technology assessment (HTA), which relates to the effectiveness, costs and broader impact of all interventions used by health professionals to promote health and to prevent and treat illness (Department of Health, 1993b). This policy document placed greater emphasis upon development initiatives, particularly those related to information systems, which include a national register of health services research in the UK and The Cochrane Collaboration, established in 1993, which is an international initiative to systematically examine the research evidence for health care and to disseminate this information electronically in the form of systematic reviews. It was also recognised that the systematic transfer of information within the health service to purchasers and providers was important and the NHS Centre for Reviews and Dissemination was set up at York. This Centre has the remit to not only compile reviews on the research evidence for health care but to also make this information accessible and to test methods for their successful dissemination and implementation in practice. The idea behind this is that effective methods for health care will be more rapidly introduced into the health service and that unwanted health interventions which waste resources will eventually cease. This strategy certainly went further in recognising and addressing issues related to the dissemination and implementation of research evidence with a view to improving the effectiveness of health care, particularly in relation to the targets identified within the Health of the Nation strategy (Department of Health, 1992).

In 1992 a taskforce was set up to specifically advise on a strategy for research in nursing, midwifery and health visiting. Recommendations were made to integrate research by the nursing professions and research into nursing issues within the NHS R and D strategy (Department of Health, 1993a). It was also recognised that these recommendations would have relevance for physiotherapy, occupational therapy, and speech and language therapy. The strategy specifically looked at the structure and organisation of the NHS R and D in order to ensure that research in nursing was fully taken into account when establishing structures, networks and information systems for setting priorities, disseminating findings and promoting research-led developments. Education and training, funding of research and integrating research, development and practice were also addressed. Dual objectives of the strategy were to improve the research skills and training of nurses and to extend and improve the research base of nursing, with the wider context of research in nursing being firmly located in the broader perspective of health services research (Department of Health, 1993a).

Nursing has long deliberated over the dissemination and utilisation of research findings into clinical practice (Closs and Cheater, 1994) and the terms dissemination and development have been defined within the Strategy for Research in Nursing, Midwifery and Health Visiting (Department of Health, 1993a: Appendix 2). This is a key policy document because it clearly addressed these terms, which had not been included in the main NHS R and D strategy, *Research for Health* in 1991 or 1993 (Department of Health, 1991; Department of Health, 1993b) and because it reflects the nursing profession's pioneering focus on developments within clinical nursing practice.

Developments and dissemination in clinical nursing practice

The development of clinical nursing roles, a clinical career structure and clinical nursing practice have been features of the Nursing Development Units (NDUs), originating in Burford, Tameside and then Oxford (Pearson, 1983, 1988; Pearson et al., 1992; Black, 1993). The formative thinking around the NDUs in Burford and Tameside was based on an analysis of the nursing literature that contributed to developments in the structure, organisation and practice of clinical nursing. Some of the key developments that arose were the establishment of nursing beds (in-patient beds for patients who need mainly nursing care which nurses admitted to and discharged from) (Pearson, 1988) and primary nursing (a named nurse accountable for individual patient care) (Ersser and Tutton,

1991). In 1989 a nursing developments programme was launched by the King's Fund to provide pump priming money and support for four NDUs at Brighton, Camberwell, Southport and West Dorset over a three-year period. The aim of the programme was to establish a focus for excellence in nursing and to improve patient care by developing nurses and nursing (Turner Shaw and Bosanquet, 1993). The Department of Health went on to fund the evaluation of these four NDUs, along with funding another 30 demonstration sites (Moores, 1993). The four King's Fund NDUs were established as agencies of change and, once the units were established, set about activities and outcomes related to clinical practice and the development of nursing staff. Turner Shaw and Bosanquet (1993) looked at the outcomes of these activities along with the costs and resources of NDUs in relation to other wards, the development of nurses and nursing and lessons for dissemination.

A recognised criticism of the early NDU developments in clinical nursing was the lack of any rigorous evaluation using research methods to measure their success and the impact of any change that had occurred. This was rectified by the evaluation commissioned from Turner Shaw and Bosanquet (1993). They found that NDUs provided a way of developing nurses and their practice to improve and individualise patient care and that they needed to be championed and supported by senior management. They required a minimum of two years to be established and recognised that the systems evaluated did not enable precise costings to be undertaken. Turner Shaw and Bosanquet also concluded that for NDU developments to be accepted in other wards and situations they had to function within the same budgets. Some of the earlier studies have now been replicated and evaluated using the appropriate research methods so that generalisable lessons can be learnt from these development initiatives for dissemination locally and nationally (Evans and Griffiths, 1994; Griffiths and Evans, 1995; Vaughan, 1996).

Dissemination and utilisation of research evidence in order to change and improve clinical nursing practice has been addressed within the United States and the United Kingdom (Closs and Cheater, 1994). In the United States, the Western Interstate Commission for Higher Education (WICHE) Regional Programme for Nursing Research Development established change agents (a clinical nurse and a nurse educator who had participated in a workshop on critical appraisal) who identified and attempted to change clinical problems, such as use of a pre-operative teaching programme, care planning for grieving spouses and the prevention and treatment of constipation in nursing home residents (Kreuger et al., 1978). Hunt (1987), in the UK, developed a similar albeit more limited approach to manage change in relation to mouth care and pre-operative fasting within hospitals.

The Conduct and Utilisation of Research in Nursing project (CURN) looked at research utilisation as an organisational process rather than it being just the responsibility of individual nurses (Horsley et al., 1978). The CURN project undertook a synthesis of research findings that was translated into a clinical protocol which was then transformed into practice and evaluated. Research utilisation was found to be greater in the experimental units than in the controls at one year, although this difference had diminished in some of the activities at two-year follow up. A development project in Oxford looking at the dissemination of research evidence on continence care using a clinical handbook compiled from a systematic review of the literature on incontinence also found statistically significant improvements in nurses' knowledge in experimental sites compared to nurses working in control units (Williams et al., 1995). The authors concluded that use of a clinical handbook and group discussion was an effective means of disseminating research evidence.

Dissemination of research evidence via consensus guidelines is increasingly being used as a means of changing health care practice (Effective Health Care Bulletin, 1994; Deighan and Hitch, 1995). A project that looked at the management of incontinence by members of the primary health care team (PHCT) compiled a national consensus guideline, went on to implement it within one clinical setting and evaluated its impact on patients' health care and continence status (Button et al., 1996, 1998). Positive outcomes included a development in the practice's computer systems to allow information on incontinence to be collected for individual patients, as well as for some aspects of their clinical care such as assessment of incontinence and the appropriate referral of patients to other health professionals.

Research has also been undertaken to attempt to identify what are the barriers to research utilisation in the United States (Funk et al., 1989; Funk et al., 1991) and has been replicated in the United Kingdom (Dunn et al., 1997). All these studies briefly demonstrate key work that has looked at developments within clinical nursing practice, along with dissemination and utilisation of research evidence and evaluation of their impact using appropriate research techniques. This serves to demonstrate that nursing has been addressing the development aspect of research within health care and health services in general for quite some time.

The present day context

It is now generally recognised that it is essential to transfer the research evidence on effective health care into practice in order to improve both patient care and health service delivery and to reduce any wasteful expenditure incurred by unnecessary practices (Department of Health, 1995). Within nursing it has also been recognised that not all nurses will undertake research or pursue a career as researchers, although nurses, midwives and health visitors are required to use research evidence to inform their clinical practice (Department of Health, 1993a: 12–13, 16). It was this recognition within nursing of the importance not only of undertaking research but ensuring that the findings were disseminated and utilised within clinical practice (Closs and Cheater, 1994) which led to a focus on development and evaluation. The nursing professions within the United States and the United Kingdom have focused their attention on the development aspects of research and appear to have embraced both research and development ahead of central NHS R and D policy (Department of Health, 1991, 1993b).

Current NHS policy is aimed at strengthening the research capacity of health professionals within provider units, with the focus for research and development being undertaken and managed within hospital and community trusts or by general practitioner fundholders (HMSO, 1994). Methods to promote implementation of research findings within health services have also been made a priority for evaluation (Department of Health, 1995). Priorities for all purchasers and providers within the NHS (NHSE, 1996) include ensuring that health care is based upon evidence of clinical effectiveness and also care based upon unsound custom and practice is eradicated. It is envisaged that dissemination and use of systematic reviews on the evidence for health care (The Cochrane Library, 1996) will assist with these initiatives. Research and development within clinical nursing practice, although specific to the nursing professions, forms part of this wider focus on evidence-based health care and health services research.

Summary

The establishment of research in nursing shows similar development in both the United Kingdom and the United States. The brief documentation of R and D presented in this chapter demonstrates that nursing has not only an established and developing track record in undertaking research but has already made headway with the issues of dissemination and utilisation of research evidence and development and evaluation within clinical nursing practice. It serves to set the scene for the following chapters and has set research and development within clinical nursing practice in the wider context of national policy on health services research and its focus on developments within health care based upon dissemination, utilisation and evaluation

References

Abdellah FG, Levine E (1965) Better Patient Care Through Nursing Research. London: Macmillan.

Black M (1993) The Growth of Tameside Nursing Development Unit: An Exploration of Perceived Changes in Nursing Practice over a Ten-Year Period. London: King's Fund.

Button D, Roe B, Webb C, Frith A, Colin Thome D, Gardner L (1998) Consensus Guidelines for the Promotion and Management of Continence by the Primary Health Care Team. London: Whurr Publishers

Button D, Roe B, Webb C, Frith A, Colin Thome D, Gardner L (1996) The Development, Implementation and Evaluation of Consensus Guidelines for the Promotion and Management of Continence by Primary Health Care Teams. Unpublished report Runcorn, Castlefields Health Centre.

Closs S J, Cheater FM (1994) Utilization of nursing research: culture, interest and support. Journal of Advanced Nursing 19: 762–73.

The Cochrane Library (1996) Issue 2. Database on disk and CD-ROM. London: BMJ Publishing.

Deighan M, Hitch S (1995) Clinical Effectiveness from Guidelines to Cost-Effective Practice. Brentwood: Earlybrave Publications Ltd.

Department of Health (1991) Research for Health. A Research and Development Strategy for the NHS. London: Department of Health.

Department of Health (1992) The Health of the Nation. London: HMSO.

Department of Health (1993a) Report of the Taskforce on the Strategy for Research in Nursing, Midwifery and Health Visiting. London: Department of Health.

Department of Health (1993b) Research for Health. London: Department of Health.

Department of Health (1995) Methods to Promote the Implementation of Research Findings in the NHS. Priorities for Evaluation. London: Department of Health.

Dunn G, Crichton N, Williams K, Roe B, Seers K (1997) Using research for practice: a UK experience of the Barriers Scale. Journal of Advanced Nursing. 26(6):1203-100

Effective Health Care Bulletin (1994) Implementing Clinical Practice Guidelines. December 1994 (8). Leeds: University of Leeds.

Ersser S, Tutton E (1991) Primary Nursing in Perspective. London: Scutari.

Evans A, Griffiths P (1994) The Development of a Nursing-led In-patient Service.

London: King's Fund.

Funk SG, Tornquist EM, Champagne MT (1989) A model for improving the dissemination of research. Western Journal of Nursing Research 11(3): 361–7.

Funk SG, Champagne MT, Wiese RA, Tornquist EM (1991) Barriers: the barriers to research utilization scale. Applied Nursing Research 4(1): 39–45.

Goddard HA (1953) The Work of Nurses in Hospital Wards. London: Nuffield Provinicial Hospitals Trust.

Griffiths P, Evans A (1995) Evaluation of a Nursing-led In-patient Service. London: King's Fund.

HMSO (1994) Supporting Research and Development in the NHS. London: HMSO.

Horlsey JA, Crane J, Bingle JD (1978) Research utilization as an organizational process. Journal of Administration 8: 4–6.

Hunt M (1987) The process of translating research findings into nursing practice. Journal of Advanced Nursing 12: 101–10.

Kreuger J, Neldon A, Wolanin MO (1978) Nursing Research: Development, Collaboration and Utilization. Germantown, MA: Aspen Systems.

Macleod Clark J, Hockey L (1979) Research for Nursing. A Guide for the Enquiring Nurse. Aylesbury: HM & M Publishers.

Macleod Clark J, Hockey L (1989) Further Research for Nursing. London: Scutari.

Menzies IEP (1959) The functioning of social systems as a defence against anxiety: a report of a study of the nursing services of a general hospital. Human Relations 13: 95–121.

Moores Y (1993) Foreword. In Turner Shaw J, Bosanquet N (1993) A Way to Develop Nurses and Nursing. London: King's Fund.

NHSE (1996) Promoting Clinical Effectiveness. A Framework for Action In and Through the NHS. London: Department of Health.

Pearson A (1983) The Clinical Nursing Unit. London: Heinemann.

Pearson A (1988) Primary Nursing. Nursing in Burford and Oxford Nursing Development Units. London: Chapman & Hall.

Pearson A, Punton S, Durant E (1992) Nursing Beds: An Evaluation of the Effects of Therapeutic Nursing. Harrow: Scutari Press.

Polit DF, Hungler BP (1987) Nursing Research: Principles and Methods. Philadelphia: Lippincott.

Times Higher Education Supplement (1996) Research Assessments 1996. The Times Higher Education Supplement. 20 December : 1259.

Turner Shaw J, Bosanquet N (1993) A Way to Develop Nurses and Nursing. London: King's Fund.

UKCC (1986) Project 2000. London: United Kingdom Central Council for Nursing, Midwifery and Health Visiting.

Vaughan B (1996) Clinical review of 1996. Nursing Standard 11: 13–15, 39.

Williams K, Roe B, Sindhu F (1995) Evaluation of Nursing Developments in Continence Care. Report No 10. Oxford: National Institute for Nursing.

Acknowledgement

This chapter was adapted from Roe B (1997) Some observations on policy for research and development in the NHS. Journal of Clinical Nursing 6(3): 171–2.

Chapter 2
The art and science of research in clinical nursing

David R. Thompson

Introduction

In the current health service culture, largely as a consequence of the recent NHS reforms and the research and development (R and D) strategy, the emphasis is firmly placed upon evidence-based healthcare (Gray, 1997), and the rhetoric is replete with terms such as evidence, effectiveness and efficiency (Miles and Lugon, 1996). This has resulted in nurses and others increasingly being expected to justify and account for their actions in such terms. This is especially true for those nurses working in clinical practice, who make many, often rapid and complex, decisions which, directly or indirectly, determine the use of expensive resources and the outcomes of patient care.

Although perceived by some nurses and other healthcare professionals as a threat, the NHS R and D programme offers nurses an ideal opportunity to engage in truly multidisciplinary research that will lead to a scientific basis for health services. Such an arena allows nurses to demonstrate to other professionals their own unique skills and distinctive approach to research as well as learning about the methods and approaches of others. However, some degree of caution is needed in a situation where there may be inequalities in the professional power of different groups.

In order to substantiate claims of effective (including cost-effective) and efficient practice, nurses must continually strive to subject the art of nursing to scientific scrutiny and revision. Research must provide knowledge relevant to nursing practice if it is to contribute to the development of a science of nursing practice. In other words, the science of nursing must evolve from, and be directed towards, nursing practice. This requires that the nursing profession acknowledge and value the pursuit of knowledge through scientific endeavour, that it has access to the findings and that it has mechanisms for implementing them where appropriate.

Art and science of research

Scientific research is directed towards solving problems and generating new knowledge. However, the method of science is itself actually a mixture of art and science. For example, although the technicalities of research are scientific, in the sense that science demands objectivity and rationality, the identification of the problem, the formulation of the questions and the generation of hypotheses are an art that depends upon the creativity and imagination of the scientist. The real life of science is on the boundary between knowledge and ignorance commonly called the research frontier. The art of doing exciting and innovative research is to know what sort of questions to ask, and this involves creativity, curiosity, and a willingness to take risks.

Science is about the search for understanding. It is a rational endeavour by virtue of its critical attitude: scientific knowledge is public in nature, representing a consensus of rational, informed opinion (Ziman, 1978). Although the significance of science has been undoubtedly exaggerated and its limits not always acknowledged (Appleyard, 1992), popular views about the nature of science and scientific activity contain serious misconceptions that were discarded long ago by most historians and philosophers of science (Bauer, 1992). Unfortunately, these misconceptions about science abound in nursing (Schumacher and Gortner, 1992) and it is not uncommon for nurses to display ignorance, misunderstanding or even hostility towards science. Much nursing literature still refers to traditional science (i.e. scientific work that has evolved from the natural sciences) as being reliant on theory-neutral facts, quantitative data and the search for universal laws, yet as Schumacher and Gortner (1992) eloquently argue, this depiction of science is incongruent with contemporary thinking. They point out that in many instances nurses use terminology that is often poorly clarified, and continue to use labels such as 'logical positivism', even though logical positivism is generally considered to be redundant as a philosophical movement.

A compounding issue is the tendency to confuse definitions of science with concepts of technology. Whilst technology may be a product of scientific knowledge, it is very much older than science

(Wolpert, 1992), and the growth of technology has different social effects from the growth of science.

Science is often depicted as a cold, lonely, calculating endeavour bereft of human spirit, and frequently it is described in terms of being reductionist, mechanistic, and dehumanising. Yet humans are not naturally objective, disinterested and sceptical, and many people fail to recognise that although science is an activity of individuals, it is pursued within a community. Nor do some seem to appreciate the beauty, elegance and importance of science and the creativity, originality and inspiration that characterise the good scientist (see Carey, 1995).

Social factors do, of course, operate in science and they can certainly advance or retard the progress of scientific knowledge, but they do not determine what that knowledge shall be. Thus, although science is socially influenced it is not socially constructed (Polkinghorne, 1996).

The scientific method

One of the myths which pervades science is that of the so-called scientific method. Bauer (1992) has cogently argued that the scientific method is an ideal, not a description of what is actually practised. This myth is compounded by the forms and conventions of scientific publications, which convey a false impression about the way in which science is conducted in reality. Medawar (1990) has described how, three decades ago, he labelled the scientific paper a fraud because it misrepresents the process of thought that accompanies or gives rise to the work described. He suggested that the traditional inductive format of the scientific paper should be discarded, and recommended that the 'discussion' section should be moved from its customary place at the end of the paper to the beginning and that the 'scientific facts and acts' should follow the discussion.

Art versus science

Whereas many argue that nurses practise a mixture of art and science, some tend to come down in favour of one or the other. This is reminiscent of the two cultures debate over three decades ago (Snow, 1961) and there is a danger that if nurses adhere to one of the two separate cultures – one relating to science and the other to the arts and humanities – nursing will become polarised. Of course, the reality is that nursing straddles both cultures, but the potential for polarisation probably reflects the educational background from which the nurse emanates. Many nurses who have graduated have done so primarily in the arts and humanities and it would appear that comparatively few have had a good education or training in science. As the former group is in the majority it is no coincidence that nursing and nurses have concentrated efforts on areas such as the social, ethical, educational and managerial aspects of nursing. This has resulted in a comparative neglect of, for example, the biological and psychological aspects. This has had the consequence of distancing many clinical nurses from other clinical professions, notably medicine. This is not to argue that science is a panacea, and that every nurse should be trained in science. Rather, it is a clarion call to nurses to appreciate the merits and importance of different types of knowledge. However, it is important to acknowledge that clinical nursing, as a practice-based discipline, requires a scientific basis (Neyle and West, 1991).

Another potential source of polarisation relates to the adherence professed by some nurses to one particular research paradigm. Some nurses perceive the methods and approaches of social science research as woolly and soft, when in fact the social sciences have their own systematic and rigorous practice. Others assume erroneously that traditional scientific research disallows the use of qualitative data, when in fact there is no philosophical or historical basis for this (Schumacher and Gortner, 1992). In field work or naturalistic research with people it is necessary to use interviews to elicit experiences, perceptions and meanings. Each research method and approach is, by itself, unlikely to satisfy most research questions. What is potentially exciting in clinical nursing is the use of a range of research methodologies that generate qualitative and quantitative data that enrich and increase the scope of evidence. The type of evidence used by the scientist should depend on the phenomenon under investigation and the specific research question.

Working together

Nurses, like scientists, are inheritors of a tradition and members of a community. As well as working with other nurses they have to work with many other community members. The current health services research culture places great emphasis on multidisciplinary proposals and collaboration. There is a danger that, either through ignorance, naivety or nursing imperialism, clinical nurses may alienate themselves from their closest clinical colleagues. This may result, not only in nurses being excluded from collaborative ventures, but also in a possible lack of recognition being given to their own unique and valuable contribution. In the current scenario, many disciplines are likely to utilise the traditional and received 'scientific' research methodologies, and nurses need to understand scientific principles in order to elicit the cooperation, support and understanding of these other disciplines, to be cognisant of their methods and to be respectful of their backgrounds and contributions (Thompson, 1993).

One of the ways around this potential problem is to offer research training and support programmes for a variety of staff representing a range of disciplines and which teach students not only about the relative merits of the different research methods and approaches but to constantly develop the theoretical framework within which nursing and other research is carried out. This is likely to generate more mutually respectful and harmonious working relationships.

Novice researchers must not only immerse themselves in the literature but must begin to serve an apprenticeship to learn the way in which research is done. This involves much more than acquiring necessary techniques, whether they be observational or experimental, but also the attitudes of commitment and relentless curiosity. These come from the observation of how other, more experienced and wiser, researchers pursue their investigations. Helping and supervising the novice researcher require careful judgement, sensitivity and tact. Initially, the novice will often be assigned a specific task which, on its own, may seem minor and mundane but which may provide an important contribution to the overall product. It is important at the outset for the novice to appreciate that most research involves long periods of toil and frustration. As Polkinghorne (1996) pointed out so eloquently, it is not a process of smooth onward and upward advance but rather an untidy trail of insight and error.

Science is a highly competitive activity where it is often difficult to gain a balance between rivalry and collaboration. Competition for access to limited funds and resources and the race to achieve personal recognition and esteem often result in fairly ruthless behaviour. The ideal is to be able to have a team of individuals sufficiently different to complement each other. It is a question of the whole being more than the sum of the parts. The hallmark of a good research team is that it has an ethos of openness, creativity, flexibility, a healthy scepticism and a willingness to question the status quo or accepted conventions.

The practice of science and research depends upon the acceptance of certain moral values and the operation of ethical codes within the community. These include honesty in the reporting of findings, acknowledgement of the contribution of others and openness in making methods and results available to others for scrutiny.

Summary

Nursing is essentially an applied discipline with unclear boundaries, broad and loosely defined problems, a vague theoretical structure and numerous overlaps with other disciplines. In an era of evidence-based healthcare, clinical nursing research has an important and distinct contribution to make, both to the profession and to the health service but to be successful it needs to develop and promote a wide range of methods and approaches. Nurses undertaking research need not only to adhere to scientific principles but to have curiosity and creativity.

References

Appleyard B (1992) Understanding the Present. Science and the Soul of Modern Man. London: Pan Books.

Bauer HH (1992) Scientific Literacy and the Myth of the Scientific Method. Urbana: University of Illinois Press.

Carey J (Ed) (1995) The Faber Book of Science. London: Faber and Faber.

Gray JAM (1997) Evidence-Based Healthcare. Edinburgh: Churchill Livingstone.

Medawar PB (1990) The Threat and the Glory. Reflections on Science and Scientists. Oxford: Oxford University Press.

Miles A, Lugon M (Eds) (1996) Effective Clinical Practice. Oxford: Blackwell Science.

Neyle D, West S (1991) In support of a scientific basis. In Gray G, Pratt R (Eds) Towards a Discipline of Nursing. Melbourne: Churchill Livingstone. pp. 265–84.

Polkinghorne J (1996) Beyond Science: The Wider Human Context. Cambridge: Cambridge University Press.

Schumacher KL, Gortner SR (1992) (Mis)conceptions and reconceptions about traditional science. Advances in Nursing Science 14(4): 1–11.

Snow CP (1961) The Two Cultures and the Scientific Revolution. Cambridge: Cambridge University Press.

Thompson DR (1993) Science and clinical nursing. Journal of Clinical Nursing 2: 327–8.

Wolpert L (1992) The Unnatural Nature of Science. London: Faber and Faber.

Ziman J (1978) Reliable Knowledge: An Exploration of the Grounds for Belief in Science. Cambridge: Cambridge University Press.

PART TWO:
RESEARCH METHODS

Chapter 3
Qualitative research: definitions and design

Anne Williams

Introduction

Qualitative research is a term used widely in the research methods literature. It is typically used to define a set of ideas and practices that are contrasted with an opposing set of ideas and practices termed *quantitative research* (Bryman, 1988). Some theorists see the opposition between the two approaches as irreconcilable insofar as they rest on completely divergent ideas about the study of societies and social life (Guba and Lincoln, 1982). Others take the view that positivism does not necessarily equate with quantitative research just as naturalism does not necessarily equate with qualitative research. Indeed, as Hammersley and Atkinson (1983, 1995) suggest, some classic and more recent qualitative research studies are based on positivist assumptions about reality. As Stanley and Wise point out, there are different versions of both positivism and naturalism that challenge conventional ideas about theory preceding research in positivism and theory emerging from research in the naturalist account (Stanley and Wise, 1993: 151).

These comments are offered to counter easy assumptions about the coherence and uniformity of qualitative research. It is difficult to define, and it nearly always requires further qualification, for example as 'ethnography', 'fieldwork', 'qualitative interviewing'. And even these categories may be differentiated (e.g. feminist ethnography, ethnographic interviewing). In the first section of the chapter, I comment on the diversity of definition as reflected in some key texts. However, the term, 'qualitative research' is helpfully unifying as it allows for a consideration of themes broadly common to a diversity of approaches, namely the purpose of qualitative

21

research, its relationship to theory and researcher–researched relationships. In the second section of the chapter, these themes are
considered in relation to sampling, selection and ethics. Examples
are drawn from current research in nursing in order to give
substance to the debates and issues discussed.

Definition and diversity

It is hard to be definitive about types or versions of qualitative
research. As Miles and Huberman (1994:5) point out, 'qualitative
research may be conducted in dozens of ways, many with long traditions behind them'. They add that 'to do them all justice is impossible here' (1994: 5). A brief review of textbooks on research methods
across a number of disciplines suggests that authors vary in the criteria they apply in order to define and differentiate qualitative
research. In this section of the chapter, I offer two case illustrations in
order to show diversity (and to hint at agreement, a point I take up in
the second section of the chapter) within two broad but relatively
bounded fields of qualitative research. They are, first, qualitative
research in the context of social research and second, qualitative
nursing research.

Qualitative, social research

Here, I refer to the writings of a number of UK authors – writings
that span the years 1983 to 1995, recognising that authors draw on
ideas, values and traditions that cross cultural, temporal and
geographical boundaries.

Hakim's (1987) text provides a useful example of social research
with a policy emphasis. She distinguishes qualitative research from
sample surveys, research reviews, case studies, regular surveys and
experimental social research. However, she uses the term qualitative
research to refer to 'a specific research design rather than as a
general term for non-quantitative research methods' (1987:26). She
describes qualitative research as 'richly descriptive', the most
common method being the in-depth interview of variable length,
which may take up to five hours (1987:26). She also identifies 'group
discussion' as a frequently used method. She emphasises that
'although qualitative research is about people as the central unit of
account, it is not about particular individuals per se; reports focus,
rather, on the various patterns, or clusters, of attitudes and related
behaviour that emerge from the interviews' (1987:26). Hakim's

undifferentiated account of qualitative research makes sense in the context of the tradition of policy research where the social survey predominates.

In contrast to Hakim's unidimensional description of qualitative research, there is considerable diversity in terminology in textbooks written from a broadly sociological perspective. For example, Burgess (1984) and Silverman (1992) have used the term 'fieldwork'. Hammersley and Atkinson (1983,1995) use the term 'ethnography' in a liberal way, which as Silverman (1992) points out, shares some properties with Bryman's (1988) use of the term qualitative research. Burgess describes qualitative research as one of a number of approaches relying principally on observation and which derive from the tradition of social anthropology. In this context, qualitative research is one of a number of terms: 'fieldwork, ethnography, case study . . . interpretive procedures and field research' (1984: 2).

Sociologists regard observation as being central to qualitative research. Bryman (1988: 46) suggests that participant observation is 'probably the method of data collection with which qualitative research is most closely associated'. Although he notes that the term 'qualitative research' is used to refer to a range of methods including in-depth, unstructured or semi-structured interviews (Bryman 1988: 2). Hammersley and Atkinson, with reference to ethnography, write:

> In its most characteristic form it involves the ethnographer participating, overtly or covertly, in people's daily lives for an extended period of time, watching what happens, listening to what is said, asking questions – in fact, collecting whatever data are available to throw light on the issues that are the focus of the research (Hammersley and Atkinson, 1995: 1).

Sociological discussions of qualitative research feature a concern with its intellectual bases, which are variously cited as phenomenology (e.g. Bryman, 1988; Miles and Huberman, 1994), symbolic interactionism (e.g. Burgess, 1984; Bryman, 1988; Silverman, 1993), functionalism (Silverman, 1993), structural functionalism and Marxist influences in social anthropology (Burgess, 1984). Hammersley and Atkinson in the second edition of their by now classic text *Ethnography* (1995) acknowledge the influence of the 'diverse' movement of post-structuralism and point out that 'while realism has not been completely abandoned', there is now a rejection of the idea that ethnographic accounts can represent reality unproblematically and 'doubt has been thrown on the claims to scientific authority associated with realism' (1995: 14). Hammersley and Atkinson are keen to challenge some qualitative researchers' claims that data 'collected' in 'natural' settings are somehow more authentic than data 'collected' in 'experimental' settings. They point out that 'naturalists share with "positivists" a commitment to producing accounts of factual matters that reflect the nature of the phenomena studied rather than the values or political commitments of the researcher' (1995: 14). Indeed they stress that:

> The language used by ethnographers in their writing is not a transparent medium allowing us to see reality through it, but rather a construction that draws on many of the rhetorical strategies used by journals or even novelists. (Hammersley and Atkinson, 1995: 14)

They are referring here, at least in part, to the idea of ethnographic authority (Clifford, 1983), which is the idea that the ethnographer or qualitative researcher draws on textual devices designed to persuade the readership of the authenticity and validity of the account. However, while Hammersley and Atkinson suggest that 'the scholarly and scientific authenticity of a text is not enhanced by the elimination of analogy or simile', they add a cautionary note: 'this is no recommendation of absolute licence. A recognition of the power of figurative language should lead also to recognition of the need for disciplined and principled usage' (1995: 246).

A feature of qualitative research as discussed by sociologists is the emphasis on critique. Processes of critique and counter-critique allow for exploration of difference while pointing to ways in which versions of qualitative research overlap. One example of such a process was the exchange of criticism and ideas in relation to feminist methodologies in the journal *Sociology* (Hammersley, 1992b; Ramazanoglu, 1992; Gelsthorpe, 1992; Williams, 1993; Hammersley, 1994). Similarly, contributors to textbooks on qualitative research constructively challenge each other on varying points of debate. As indicated, Hammersley and Atkinson take a critical perspective on classic and more recent exponents of ethnography. Readers of this present volume might find it useful to read Silverman (1993) who looks critically at the versions of qualitative research put forward by Bryman (1988), Hammersley (1990), Hammersley (1992a) and Hammersley and Atkinson (1983) and offers his own version, which, as he notes, contains simplifications that can be criticised (1993: 28–9).

Qualitative nursing research

Here I refer to commentary contained mainly, although not exclusively, within a particular volume of work *Qualitative Nursing Research*

(Morse, 1991). The contributors (from the USA and Canada) to the volume met at a two-day symposium in Chicago in 1987 to discuss 'sticky issues' in qualitative research.

The preface to the book signals a number of versions of qualitative research insofar as the contributors are categorised as 'phenomenologists', 'grounded theorists' and 'ethnographers'.

As the book proceeds, it becomes clear that this kind of categorisation implies a process of specialisation of research within nursing in North America at the time of publication. Morse criticises mixing of methods. Referring to a piece of work that was described as a unique blending of phenomenological, grounded theory, and ethnographic methodologies, she writes:

> Such mixing, while certainly 'do-able' violates the assumption of data collection techniques and methods of analysis of all the methods used. The product is not good science, the product is a sloppy mishmash. If the goal of a study is phenomenological, then clearly phenomenological methods must be used if the goal is to be attained. As ethnoscience methods of data collection have been developed to elicit a particular kind of structured data, and grounded theory methods of analysis have developed yet another type of question, any mixing or adapting of these methods runs the risk of producing other than the desired results. (Morse, 1991: 15)

This comment is set against other comments that suggest that 'nursing problems and situations for which nurses use qualitative methods generally differ from the situations and contexts found in the disciplines in which they (the qualitative methods) were developed' (1991: 17). Morse compares 'traditional ethnography' with 'nurse-ethnographers'. Where, for the former, 'the unit of analysis may be a village', for the latter it may be 'a health care unit' or 'a hospital unit or ward' (1991: 17). Morse suggests a difference between exploring the culture of a village for which she uses the term 'culture as a whole' and work that is more focused. She poses the question, 'do these types of ethnography need to be differentiated?'(1991: 17).

Whether or not one finds Morse's comparison helpful, or whether or not one agrees with Morse that anthropologists study 'whole cultures', most of the contributors to the volume appear to grapple with the tension between, on the one hand, remaining 'true' to a specific tradition and, on the other hand, seeing and utilising the tradition as research for nursing. This latter position could mean mixing of methods, a theme to which Morse and others return both in the text of chapters and as a recurring theme 'between chapters' in what Morse describes as 'dialogues between chapters'.

The theme of mixing methods is taken up in Anderson's (1991a) chapter, 'The Phenomenological Perspective'. Citing Giddens (1976), she draws attention to the point that phenomenology is not a unified philosophical tradition (Anderson 1991a: 25), and she notes that there are several versions of phenomenological research, including links with reflexive sociology, ethnomethodology and conversational analysis (1991a: 33). She makes the point that 'the intent of the method' about which she writes, phenomenology, is 'not to build grand theories of nursing but to understand the lived experience of people (e.g. what it means to be a patient or to be a nurse)'. Indeed her own work exemplifies this latter position (e.g. Anderson, 1991b).

May and Brink take up the theme of mixing methods in a 'dialogue between chapters' (Morse, 1991: 125) with respect to phenomenology and grounded theory. May comments:

> Nurse scientists have deviated considerably from the original 'analytic drivers in grounded theory', so that I can talk to Benner and understand what she does with data as a phenomenologist, and she understands what I do with data as a grounded theorist. She tells me that I think more like a phenomenologist than a grounded theorist, and I ask: 'Why should that surprise you?' (May, as quoted by Morse, 1991: 125)

May fails to elaborate on why it should not be surprising. From one perspective, it is hardly surprising given that phenomenology as philosophy has considerably influenced social theorists who have tried to look beyond orthodox science in order to understand the social world. For example, Schutz (1973), crudely summarised, took Weber's ideas about *Verstehen* (interpretive understanding as opposed to understanding a scientific fact) and linked them with Husserl's phenomenology (notably the 'bracketing' – setting aside – of prior assumptions about a situation in order to grasp subjective experience in its purest form) and looked at their relevance for social science. Schutz was particularly interested in how social theorists question their own culture and with questions concerning the self and its relationship with others. These questions have subsequently informed social theorists' work, for example Berger and Luckman (the latter a student of Schutz), who argued that reality is socially constructed and that a sociology of knowledge must analyse the process in which this occurs (Berger and Luckmann, 1973: 13). These ideas have found resonance in the various methodologies that have evolved across disciplines and specialities where researchers aim to understand social reality that is grounded in people's experience of that social reality (Bryman, 1988: 52).

From another perspective, May's comments are not surprising insofar as one would expect some common ground between researchers in the field of nursing. However, Brink's response to May is interesting as it reflects a tendency towards prescription, which, incidentally, is not exclusive to nursing. Silverman (1993: 29) also offers 'a prescriptive model of qualitative research'. Brink comments:

> I think we should develop a standardised system of labels for the phenomena we study that is (sic) uniquely nursing. We could then train the rest of the nursing world about what qualitative methods are. I think we do a different kind of qualitative method than what other people do. For example, more qualitative studies (in other disciplines) are studies of content that look at a single phenomena (sic), at a single moment in time. In nursing we look at process variables. We look at how people respond to illness, and that's a process! (Brink, as quoted by Morse, 1991: 105)

It is not hard to imagine these words uttered ironically in a small group of nurse researchers. Even if they were offered in serious tone then, as Morse comments, the 'taped transcripts were, unfortunately, more revealing than our scholarly analysis' (Morse, 1991: 10). Nevertheless, the words have been included within the covers of a text for the scrutiny of the 'advanced graduate student' if not recommended for 'the beginning qualitative researcher' (1991: 10) and, as such, are available for critical comment. The idea that nurses do a different kind of qualitative research from researchers in other disciplines, in juxtaposition with the words 'standardised labels' and 'uniquely nursing', does suggest an essentialism and narrowness of perspective that could stifle innovation in research, especially when linked to an imperative to 'train the rest of nursing about what qualitative methods are'.

Divergence between case illustrations

The work contained within the volume edited by Morse (1991) offers a number of versions of qualitative research. In turn, there are differences between Morse and her colleagues' treatment of qualitative research and the work that I have classified as qualitative social research in the UK tradition. A notable difference turns on the use of the term 'phenomenology'. In the volume edited by Morse, phenomenology is seen as research methodology (as it is in other nursing research texts – see Burns and Grove, 1993; Polit and Hungler, 1990), whereas most authors writing from a social science perspective refer to phenomenology as part of the intellectual tradition underpinning qualitative research. Both understandings of phenomenology are used by researchers in nursing in the UK. The focus of phenomenology on understanding the lived experience of people (e.g. what it means to be a patient or to be a nurse) has driven 'phenomenological studies' in clinical and related research which include, for example, Koch's inquiry into what matters to older patients (Koch, 1993) and Hallett's phenomenological study of a Project 2000 placement (Hallett et al., 1996). More often, phenomenology 'as a philosophical tradition which has influenced research' hovers between the lines of qualitative research, occasionally brought to the fore to make a point, as, for example, in my own research where I trace the imperative not to take received notions for granted back to Schutz's treatment of Husserl's phenomenology (Williams, 1989: 173).

Despite divergence within and between versions of qualitative research, there is some hint of concern for issues that cut across versions. In both the case illustrations discussed above, the term 'qualitative research' is an artefact of disciplines where researchers have sought methodologies in order to solve research problems and questions that quantitative methodologies cannot solve. The problems and questions are closely linked to the purpose of qualitative research, which is to gain an understanding of how people interpret their experiences – not simply through the exploration of individual accounts, however compelling, but, rather, the exploration of ideas, values and beliefs and how these relate to structural elements like power. Problems and questions link to a theoretical interest in how reality is constructed not only by those who are being researched but also through the accounts of qualitative researchers. There is a strong concern for maintaining the integrity of those who are being researched. These issues are discussed in the following section.

Qualitative research design and related issues

Following a brief comment on the idea of research design as it relates to qualitative work, issues broadly common to the various approaches outlined above are considered. I discuss the purpose of qualitative research and its relationship to theory, insofar as there are implications for sampling and selection strategies. I then consider researcher–researched relationships, with special reference to ethical implications. Needless to say, the two areas of discussion overlap.

A comment on research design

The term 'research design' is not without problems. Burns and Grove (1993: 261) write that the term is used in two ways: first to refer to the entire strategy for an individual study, from identifying the research problem to final plans for data collection and second, as a 'blueprint' or broad pattern or guide that can be applied to many studies. Hakim writes that research design deals 'primarily with aims, uses, purposes, intentions and plans within the practical constraints of location, time, money and availability of staff'. She adds that 'it is also very much about style . . . preferences and ideas' (1987: 1).

Very often, textbooks that cover both quantitative and qualitative research seem to be unable to treat qualitative research seriously in design terms. The format for design choices is never completely uniform, but it is restricted to quantitative approaches. For example, compare Burns and Grove (1993) with Polit and Hungler (1990). The former present the options as follows: descriptive designs, correlational, quasi-experimental and experimental (Burns and Grove, 1993: 287–330) whereas the latter present the options as experimental design, quasi-experimental research and non-experimental research. Qualitative research, while not ignored, seems to be placed outside the framework. Hakim, by contrast, treats qualitative research 'as a design' alongside, for example, surveys, case studies and experiments. However, even this concession is unsatisfactory given that the diversity and complexity of qualitative research remains unacknowledged.

In contrast, texts dealing with specific types of qualitative work, although they may or may not use the term 'research design', discuss in detail the plans, purpose, problems and people to be involved. They are mindful of the relationship of the research to theory and the relationship between researcher and researched. Burgess (1984: 6), writing about 'field research', suggests that it depends on a complex interaction between the research problem, the researcher, and those who are researched. It is on this basis that the researcher is an active decision-maker who decides on the most appropriate conceptual and methodological tools' (Burgess, 1984: 6). Hammersley and Atkinson, writing about ethnography, do use the term 'research design', advising against the notion that ethnography is so 'open-ended' that research design is superfluous. Rather they stress the need for preparation and for the researcher to guard against haphazard behaviour. They write, 'the research design should be a reflexive process which operates throughout every stage of a project' (1995: 24). I take their use of the term reflexivity in this context to mean a questioning of research processes so that certain practices and ideas are not taken for granted as correct in every situation.

Given the differentiation within qualitative research as discussed in the previous section, it is not surprising that, while certain authors discuss specific methodologies in fairly broad design terms and indicate the relevance of their discussions to the wider field of qualitative research, some methodologies have evolved within fairly narrow design parameters, for example the ethnographic interview as described by Spradley (1979), and grounded theory as described by Glaser and Strauss (1967), although the latter has been interpreted and reinterpreted to produce forms not first envisaged by their authors (e.g. Glaser, 1978; Strauss, 1970, 1993; Strauss and Corbin, 1990). Further, theoretical sampling, a key aspect of grounded theory, is used without recourse to the total package (Burgess, 1984: 55; Hammersley and Atkinson, 1995: 138) as is the term ethnographic interviewing (Hammersley and Atkinson, 1995).

It is against this backdrop of differentiation and complexity that I next turn to consider issues that cut across the variation and which have implications for decisions made about the design and subsequent process of qualitative research.

The purpose of qualitative research and its relationship to theory: implications for sampling and selection

What is the purpose of qualitative research? Although there is no consensus on what constitutes 'meaning' (Silverman, 1993: 25), there does appear to be agreement between researchers that the purpose of qualitative research is to produce work that will say something about the meanings people attach to their experiences (e.g. Bryman, 1988; Hammersley, 1990, 1992a; Hammersley and Atkinson, 1995). For example, Brown (1993) in a study exploring women's experiences of rheumatoid arthritis was concerned to examine the meanings women attributed to 'having rheumatoid arthritis'. A paper based on the study (Brown and Williams, 1995), looked at meaning related to cause of disease:

> Despite considerable biomedical research, the cause of rheumatoid arthritis remains unknown. The women in the present study had picked up on this, and had considered a multiplicity of potential factors in attempts to make sense of their illness. Their individual theories included aspects of biomedical hypotheses; for example, possible influences of environmental factors, occupational factors and auto-immunity.

> However, each account had a personal component in that each woman related how events in her past might have a bearing on her disease. For example, one woman firmly believed that her illness was due to her cutting her foot on the beach. For this woman, the initial symptoms commenced shortly after this event . . . Another woman felt the stress of a violent marriage was an important causal factor. (1995: 698)

As indicated by the words 'their individual theories', meaning is not merely assessed by eliciting feelings and opinions. Rather, it is assessed through an examination of the ideas to which people appeal in order to make sense of their lives and in order to give structure to their experiences. For example, in the same study, the women 'reported that their initial symptoms had been mild, vague and non-disabling, and that it had been difficult for them to interpret what was happening to them'. It is suggested that, 'In trying to explain what the symptoms meant, they [the women] employed a range of common sense explanations such as minor trauma and over exertion' (1995: 698).

Silverman (1993) provides a slightly different perspective on the problem of meaning. He writes that in order to show meaning, it is important to consider the function of what people say (1993: 25). For example, in relation to the words cited above we could ask what is the function of the meanings attributed by the women to their disease? We could say that it was important for the women to see some sort of cause–effect link between two events. We could then go on to conjecture that establishing such a link provides an element of certainty, as indeed the authors go on to suggest, explaining that the causes cited by this woman, and other women in the study, tend to serve the function of dealing with the uncertainty of the disease which, they write, is demonstrated not only by 'textbook descriptions of rheumatoid arthritis' (Thomson, 1982; Grennan, 1984), but which is also demonstrated by the women's accounts of the variable and unpredictable nature of day-to-day experiences of the disease (1995: 699). One example given is of a woman who said, 'I dread going to bed at night, because I don't know how I'm going to be when I wake up' (1995: 699).

Relationship to theory

As indicated, in order to elucidate meaning, it is important to identify ideas, values and beliefs and to show how people draw on them to give sense to situations, actions and processes that impinge on their lives. In short it is important to get a sense of the cultural context of what one observes and hears as a researcher. In this way a researcher not only gets a sense of differences between people but also a sense of what unites people in their experience. The suggestion made by the researchers in the study cited above is that uncertainty is a common feature of women's experiences of rheumatoid arthritis.

As a researcher one might then ask the question, 'how does my interpretation of my participants'/respondents' experiences challenge or confirm other researchers' interpretations?' In the example cited above, the authors point out that uncertainty is identified as a recurring theme in analyses of chronic illness (Davis, 1963; Bury, 1982; Charmaz, 1983; Nyhlin, 1990). A paper (Callaghan and Williams, 1995) based on a study by Callaghan (1993), which addresses the concerns of people who live with diabetes mellitus, makes the following comments:

> uncertainty is evident in participants' expressed concerns regarding their illness trajectory, with the threat of long term complications being prominent. Some look to a future of ageing which is compounded by the complications of diabetes. Others expressed fear of becoming a burden on their families. Minor 'aches and pains' became suspected beginnings of long term complications . . . All married participants in the study were found to have children, and an uncertainty emerged relating to the tendency for familial occurrence of diabetes. People worried about the risks for their children. (Callaghan and Williams, 1995: 135)

The authors then comment on the relationship of these study findings to ideas developed in the literature about uncertainty, underlining that 'these concerns echo the everyday symptomatic uncertainty described by Conrad (1987)'. In commenting this way, albeit briefly at this point in their discussion, the authors engage in what has come to be known as theory building. This is a process that is sometimes crudely contrasted with theory testing, a process associated with the testing of hypotheses in quantitative research, although not exclusive to quantitative research (Hammersley and Atkinson, 1995).

Implications for selection and sampling

The questions now raised are: how do you select from populations and employ sampling strategies so that you are able to make statements about meaning with some authority? And what are the implications of theory building for the sampling and selection processes?

It is important to note that rules that apply to sampling within a measurement framework of analysis do not of necessity apply to qualitative research. It is not the purpose of qualitative research to produce statistically significant or mathematically generalisable data based on a sample drawn in such a way as to remove all possible trace of 'bias' through employing probability sampling strategies. These sampling strategies may be employed in qualitative research designs for convenience or fairness, but they are not essential to the purpose of qualitative research.

To reiterate, the purpose of qualitative research is to explore a topic in such a way as to be able to comment on meaning and to contribute to understanding the theoretical basis of particular problems. As indicated by the examples above, in clinical nursing research, qualitative research is employed, for example, in instances where it is important for those involved in care and treatment to know what effects interventions have, not only in clinical terms, but also in terms of an individual's life (Gerhardt, 1990).

When thinking about selection and sampling, it is important to consider the question, 'Who are the people most able to assist the researcher with an exploration of a research question?' In the example of the problem of understanding women's experiences of rheumatoid arthritis, selection has already occurred, as the authors recognise when they write how there is 'a need to develop gender specific studies of how disease is experienced' (Brown and Williams, 1995: 697). Thus, the target population is women, but other considerations may apply. For example, a preliminary reading of the literature may suggest that length of duration of the disease has an impact on how it is understood and the meaning it has for those who live with it. It might, therefore, be useful to select women who have lived with the disease for some length of time, and to compare their experiences with the experiences of women who have recently been diagnosed as having rheumatoid arthritis.

To take another example (from research in progress), if the research problem is to explore how women conceptualise risks associated with taking hormone replacement therapy (HRT), then knowledge of the field and associated fields of study is likely to suggest that factors such as geographical location, class and ethnicity may make a difference to how risk is conceptualised. These factors need to be considered in the initial selection of research participants. Where they are considered, sampling is referred to as 'judgement sampling' (Burgess, 1984). However, it may be the case that, as research progresses, other factors arise that might suggest that further selection would strengthen the research (e.g. in the case of HRT, age and duration of 'treatment'). Again, selection is guided strategically and may be understood as 'judgement sampling' (e.g. Burgess, 1984).

However, it is also useful to note that a process where ideas or 'knowledge of the field' guide the selection of people (or events or situations) can be read as theoretical sampling. This process is a feature of Glaser and Strauss's (1967) 'grounded theorising', where theory is developed out of data analysis, and subsequent data collection is guided strategically by the emergent theory (see also Hammersley and Atkinson, 1995). Burgess comments on this strategy:

> Data collection is controlled by the emerging theory and the researcher has to consider: what groups or subgroups are used in data collection? For what theoretical purpose are the groups or subgroups used? Theoretical sampling therefore involves researchers in observing groups with a view to extending, modifying, developing and verifying theory. (Burgess, 1984: 56)

Burgess's words 'theoretical sampling involves researchers' are telling insofar as they highlight another aspect of research, mentioned earlier, which is that researchers cannot ignore how their own interests affect interpretation of data generated by research (Gouldner, 1970; Stanley and Wise, 1993, Hammersley and Atkinson, 1983; Williams, 1991, 1993). The researchers' interests are part of 'extending, modifying, developing and verifying theory' – otherwise understood as processes of theory building. In clinical nursing, interests will include professional nursing concerns, of course. As in all stages of the research, it is important to explain the concerns that affect processes of selection and sampling.

Thus one gets a sense of how certain sampling strategies contribute, at least in part, to providing a basis upon which the validity and relevance of research may be assessed. Other sampling strategies may be employed and they are discussed in detail in the research literature (e.g. Becker, 1979; Burgess, 1984; Hammersley and Atkinson, 1995). What becomes apparent is the importance of the researcher–researched relationship to this aspect, as well as other aspects, of the research process. If qualitative research is about the exploration of meaning, which in turn involves an examination of the ideas to which people appeal in order to make sense of their lives and in order to give structure to their experiences, then no matter what strategies are employed to retain critical distance, the researcher will need to engage with participants.

Researcher–researched relationships and ethical implications

Those who undertake research across disciplines that include anthropology and sociology, as well as applied disciplines such as nursing, have been preoccupied by ethical issues concerning how researchers engage with those they encounter in their research. As Burgess (1984: 197–200) records, classic debates include the exchanges between US researchers Erikson (1967, 1968) and Denzin (1968) and UK researchers, notably Homan and Bulmer (e.g. Homan and Bulmer, 1982) on the issue of covert ethnographic research. Burgess comments on how discussions about this issue tend towards over-simplification, exhorting ethnographers to consider and then to choose whether their research will be overt or covert. Burgess himself suggests that the boundaries between overt and covert research are more problematic than some writers suggest. In this respect, Burgess follows other researchers who usefully discuss the complexity of issues that pertain to how open researchers should be about their research, and how much information they should make available to their subjects. The point stressed is that researchers make decisions according to situational limitations and opportunities (Roth, 1962; Schatzman and Strauss, 1973).

Researchers within nursing have drawn on aspects of the debates as discussed within the context of social research. Two major areas of concern in the design phases of qualitative research are the linked issues of informed consent and confidentiality.

Informed consent

May (1979), an early commentator on informed consent within the context of nursing, drew attention to the difficulties of informed consent in relation to the multiple roles held by nurses who undertake research in clinical contexts. She was concerned that patients may misinterpret the roles of a person who approaches them to enter a research study when they know the person to be a nurse, but who is asking 'as a researcher' for them to consent to be part of the study. She asks to whom has the research subject given consent, the nurse or the researcher? (May, 1979). Subsequently, the point has been taken up by other researchers in the context of nursing. Merrell, referring to the unpaid volunteers who were participants in her research about well woman clinics, asks 'Were they (the volunteers) consenting to me as co-volunteer . . . or as a researcher?' (Merrell and Williams, 1970: 169).

The complexity of multiple roles and agendas and how they relate to informed consent and other ethical issues is a problem that I have discussed in relation to my own research (Williams, 1991, 1995). One of the examples I have taken from my research to illustrate the problem refers to a nurse who once recounted to me a painful experience about a drug overdose (Williams, 1989, 1991, 1995).

At the time I was working as a clinical teacher while doing ethnographic research. I was both a participant and an observer. The nurse was aware of my research and she had consented to being a participant. I wrote about the details of our conversation in my fieldnote book. However, when I came to the point of writing about the incident for a thesis and publications, I realised that I was uncertain about whether she had told 'me as researcher' or 'me as a colleague' or even 'me as friend' about the incident. I therefore decided not to recount the details of her experience as an example of a problem encountered by nurses. Rather I decided to use her words in an edited and abbreviated version to make a methodological point about the complexities of multiple roles as they relate to informed consent and confidentiality (discussed in detail in Williams, 1991). In short, I moved the focus of discussion to explore the question posed above, namely: to whom has the participant given consent? However, with the issue of informed consent in mind, one could question whether or not the nurse had consented to the use of her recorded experience as an example of a methodological point.

Confidentiality

From one perspective, the decision to use the incident in order to explore the question of consent was made in order to maintain confidentiality. I write that Pamela (a pseudonym) talked to me about her experiences following the drug overdose. The talk was included in time spent off the ward discussing 'private' matters. I read it now as an instance where a friend and a colleague confided in me about something that had upset her greatly. If I had not been doing fieldwork, it would not have occurred to me to talk about it with anyone else, let alone write about it (Williams, 1991: 78).

Ways of dealing with the problem of 'what are to be considered data for publication?' are addressed by contributors to the action research literature. Meyer (1993) handed back transcripts of interviews to those she interviewed, asking them to change any aspect they did not feel comfortable sharing with others. This is a courageous gesture as it might mean the deletion of data that the researcher considers valuable. However, even this gesture does not deal with the problem in an entirely satisfactory way, as I suggest elsewhere (Williams, 1995). There is still the question: what if the interpretation of the remaining data leaves participants feeling uncomfortable about what is being suggested in the account given by the researcher?

Questions such as 'to whom does a research subject give consent?' and 'to what are research subjects consenting?' and 'against what criteria are researchers assuring confidentiality?' are artefacts of the complexity of researcher–researched relationships. It is of interest that they tend to be questions posed by researchers in the context of qualitative research where researchers acknowledge the uneven distribution of power in researcher–researched relationships. Increasingly, researchers in nursing, whether undertaking, for example, qualitative interviewing, ethnographies or action research, are aware that since they hold multiple roles they will encounter people not only as researcher to researched, but also as nurse to patient, woman to woman, man to man, ward sister to staff nurse, tutor to student, clinical manager to first-level nurse, and so on. As I write elsewhere (Williams, 1995), a corollary of the multiple roles held is that researchers are likely to justify their practice not only by appeal to research codes of ethics (e.g. British Sociological Association, BSA, 1993) but also to professional codes (e.g. UKCC, 1992). Indeed some codes may not be written down anywhere, but they arise out of personal conviction.

Summary

Qualitative research is a term that defies specific definition. In this chapter, I have attempted to give an overview of possible versions and to show that where there is diversity there is also correspondence between versions in relation to research design. The chapter does not contain prescriptions for the design of qualitative research. However, it does show that there is a logic to qualitative research, one that rests on a fundamentally systematic and critical approach to understanding the purpose of qualitative research, to elucidating its relationship to theory and to showing how researcher–researched relationships have consequences for the ethical conduct of research.

References

Anderson J (1991a) The phenomenological perspective. In Morse JM (Ed) Qualitative Nursing Research. Newbury Park, CA: Sage. pp. 25–38.

Anderson J (1991b) Immigrant women speak of chronic illness: the social construction of the devalued self. Journal of Advanced Nursing 16: 710–17.

Atkinson P (1990) The Ethnographic Imagination. London: Routledge.

Becker H (1979) Practitioners of vice and crime. In Habenstein RW (Ed) Pathways to Data. Chicago: Aldine. pp. 30–49.

Berger P, Luckmann T (1973) The Social Construction of Reality: A Treatise in the Sociology of Knowledge. Harmondsworth: Penguin Books.

Brown S (1993) Women's Experiences of Rheumatoid Arthritis: A Qualitative Study. Unpublished MSc thesis, University of Manchester.

Brown S, Williams A (1995) Women's experiences of rheumatoid arthritis. Journal of Advanced Nursing 21: 695–701.

Bryman A (1988) Quantity and Quality in Social Research. London: Unwin Hyman.

BSA (1993) Statement of Ethical Practice. Produced by the British Sociological Association. Durham: BSA Mountjoy Research Centre.

Bulmer M (1982) Social Research Ethics: An Examination of the Merits of Covert Participant Observation. London: Macmillan.

Burgess R (1984) In the Field: An Introduction to Field Research. London: George Allen & Unwin.

Burns N, Grove SK (1993) The Practice of Nursing Research. Philadelphia: WB Saunders.

Bury M (1982) Chronic illness as biographical disruption. Sociology of Health and Illness 4(2): 165–82.

Callaghan D (1993) Living with Diabetes: A Qualitative Analysis. Unpublished MSc thesis, University of Manchester.

Callaghan D, Williams A (1994) Living with diabetes: issues for nursing practice. Journal of Advanced Nursing 20:132–9.

Charmaz K (1983) Loss of self: a fundamental form of suffering in the chronically ill. Sociology of Health and Illness 5(2): 168–95.

Clifford J (1983) On ethnographic authority representations 1: 118–46.

Conrad P (1987) The experience of chronic illness: recent and new directions. In Roth JA, Conrad P (Eds) Experience and Management of Illness: Research in the Sociology of Health Care, Vol. 6. Greenwich, CT: JAI Press.

Cook P (1996) An Examination of the Research Basis of Clinical Nursing Practice. Unpublished MSc dissertation, University of Manchester.

Davis F (1963) Passage Through Crisis. Indianapolis: Bobbs Merrill Publishing.

Denzin N (1968) On the ethics of disguised observation. Social Problems 15(4): 502–4.

Erikson KT (1967) A comment on disguised observation in sociology. Social Problems 14(4): 366–73.

Erikson KT (1968) On the ethics of disguised observation: a reply to Denzin. Social Problems 15(4): 505–6.

Gelsthorpe L (1992) Response to Martyn Hammersley's paper, 'On Feminist Methodology'. Sociology 26(2): 213–18.

Gerhardt U (1990) Qualitative research on chronic illness: the issues and the story. Social Science and Medicine 30(11): 1149–59.

Giddens A (1976) New Rules of Sociological Method. London: Hutchinson.

Glaser B (1978) Theoretical Sensitivity. Mill Valley, CA: The Sociology Press.

Glaser B and Strauss A (1967) The Discovery of Grounded Theory: Strategies for Qualitative Research. Chicago: Aldine Publishing.

Gouldner A (1970) The Coming Crisis in Western Sociology. New York: Basic Books.

Grennan D (1984) Rheumatology. London: Ballière Tindall.

Guba E and Lincoln YS (1982) Epistemological and methodological basis of naturalistic enquiry. Educational Communication and Technology Journal 30(4): 233–52.

Hakim C (1987) Research Design: Strategies and Choices in the Design of Social Research. London: Allen & Unwin

Hallett C, Williams A, Butterworth T (1996) The learning career in the community setting: a phenomenological study of a Project 2000 placement. Journal of Advanced Nursing 23: 578–86.

Hammersley M (1990) Reading Ethnographic Research: A Critical Guide. London: Longman.

Hammersley M (1992a) What's Wrong with Ethnography: Methodological Explorations. London: Routledge.

Hammersley M (1992b) On feminist methodology. Sociology 26(2): 187–206.

Hammersley M (1994) On feminist methodology: a response. Sociology 28(1): 293–300.

Hammersley M, Atkinson P (1983) Ethnography: Principles in Practice. London: Routledge.

Hammersley M, Atkinson P (1995) Ethnography: Principles in Practice. 2nd ed. London: Routledge.

Homan R, Bulmer M (1982) On the merits of covert methods: a dialogue. In Bulmer M (Ed) Social Research Ethics: An Examintion of the Merits of Covert Participant Observation. London: Macmillan. pp. 105–21.

Koch T (1993) Towards Fourth Generation Evaluation: Listening to the Voices of Older Patients. Unpublished PhD thesis, University of Manchester.

May KA (1979) The nurse as researcher: impediment to informed consent? Nursing Outlook 27: 36–9.

Merrell J, Williams A (1995) Participant observation and informed consent: tactical decision making in nursing research. Nursing Ethics 1(3): 163–72.

Meyer J (1993) New paradigm research in practice: the trials and tribulations of action research. Journal of Advanced Nursing 18: 1066–72.

Miles MB, Huberman AM (1994) Qualitative Data Analysis. Newbury Park, CA: Sage.

Morse JM, (1991) Qualitative Nursing Research: A Contemporary Dialogue. Newbury Park, CA: Sage.

Nyhlin TK (1990) Diabetes patients facing long term complications: coping with uncertainty. Journal of Advanced Nursing 15: 1021–9.

Polit DF, Hungler BP (1990) Essentials of Nursing Research. 2nd edn. Philadelphia: JP Lippincott.

Ramazanoglu C (1992) On feminist methodology: male reason versus female empowerment. Sociology 26(2): 207–12.

Roth JA (1970) Comments on secret observation. In Filstead WJ (Ed) Qualitative Methodology: Firsthand Involvement with the Social World. Chicago: Markham. pp. 278–80.

Schatzman L, Strauss AL (1973) Field Research: Strategies for a Natural Sociology. Englewood Cliffs, NJ: Prentice-Hall.

Schutz A (1973) Collected Papers 1. The Problem of Social Reality. The Hague: Martinus Nijhoff.

Silverman D (1992) Applying the qualitative method to clinical care. In Daly J, McDonald I, Willis E (Eds) Researching Health Care: Designs, Dilemmas, Disciplines. London: Tavistock/Routledge. pp. 176–88.

Silverman D (1993) Interpreting Qualitative Data: Methods for Analysing Talk, Text and Interaction. London: Sage.

Spradley J (1979) The Ethnographic Interview. New York: Holt, Rinehart & Winston.

Stanley L, Wise S (1993) Breaking Out Again: Feminist Ontology and Epistemology. 2nd edn. London: Routledge.

Strauss A (1970) Discovering new theory from previous theory In Shibutani T (Ed) Human Nature and Collective Behaviour: Essays in Honor of Herbert Blumer. Englewood Cliffs, NJ: Prentice-Hall.

Strauss A (1993) Continual Permutations of Action. New York: Aldine de Gruyter.

Strauss A, Corbin J (1990) Basics of Qualitative Research: Grounded Theory Procedures and Techniques. Newbury Park, CA: Sage.

Thomson G (1982) Rheumatoid Arthritis. London: Arthritis and Rheumatism Council.

United Kingdom Central Council for Nursing, Midwifery and Health Visiting (1992) Code of Professional Practice. London: UKCC

Williams A (1989) Interpreting an Ethnography of Nursing: Exploring the Boundaries of Self, Work and Knowledge. Unpublished PhD thesis, University of Manchester.

Williams A (1990) Reflections on the Making of an Ethnographic Text. Studies in Sexual Politics. Monograph 29, Department of Sociology, University of Manchester. pp. 1–60.

Williams A (1991) Practical ethics: interpretive processes in an ethnography of Nursing. In Aldridge A, Griffiths V, Williams A Rethinking: Feminist Research Processes Reconsidered. Feminist Praxis Monograph No. 33, University of Manchester. pp. 61–83.

Williams A (1993) Diversity and agreement in feminist ethnography. Sociology 27(4): 575–89.

Williams A (1995) Ethics and action research. Nurse Researcher 2(3): 49–59.

Acknowledgement

I would like to take this opportunity to thank all past and present postgraduate students with whom I have discussed the issues covered in this chapter. Our work together, over the past seven years, confirms for me the strength of the contribution of qualitative research to nursing.

Chapter 4
Data collection in qualitative research

Heather Waterman

Introduction

This chapter offers theoretical and practical advice and guidance to neophyte qualitative researchers and offers a basic introduction to the validity of interviews and participant observation. It takes the reader through the process of interviewing, discussing its purpose, preparation and conduct and, finally, its closure. A similar step-by-step guide is presented with regard to participant observation. It reveals the messiness or complexity of these research methods and briefly considers ethical issues.

Interviews

> It is much easier for the field worker to make use of selected informants skills and insights by giving these informants free rein to describe the situation as they see it. The field worker frequently wants his (sic) informants to talk about what they want to talk about; the survey researcher has to get them to talk about what he wants. (Dean et al., 1969: 23)

This quotation draws attention to the style of qualitative interviewing, which makes it a very successful technique for acquiring new knowledge. Interviewing is the most popular method of data collection employed by nurses undertaking qualitative research. The majority of objectives of qualitative nursing research focus on a desire to explore and understand patients' and others' experiences of health and disease. Clearly these preoccupations are best answered by interview rather than observation. In my study of visual impairment (Waterman, 1994), for example, I was keen to identify patients' perceptions of loss of sight. Observing them would not provide the information required and I concluded that the population concerned had to be questioned directly.

Interviews give researchers and patients opportunities to discuss affective, cognitive and normative aspects of life. Patients told stories of the distress they had felt on learning that sight loss was permanent. Some recalled how they had reorganised their lives so that their impairment would not take over. Others described how they tried to balance requesting help against appearing too demanding (Waterman, 1994).

Essentially, the aims of qualitative interviews are to understand the underlying assumptions, ideas and actions of life. Qualitative interviews draw on the qualities of everyday conversation in order to investigate the research problem. It is accepted that the 'rules and behaviour' of day-to-day conversation are a part of qualitative interviewing, in so much as the interviewer and interviewee have to make sense of what is being asked and explained through shared assumptions and common knowledge. In doing so, the context of the interview is not stripped away. As Mischler (1986) argues, the interview should not be viewed simply as a technical event and speech should not be taken at face value. Rather, speech should be seen as problematic and its meaning explored through interview.

A fair amount of planning is needed to be a successful interviewer. The first, but often underestimated, problem concerns how the study population is to be located. In my study, I had few obstacles in approaching patients at a local eye hospital. In contrast, Rose (1996) reports tremendous difficulties in trying to gain access to a sample of carers of people who were dying. Rose (1996) suggests that some of her problems arose because community nurses were excessively cautious in referring people to her. Difficulties in access can seriously extend the length of a study or jeopardise the sample size. Ease of access should be estimated, if possible, while the study is being designed, to prevent slippage at a later stage.

Part of the preparation for an interview involves listing general areas for discussion. Depending on the purpose of the interview and the confidence of the interviewer, these may be phrased as questions or listed as key words. However, they exist as a guide and are not administered in a strict predetermined manner, as in structured interviews. Questions are usually open-ended, giving interviewees the chance to express their perspectives and feelings. Marshall and Rossman (1989) argue that the willingness to explore research participants' views rather than those of researchers is one of the strengths of qualitative interviewing. This approach is termed 'emic' because the constructs of participants are used to frame and understand the data. An alternative is the 'etic' approach, which refers to the use of structures and ideas external to participants to gather and analyse data (Kane, 1985; Boyle, 1994). Etic studies can help to consider concepts over a range of situations; for example, instead of using nurses' categories of expert nurses to analyse interviews, researchers might use Benner's (1984) theory, so that it could be studied across several countries.

Novice qualitative researchers may feel that it is useful to have a 'dummy run' at interviewing. This can increase confidence in asking questions and operating the tape-recorder. I found it helpful at the start of my PhD work to play a recording of an interview to my research supervisors to seek reassurance and tips on technique.

Pilot studies in the conventional sense are unwarranted in qualitative interviewing. They generally serve to assess the reliability of quantitative data collection tools, such as questionnaires, as well as to check the feasibility of a full study (Polit and Hungler, 1995). In qualitative research a rigid and standard application of a list of questions would not enhance the exploration and development of issues. However, the first few interviews will give some indication of whether question areas will elicit the responses anticipated. It is likely that research participants will identify additional areas not previously recognised as important. Areas for questioning continue to be added or reworded throughout the period of data collection as people raise slightly different issues. The data that I gained from the initial interviews were not rejected as unreliable but were included in the analysis because they still contained detailed and clear descriptions of people's experiences of loss of sight (Waterman, 1994).

Occasionally, direct questions are proposed and may become more frequent as concepts or theoretical frameworks are refined. I began my study with little awareness that perceptions of prognosis and functional disability would be important concepts in people's perceptions of visual impairment. Later in the project, I realised that 'hope' played an important role in helping some people cope, but not everyone mentioned it, so in some instances I enquired about it directly. Van Maanen (1983) recalls that he missed a vital piece of information about one policeman he had been studying simply because he failed to ask.

The next, but related, issue is that of gaining the consent of research participants to be interviewed. Letters of introduction about the study and consent forms have to be ready in advance, and in most instances must be approved by a local ethics committee. Ethics committees may take up to three or four months to approve a study. This potential delay should be accounted for in a study timetable. Consideration ought to be given to the ease with which potential participants are able to read the letter and consent form, and the degree to which they understand them. If patients cannot read, I record their oral consent on a tape-recorder at the beginning of an interview.

Even well thought-out strategies can sometimes lead to unintended complications that may prevent an interview from taking place. In my first experience of interviewing (Waterman and Webb, 1992) an elderly woman became upset when she thought I was asking her to sign a bank form. Despite my explanation, she had not understood the purpose of the consent form or the study. The interview had to be abandoned.

Once consent has been given, the date, time, and place of interview can be arranged. After a few near disasters when I forgot to take either a participant's address or the interview schedule, I drew up a list of everything I needed and referred to it immediately prior to going on any interview (see Table 4.1). I also find it absolutely necessary to orientate my mind to the interview that is about to be carried out. To arrive at interviews with irrelevant mental baggage can be distracting and a waste of time. So, be it on a bus or train, I refresh my memory of the topics to be explored. This is essential for a smooth interview and for the collection of relevant data.

Table 4.1: Packing list

---

tape recorder
2 batteries
2 C90 tapes
interview schedule
reflexive journal
pen and pencil
diary
notepad
clipboard
travel timetable
town plan (A-Z)
interviewee's address
interviewee's telephone number
small change or telephone card

Due consideration also needs to be given to the choice of equipment needed for data collection. Tape-recorders are excellent for collecting reliable data and also allow for freer-flowing conversation. Small discrete tape-recorders that are handy and light to carry around, are often recommended. It is not advised to conduct interviews with a hefty bright red 'ghettoblaster' of the type that I used whilst carrying out my first set of interviews as an undergraduate. However, it did serve as an ice-breaker at those potentially awkward moments at the beginning of an interview. My budget precluded the purchase of a new recorder.

A restricted budget can also limit the travelling distance for interviews and consequently possibly affect the sample size and sample characteristics. Overnight visits can incur hotel fees and can considerably raise the cost of a study. Some research participants may expect something in return for granting an interview, such as a free lunch.

The setting of an interview may also affect its outcome. A busy room or office with people passing and telephones ringing will serve to interrupt the concentration of interviewee and interviewer. The participant may be called away and the interview consequently have to be aborted. To counteract these problems I arranged to interview patients at home. However, I have learned that home interviews can occasionally be equally distracting as people 'pop' in and out and offer their contributions to questions posed. When arranging interviews now I suggest, as tactfully as possible, that the interview should take place on a day and at a time when interruptions will be at a minimum. Some participants will not want an interviewer to visit them at home and alternate arrangements should be available.

Interviews are often treated by participants as significant social occasions and most will do their utmost to welcome the researcher. I was frequently treated as a guest of honour, being collected from the local station and having cakes baked in preparation for the interview. I have been touched by the generosity of patients and have been worried about how to repay their kindness. This I did in less obvious ways like giving information about their eye condition when they asked or offering to get booklets for them. Some qualitative researchers argue that the process of interviewing allows interviewees the attractive opportunity not normally available in everyday life to talk at length about themselves:

> Almost without exception respondents proved more durable and energetic than their interviewer. Again and again I was left clinging to consciousness and my tape-recorder as the interview was propelled forward by respon-

> dent enthusiasm. Something in the interview process proved so interesting
> and gratifying that it kept replenishing respondent energy and involvement.
> (McCracken, 1988: 27)

Researchers have to be aware that they could take advantage of participants unfairly in this situation, for example patients could be emotionally exploited.

In nursing research generally, the focus of interviews is often on sensitive or taboo topics, such as cancer or loss of sight, or interviewees are from vulnerable groups, for example the elderly, who possess relatively little power in society. As with more traditional forms of quantitative research, due regard and attention should be given to actual or potential ethical implications of qualitative research. It can not be assumed that because no interventions are introduced in the course of the study that ethical issues are of no consequence. Neither can qualitative researchers claim smugly that, because participants are allowed to voice feelings or opinions at length, qualitative interviews are therapeutic (Hutchinson and Wilson, 1994). The principles that researchers should do no harm to the patient, be respectful and maintain patients' dignity still apply to qualitative interviews, although the way in which these issues are observed is different.

It is not uncommon to find reports of qualitative research in which researchers describe and justify how they dealt with participants who broke down during an interview. Jones (personal communication, 1997) discusses how some patients burst into tears and were upset during interviews about communication on a rehabilitation ward. She considered whether to abandon the study because of the distress it aroused. However, she concluded that the interviews were not the cause of the patients' anguish but rather that they were the medium through which it was revealed. She persisted with the interviews, preparing herself for those who might break down and passing any appropriate information on to nursing staff.

Following an interview, research participants may be left alone with strong emotions that they may never have seriously considered before and with which they may be ill-equipped to cope. It is general practice to debrief people at the close of interview by bringing the conversation back to innocuous everyday topics, like the weather. This can prevent untoward and irrational behaviour after interviews.

Finch (1984) highlights how the nature of qualitative interviews may lead the research participants to divulge more than they had anticipated and afterwards they may regret their candour. To overcome this problem in a study of nurses who worked in an ophthalmic out-patient department, I returned the interview transcript and gave them the opportunity to withdraw ill-advised statements. However, no one wished to alter his or her transcript and most people were more concerned about the seemingly disjointed nature of the interview as it appeared in transcript form.

Some interviewees might behave in an offensive manner or have racist, sexist or ageist tendencies, which might make the interviewer feel uncomfortable. This can place interviewers in a dilemma. If researchers were to reveal their own perspective the interviewee might withhold further information, yet by remaining silent they are effectively negating the value of their own views. The researcher has to assess each situation and attempt to determine whether a passive or active approach is likely to be acceptable and whether it is safe to admit to a different point of view. It is usual during ordinary conversations to seek out other people's opinions and frequently interviewees carry on this practice in interviews. If research participants ask for my view I give it, but avoid elaboration unless it is requested.

The issue of privacy is closely linked to that of confidentiality. It is common practice to assure interviewees that no one apart from research personnel will have access to their interview tape and that all data will be kept secure in locked filing cabinets. Participants are told that they will not be identified in the final report. However in some instances, interviewees may wish their identities to be revealed. Light and Kleiber (1978) argue that women who participated in a study at a Women's Health Collective in North America wanted others to know and read about what each had said at interviews. They were adamant that anonymity contradicted the operational philosophy of openness and honesty of their clinic, minimised their contribution to the research and propagated the power differential felt between the researched and researchers. Light and Kleiber found that the sharing of data assisted in the research aims of understanding the organisation of the collective.

As intimated earlier, qualitative interviewers are expected to probe interviewees to glean relevant information. They develop skills that encourage people to speak openly and often have to rely on their own wits and experience in order to know how and which points to follow up. Interviewers and interviewees obviously contribute to the course, depth and range of an interview, both parties shaping the interview's process and outcome. I remember explaining something innocuous to one patient about her eye condition but she misheard and accused me of misrepresenting the truth.

She kept making references throughout the interview to this unfortu-nate episode and the data thus collected did not seem as informative as other interviews where proceedings had gone smoothly. Different interviewers inevitably gather slightly different data at qualitative interviews and proceed to emphasise differing aspects of people's lives in their reports and theories. On the other hand, some similari-ties in data and analysis will be detected between interviews because it is likely that people involved will have come from similar cultures and be of the same generation. Qualitative interviewers therefore cannot demonstrate validity in the same way as their quantitative counterparts.

Researchers inevitably influence research. Researcher neutrality and independence of interview settings are generally disputed in quali-tative research. Rather than pretending to be objective and claiming minimal interference, some qualitative researchers prefer to take a reflexive stance. This involves examination and analysis of all aspects of the research process, including how they have contributed to the research question, data collection, analysis and report writing. Reflexivity requires a sense of awareness of behaviour, culture and feel-ings and allows researchers to come to some understanding of how they have reached their conclusions. For example, researchers could explain why particular subject matter is of interest to them, or why they chose certain questions at interview. They could divulge those ideas that have influenced them in the course of their studies. Reflexivity also allows them to challenge any deep-rooted preconceptions they have and open them up to other forms of analysis. This attitude takes the position that if researchers cannot be strictly objective they should at least attempt to understand how they are contributing to the research process by being 'upfront' about their biases. Revelation does not remove biases but it does open them up for critical analysis.

Validity, put simply, whether from a quantitative or qualitative perspective, refers to whether researchers have achieved what they set out to achieve. For example, did I manage to grasp the meaning of visual impairment as described to me by the research partici-pants? Validity cannot be proved because it is a subjective judge-ment, but researchers can demonstrate how they have been rigorous in several ways, including revealing the nature of the interview and interview schedule to show how it developed and how new questions were added. Quotations from the interview transcripts could be included in the report, thus showing the depth of discussion and illustrating the main points. The number and length of interviews should be discussed in relation to the quality of data gained.

Mackenzie (1994) argues that researchers need to be in the field for sufficient time to understand the culture of interest. Clarification by the interviewer of interviewees' statements at the time of the interview is obvious and is termed 'member checking' by some researchers (Sandelowski, 1986). Researchers can also show how they have attempted to include a range of people who give varying perspectives on the subject matter and those who can offer alternate experiences to the norm. Glaser and Strauss (1967) describe this as negative case analysis.

Another debate within qualitative research concerns whether traditional research ideas about reliability can be transferred to qualitative research. To be reliable means to collect data in a consistent manner (Polit and Hungler, 1995). However, as just demonstrated, qualitative interviewers use their own initiative as much as the questions written down to extract the information they need; they have a part to play in the construction of knowledge as much as the interviewee. To be consistent in the application of questions between interviews would be detrimental to the collection of qualitative data. From my experience it is important to be prepared and systematic but flexible in one's approach. Qualitative interviewers should be prepared to demonstrate how they have achieved this.

Qualitative researchers favour familiar and lengthy contact with research participants; however, such research relationships are not easy to close. As described previously, the interview becomes a social occasion and the interviewer is treated as a guest and friend. Rose (personal communication, 1997) describes such a situation with a group of elderly patients in which the interviews became a setting for company and solace, making the closure of such meetings a delicate task. Some were lonely and it was clear that the interviews provided an opportunity for rare social interaction – she was asked to read poetry by one and sent postcards by another. She did not refuse or reject these requests, arguing that the interview should be seen as a reciprocal arrangement. This, she argues, will also give rise to better data because as interviewees' concerns are valued they will feel more inclined to help the researchers with theirs. However, it does mean that the closures of interviews will be more difficult. Rose (personal communication, 1997) suggests that researchers could make the interviewee aware of the number of visits to be made at the first interview, and she argues that some participants may need to be reminded of this gently at later visits. However, withdrawal after the last interview is not easy and feelings of loss may be felt within both parties and may need to be addressed. Some kind of contact may be kept through letters or cards. Occasionally, true friendship is struck and interviewer and interviewee may continue to see each other long after the research is ended.

Qualitative interviewing can lead to mutual understanding and better communications amongst patients and health professionals. However as a method it should not be relied upon exclusively for it can only give one perspective. To gain a rounded picture of social life it is important to observe it as well.

Participant observation

Participant observation is the other key method of data collection used by qualitative researchers. As Kahn and Mann (1969) argue:

> The academic stereotype places the professor in the library for research purposes, or if his [sic] field of endeavour requires it, in a laboratory populated either by white mice or sophomores. In recent years a good deal has been done to change this stereotype. Increasing numbers of social scientists have come to see the importance of studying functioning organisations. Many of the more complex problems which social scientists are presently tackling yield themselves only to imperfectly to laboratory treatment. As a result, it is sometimes safer to generalise from studies of real life situations than from the laboratory . . . (Kahn and Mann, 1969: 45)

Participant observation can provide insight into the cultural milieu of everyday life, of how people make sense of their lives and the assumptions or 'taken-for-granted' aspects of work and other activities that are simply too difficult to study in any other way. It gives access to parts of life that may not be explicitly mentioned during an interview or are too complex to explain adequately, or to those elements that are habitual or are passed by unnoticed. I carried out participant observation with ophthalmic out-patient nurses when I realised that interviewees had difficulty explaining contextual factors that inhibited their professional development, and when I had problems conceptualising what it was they were trying to tell me. Once I had observed and experienced nursing in the clinic I was in a better position to understand.

Gold (1969) distinguishes between four different observer roles, which are dependent on the degree of participation and awareness of the research of those studied: complete participant, participant as observer, observer as participant and complete observer (for a full discussion the reader is referred to Gold's text). However, as Johnson (1993) argues, participants' roles are not as clearly defined as Gold suggests, being much more 'fluid' and variable. The level of participation depends on the people being observed and those observing, the purpose and stage of the research. The researcher may passively watch or actively participate within one hour of observation. I found that initially I participated readily in the treatment room but held back and observed in the waiting and consulting area of the clinic, for I did not have sufficient understanding of how the clinic functioned to take part safely and properly (Waterman, 1994).

Gold (1969) highlights that observation may be covert or overt, which refers to whether researchers are honest with those being studied about their intentions to study, and whether they seek their consent to be observed. Field (1989) describes a study about 'nursing the dying' that was completed through covert observation. A researcher posed as a health care assistant whilst collecting data and did not reveal her other occupation. Deceptive research such as this has been criticised by Johnson (1992), who advocates the teaching and undertaking of non-deceptive work. Roth (1962) points out that it is impossible to tell everything to everyone about a study. The degree of researcher revelation is linked to the issue of access. Homan (1980) argues that a covert stance is necessary in situations where access is not permitted.

Whether covert or overt, observation requires careful planning and execution. Clarity of purpose is essential to avoid feelings of being overwhelmed by the sheer extent of what might be observed, and the frustration of being physically unable to access everything relevant. Novice researchers are frequently advised to enter the setting with a broad topic area in mind. For example, I sought to understand roles of nurses in an out-patient department and at first logged every kind of activity that they undertook, but then proceeded to study the contextual constraints on their practice. The point at which researchers 'home in' on certain issues is dependent upon their confidence and the matter to be investigated.

Events, social groupings, geographical lay out, language, formal and informal relationships are a few subjects for study. I shadowed all nursing and auxiliary staff to grasp the complexities of their roles (Waterman, 1994). I attempted to learn and understand the significance of the differing aspects of their work and, in particular, the intricate system of the movement of notes and people around the out-patient department. As the project progressed I concentrated on the contextual and organisational constraints on nurses and how these impinged on their roles.

This method of data collection relies heavily on the researcher to take note of matter relevant to the research question. I would carry a pocket-sized notebook in which I jotted key words regarding my observations. After working a morning or afternoon shift, I went back to the office and used the references in the book as a framework to type up my field notes, which included descriptions of incidents, my experiences, feelings, methodological and theoretical ideas, and analytical commentary. Anything that occurred to me regarding the topic in hand I included in my fieldwork diary. Some researchers prefer to separate these various aspects into different sections in a diary or books (Kane, 1985). The entries in a fieldwork diary are the equivalent of interview transcripts – that is, they are data.

Researchers need to be equally aware when conducting participant observation, as when interviewing, of whether their ideas or categories or frameworks for understanding the situation are externally generated, that is etic in origin, or whether they arise from those under study, that is are emic. It is essential according to Van Maanen (1983), that researchers can distinguish between the two types of concepts, otherwise they could make unwarranted claims about the data. I used nurses' and health care assistants' categories when describing the different nursing roles in the out-patient department – for example 'on the front' and 'in the treatment room'. As well as including their views I also employed a range of concepts from sociology and psychology to help organise and understand organisational factors that negatively impinged on their work. Researchers should be careful not to claim their interpretation of a situation to be fact (Van Maanen, 1983).

In the course of participant observation, researchers will attempt to interview those they are studying. This might involve quick snatches of conversation in the sluice or longer discussions over a cup of coffee. But these interactions tend not to be formally prearranged and are generally not tape-recorded. They function as opportunities for researchers to clarify their interpretations of situations and to test out conceptual ideas. For example, nurses in the ophthalmic out-patient department talked of being allocated to work 'on the box', which I found out after questioning them meant that they were positioned outside the consulting rooms near a grey box containing patients' notes. They ran the clinic from there (Waterman, 1994).

It is common to come across claims that informants make about their work or lives that do not appear to match reality. Nurses and health care assistants espoused the psychological care of patients but when under pressure in a busy clinic this appeared to be neglected and abandoned almost completely. I investigated whether the claims should be regarded as genuine misapprehension or read as untruths in order to protect individual or collective interests. This process gave rise to valuable information about how the nurses and health care assistants viewed themselves and conceptualised nursing. This kind of information can lead to some of the most interesting qualitative theories.

The few excerpts of participant observation offered here suggest the closeness of the relationships that researchers have to nurture in order to maintain access. Researchers have to detect and act accordingly to local and organisational senses of decorum and etiquette. I perceived that nurses related to each other in a strictly hierarchical way and thought it prudent to request that my first periods of observation were with the senior sister in charge. Once I had shadowed her, all but one of the other staff did not object to my presence.

Many of the points about the validity and reliability of qualitative interviews can be transferred to participant observation, the aim of which is to attempt to understand people's ways of life and how these are constructed and perceived. Researchers could focus on a whole variety of attributes and theoretical explanations and they have to deal with a perpetually changing research setting, although the degree of change experienced will vary. It is impossible, therefore, for researchers to claim that their analysis is absolute. There is a sense, however, that some theoretical explanations could be misguided or that researchers are not portraying a fair picture. Techniques described previously can be used to prevent these accusations: interpretations need to be checked with people being studied to avoid misunderstandings; field notes ought to written up regularly as soon as possible after observation or important material could be forgotten or written about inaccurately; all perspectives should be considered and people or events who represent the antithesis of the norm should be sought out to broaden the theory developed; and researchers should demonstrate how they immersed themselves in the setting in order to gain a thorough understanding.

Participant observers should also acknowledge that the whole process and outcome of the research is inevitably bound by the culture from which they come and their life experiences and those that were studied. A reflexive stance, therefore, is warranted in order to explore and analyse how they have influenced the research, to justify the reasoning behind their method and to reassure readers that they were attempting to be aware of how they affected the research. A reflexive diary is often kept as a record of these developments. I made entries in mine on my journey home from episodes of observation. It became, in some respects, another data resource and revealed, amongst other things, the development of ideas and their possible source. It helped me to recognise and justify why I had decided to take a particular course of analysis and highlighted areas where I could have been accused of being biased.

Some writers suggest that participant observers should take the stance of naive outsiders or learners (Strauss, 1969). This suggests that researchers should behave as unsophisticated and trusting people who do not understand the setting and the people involved. Such behaviour is thought to elicit a great deal of information from those being studied and also allows the researcher to 'see what really is going on'. Other authors argue that a prior understanding of the research setting can save time and avoid misrepresentations. The attitude of the naive outsider is inappropriate for most nurse researchers who will tend to be investigating aspects of practice within which they have some knowledge if not expertise. They are also likely to be people holding senior positions or people who are seeking to obtain academic accreditation for their research and therefore cannot either claim to be naive or an outsider. As already indicated, researchers cannot stand outside of themselves to study the world as 'it really is'. They shape the research. A reflexive stance seems to be a wise alternative.

Reactivity is problematic for those undertaking participant observation. It is something researchers have to learn to cope with and for which they have to make allowances. Participant observers could note the degree of reaction to their presence and watch how and when it alters. This allows them to make informed claims about their work. The quality and type of reaction can also provide useful information on the people being studied; for example, if they react with a lot of suspicion this may give an indication of the local management style.

The presence of researchers may serve to inhibit the work of nurses being studied. I attempted to check how much I was disturbing the work of the nurses in the out-patient department and removed myself if they or I considered that I was in the way. On the other hand, occasionally I was an asset to them and could be relied upon to run a clinic by myself and instil eye drops when they were short of qualified nurses (Waterman, 1994). The degree of integration depends on the skills of researchers and the purpose of the study.

At times researchers may inadvertently cause 'trouble' for those observed. I remember becoming involved in a conversation with a junior nurse and being surprised and disturbed when the nurse was abruptly 'told off' by the sister for being in the wrong place. I had not anticipated this and I did not want to 'harm' any of the nurses. I was also aware that if I was perceived to be interfering in the smooth running of the clinic, access to it would be withdrawn. After this incident, I was careful to conduct conversations with junior nurses and auxiliaries out of the sight of sisters. In some respects, I felt subversive but in other respects I had to recognise the needs of this vulnerable group.

I was also conscious that observation could imply criticism of their nursing practice. Readiness to 'muck in' and an open and honest approach to what I was doing assisted in the amelioration of this potential problem. I did not hide my notebook and note taking, and offered to let the staff inspect its contents. Since they had known me as a ward sister, I believe that they were more ready to accept and trust me. McCall and Simons (1969) suggests that maintaining good relationships is never easy because those being observed are:

> accustomed to life in a more or less ordinary social world ... they do not know what kind of a creature a participant observer is – what runs in his [sic] veins and his mind, how much he should count for on the scales of human goodness and worth, or how he may be evaluating them. After all, what motives, what alien causes, would lead a man to turn on his brethren with analytic eye? (McCall and Simons 1969: 28)

Unless those being studied have undertaken research or studied it, they are unlikely to fully comprehend participant observation. I believe most good participant observers nurture understanding amongst participants about the research process in order to gather appropriate data (Strauss, 1969).

Another problem nurse researchers encounter is knowing what course of action should be taken, if malpractice should be observed. As a nurse I considered that I was obliged to act according to the Code of Conduct (United Kingdom Central Council, 1992), in that I would inform appropriate persons of any circumstances in which safe and appropriate care for patients could not be provided. I was also aware that whilst observing I should not place myself in positions of responsibility for which I was not prepared, as the Code of Conduct (UKCC, 1992) also advises. However, I was a qualified ophthalmic nurse and did intervene in some situations that required my knowledge. Before observation commenced I discussed my role in the clinic with staff, but early on in the project I did not fully appreciate how the participant observation would develop and change. So as I learnt to function as a clinic nurse, I found I needed to clarify regularly my degree of participation and responsibilities. This was debated amongst staff and we managed to come to an amicable understanding.

The UKCC (1992) also recognises patients' rights to privacy and, in theory, participant observation could place a nurse in a compromising position with regard to this. It is usual to seek people's informed consent prior to observation. All persons in the research setting should be aware that they may be observed, and this includes patients, nurses, doctors and cleaners. This presents a particular problem to nurses undertaking participant observation because they may experience a high throughput of people in their research setting. Approximately 100–200 patients would pass through the out-patient department in one day when I was carrying out participant observation (Waterman, 1994). Although nurses were the main focus of my study and patients were only observed as they came into contact with nurses, I still felt they should be informed and their consent gained. Letters were distributed to patients during each period of observation as they entered the clinic in which I was working. They were informed of the study and their role therein. They were also asked to advise the nurses or myself if they did not want to be observed. Only two patients declined.

As indicated, participant observation is labour intensive and time consuming and, as a consequence, it is considered expensive. For researchers it can be physically and emotionally exhausting; they suffer a 'double whammy' in the sense that they live the experience once and then go over it again when writing up field notes. Making detailed notes is a painstaking and laborious business which takes a while to learn to do accurately. However, reliving the experience can assist in the process of 'immersion' and aid analysis.

Researchers may immerse themselves so successfully that they 'go native', that is they become unable to function effectively as a researcher. They are unable to maintain a critical eye and may find it difficult to identify with any others apart from those whom they are supposed to be studying. 'Not being able to see the wood for the trees' is a frequently applied expression in these circumstances. Researchers need to be alert to this paradox of needing, on the one hand, to get close to people under study yet, on the other hand, needing to be sympathetic to a variety of perspectives. In order to limit this problem, most researchers spend time out of the field so that they can maintain some sort of freshness in their approach.

Summary

Interviewing and participant observation are the backbone of qualitative research and are the key to the success of this approach. Both methods can be physically and intellectually demanding but the quality of data collected makes the investment of effort worthwhile.

References

Benner P (1984) From Novice to Expert: Excellence and Power in Clinical Nursing Practice. London: Addison Wesley.

Boyle JS (1994) Styles of ethnography. In Morse J (Ed) Critical Issues in Qualitative Research Methods. London: Sage.

Dean JP, Eichhorn RL, Dean LR (1969) Establishing field relations. In McCall GJ, Simons JL (Eds) Issues in Participant Observation: A Text and Reader. London: Addison-Wesley.

Field D (1989) Nursing the Dying. London: Routledge.

Finch J (1984) 'It's great to have someone to talk to': the ethics and politics of interviewing women. In Bell C, Roberts H (Eds) Social Researching: Politics, Problems, Practice. London: Routledge & Kegan Paul.

Glaser B, Strauss A (1967) The Discovery of Grounded Theory: Strategies for Quatitative Research. Chicago: Aldine.

Gold RL (1969) Roles in sociological field relations. In McCall GJ, Simons JL (Eds) Issues in Participant Observation: A Text and Reader. London: Addison-Wesley.

Homan R (1980) The ethics of covert methods. British Journal of Sociology 31(1): 46–59.

Hutchinson S, Wilson H (1994) Research and therapeutic interviews: a post-structuralist perspective. In Morse J (Ed) Critical Issues in Qualitative Research Methods. London: Sage.

Johnson M (1992) A silent conspiracy: ethical issues of participant observation in nursing research. International Journal of Nursing Studies 29(2): 213–23.

Johnson M (1993) Unpopular Patients Reconsidered: an Interpretative Ethnography of the Process. Unpublished PhD thesis University of Manchester.

Kahn R, Mann F (1969) Developing research relationships. In McCall GJ, Simons JL (Eds) Issues in Participant Observation: a Text and Reader. London: Addison-Wesley.

Kane E (1985) Doing your Own Research: Basic Descriptive Research in the Social Sciences and Humanities. London: Marion Boyars.

Light L, Kleiber N (1978) Interactive research in a health care setting. Social Sciences and Medicine 12: 193–8.

McCall GJ, Simons JL (1960) Issues in Participant Observation. London: Addison Wesley.

McCracken G (1988) The Long Interview. London: Sage.

Mackenzie AE (1994) Evaluating ethnography: considerations for analysis. Journal of Advanced Nursing 19: 774–81.

Marshall C, Rossman GB (1989) Designing Qualitative Research. London: Sage.

Mischler EG (1986) Research Interviewing: Context and Narrative. London: Harvard University Press.

Polit D, Hungler B (1995) Nursing Research: Principles and Practice. Philadelphia: Lippincott.

Rose K (1996) Caring for a Dying Relative: the Experiences of Informal Carers of Terminally Ill Patients. Unpublished PhD thesis, University of Manchester.

Roth JA (1962) Comments on secret observation. Social Problems 9(3): 283–4.

Sandelowski M (1986) The problem of rigor in qualitative research. Advances in Nursing Science 8: 27.

Strauss A (1969) Field tactics. In McCall GJ, Simons JL (Eds) Issues in Participant Observation: a Text and Reader. London: Addison-Wesley.

Van Maanen J (1983) Qualitative Methodology. London: Sage.

UKCC (1992) Code of Professional Conduct for the Nurse, Midwife and Health Visitor. London: UKCC.

Waterman H (1994) The Meaning of Visual Impairment: Developing Ophthalmic Nursing. Unpublished PhD thesis, University of Manchester.

Waterman H, Webb C (1992) Visually impaired patients' perceptions of their stay in hospital. Nursing Practice 5(3): 6–9.

Chapter 5
The preparation and analysis of qualitative interview data

Carl May

Introduction

The past two decades have seen an astonishing growth of interest in qualitative research techniques amongst British health researchers. This book, like many others, bears witness to the extent to which the health professions have sought to engage with models of data collection and analysis that lie outside of the conventional biomedical model. My brief in this chapter is to provide an outline account of the way in which interview data can be treated once they are 'gathered' in qualitative research, but before I can move on to the substantive topic of the chapter I need to offer the reader some important caveats.

Theory is important

I do not propose to deal with the theoretical underpinnings of data analysis. There is a bewildering number of theoretical models on which the collection of such data is predicated, drawn from a variety of academic disciplines. However, theory is a vital component of qualitative research at two levels:

- It is important to understand the epistemological foundations of qualitative research (that is, its philosophical basis), so that the researcher can properly limit the claims that she or he makes about the form and results of a particular project. The failure to understand the philosophical basis of this mode of data collection has led to some extraordinary outcomes and to some unfortunate failures in research.

- Theory forms the lens through which data are interpreted. In this sense, it offers the researcher a means of understanding the content of collected data in terms of interactions and processes that take place amongst people. Beyond this, theory offers a route by which connections can be made between categories of data within a study, and also between studies. Thus, common features of one set of interactions and processes can be compared and understood in relation to quite different contexts.

The important implication of these two points is that theory is an explanatory device that permits the interpretation of data. Without a set of theoretical underpinnings, qualitative research easily slides into mere description, for theory is what gives any model of research its explanatory power. As I have already noted, qualitative research techniques are derived from theoretical developments in several academic disciplines: anthropology, sociology and, increasingly, psychology. Their central feature is that they derive from a philosophical perspective that stresses induction rather than deduction, and that they explore the realm of subjective experience, rather than the objective structure and distribution of phenomena.

- **Theory is important because it provides a vantage point from which 'data' can be interpreted and conclusions drawn.**

The researcher is the research instrument

Distinctions between the collection, interpretation and analysis of qualitative data are all, to some extent, false. It is certainly true that there are practical differences between these activities but it is more important to note that they are linked by the person of the researcher. In most qualitative studies, one individual conducts the fieldwork, collates and prepares the data and undertakes the analytical procedures that lead to the publication of results. Such a model of research therefore relies on the researcher being subjectively or reflexively engaged with the topic of study in a way that other models of research practice do not. The boundaries of data collection and analysis are therefore very fuzzy, if they exist at all: in a qualitative interview the researcher is making decisions about what is or is not significant data even as the interviewee is speaking. Indeed, the researcher is structuring her or his conversation with the interviewee to precisely that end in the interview. The fundamental act of the qualitative researcher undertaking interview-based research is, however, to critically interrogate talk and text. The basic activities, therefore, are listening and reading.

- **Qualitative research relies on the researcher engaging creatively with the research topic. Although explicit procedures may be used, the boundaries between data collection and analysis are not clearly defined.**

Qualitative research cannot be automated

For the purposes of this chapter, then, the creative interpretative engagement between the researcher and the researched is the hub of all of the activities that I shall describe. But this subjective engagement is also a problem. It means that much of the work that the qualitative researcher undertakes is hidden from view, in a way that is not the case when studies are undertaken using statistical methods. More importantly, it means that it is sometimes difficult, and not always desirable, to codify precisely the activities that such interpretative analysis involves in a way that mechanically leads the researcher to move through different stages of analytic work. It is important to be clear that this does not mean that such work should be undertaken in a way that lacks structure and cannot be demonstrated to be rigorous. Both are vital to the integrity of the research (and the researcher).

If the different activities that go together to make up qualitative research should not be seen as mechanically leading one to another, this leaves the question of the extent to which computer software packages assist in the interpretation and analysis of qualitative data. There are a number of packages available to the researcher which promise to help. Perhaps the most popular is QSR NUDIST. The key point about such packages is that they can only assist in the collation and retrieval of text. They cannot analyse the data, for that is an entirely human function.

The question for the researcher, when making choices about the use of software like QSR NUDIST, is whether the effort is commensurate with the reward. These packages really come into their own when there is a large body of data, already transcribed and prepared. But most people who undertake qualitative studies are not searching through very large bodies of ready-transcribed data: instead they are students and research assistants working in quite tightly circum-scribed settings, often with relatively small bodies of data.

- **Software packages are available to assist in the analysis of qualitative data. However, they cannot analyse data in the way that some statistical packages do: instead they are valuable as a means of manipulating transcribed material.**

Objectives of this chapter

Having set out some caveats about the practice of qualitative research, I want to make it clear what this chapter is intended to deliver. Much of the interpretative and analytical work that is undertaken in qualitative studies is done in the course of fieldwork itself. The decisions that are made then and the lines of enquiry that the researcher follows within interviews profoundly shape all that follows. Similarly, the theoretical orientations of the researcher (which define the very research topic itself, and the selection of technique) are equally profound in the ways that they shape subsequent work. Given this, my objective in this chapter is to set out a simple model of qualitative analysis that will mesh with most kinds of research topic and most kinds of theoretical orientation. In doing so, I rather lay myself open to a good deal of expert criticism about epistemology and practice, but my approach is to be a guide through two types of procedures:

- The physical preparation of qualitative data for formal analysis: including transcription, and the editing and layout of transcripts.
- A simple model for defining and recording particular analytical devices within a transcript or body of transcripts.

What follows, then, is an outline of the practical procedures that are involved in a simple model of constant comparative technique (see Strauss, 1987 and Strauss and Corbin, 1990, for a more detailed account).

The kinds of interviews in which qualitative techniques are operationalised can be extraordinarily fruitful and interesting. One of the most important claims that proponents of these techniques make is that they enable the subjects of research to give voice to their authentic, and often spontaneous, perspectives on a topic in a way that brings them closer to those who ultimately make use of research reports or papers. The extent to which this is true for any particular project depends entirely on the quality of the fieldwork on which such studies are founded and the degree to which subsequent interpretation and analysis are rigorously undertaken. In qualitative studies, as in any other kind of research, no amount of analytical fervour can compensate for poorly designed and conducted fieldwork.

Converting talk into text

This section of the chapter is about the preparation of data for formal analysis. I operate from the assumption that interviews have been recorded – either on audio or video-tape – and that these tapes form the raw data from which subsequent formal analysis will be undertaken.

Transcription is not the beginning of analysis

I have already noted that the practice of qualitative research means that analytical work is being done from the moment that the first observation or interview begins. All research demands that the researcher is reflexive: that is that the significance, relevance and meaning of what research subjects say and do is critically questioned from the very beginning of the study. For this reason it is helpful to keep a research journal through which the development of the analytical framework that is used can be tracked, particular decisions about the direction of the study recorded, and ideas about emerging analytical categories can also be recorded. These initial categories – what Bernstein (1976) calls 'first order constructs' – are crucial to the development of any qualitative study: they form the framework through which subsequent data analysis is developed. Whatever specific qualitative technique is used, it is important to keep track of how your ideas develop, and how these relate to other work in the field. A research journal, therefore, permits the construction of two kinds of audit trail through the study. First, it allows the researcher to develop a practical 'history' of the project that shows who was interviewed and when, and points of interest in the interview itself. Second, it permits the development of an 'intellectual' biography of the study, showing how particular ideas about what research subjects are saying and doing emerged in the course of the study, and how these ideas influenced its development. Most importantly, it helps you, the researcher, to keep in touch with what you are thinking and to keep your ideas organised.

● **Analysis of qualitative data begins during its collection. Keep a research journal so that you have a written**

record of your thoughts about specific interviews and their results.

Technical aspects of recording the interview

In the previous chapter, the development of interview schedules or topic lists was discussed in depth. It is normally the case that an audio (or sometimes a video) recording is made of interviews in qualitative research, and that this is intended for subsequent transcription. The quality of that record depends on the way in which the tape-recorder is used during the interview. Most people use personal stereo tape-recorders, which are compact and can take a full size audiocassette. If you use a well-known brand of cassette you can be confident that the quality of sound reproduction will be good. You can also be confident that the cassette will last well into the interview if you use a 45-minute cassette (C60 – 30 minutes per side – cassettes are usually too short, necessitating frequent changes). Try not to use Dictaphone-type machines as they tend to produce poor quality sound and their cassettes have a very short duration. Always label the cassette that you use for an interview with a code letter or number and the date of interview and keep it safe. If you have promised to respect the interviewee's anonymity and confidentiality it is as important to do this with the 'raw' data that you have collected as it is to do so in the final report.

The first obstacle to the production of a quality record is the location of the tape-recorder itself: if a machine with an integral microphone (usually called a 'condenser microphone') is being used then make sure that the microphone is pointing towards the interviewee. If such a microphone is being used, then the machine ought to be placed on a soft surface otherwise the motor that drives the tapes will cause the machine to vibrate against the surface of a table or desk, causing a rumbling noise on the tape that will make it difficult to hear the interview itself. Using a conference or tie-clip microphone means that you do not have to worry about machine noise. It also has the advantage that the tape-recorder itself can be concealed from view. This helps to put the research subject at ease. The quality of subsequent transcripts to some extent depends on the technical quality of the record that you make of the interview. So:

- **Use an appropriate tape-recorder and microphone.**
- **Practise using the machine and learn where to place it to obtain the best sound quality.**
- **Label audiotapes and store them safely.**

There are occasions when it is either inappropriate or impossible to use a cassette recorder. Where this is so you will need to make short verbatim notes. If you do, remember to take the interview more slowly and do not be afraid to ask the interviewee to repeat or paraphrase things that they have said so that you can record them accurately. Always take a pen and notepad to the interview.

Transcribing tape-recorded interviews

Most researchers do not, in practice, have the luxury of having their interview tapes transcribed for them by a trained audio-typist and most end up doing this work in rather arduous circumstances. Yet this is the foundation of all subsequent work and needs to be undertaken in a physical environment that is conducive to concentration and accuracy. For the best results a purpose-designed transcription unit – like that used by audiotypists – is required, with headphones and foot-pedal controls. (This means that the person doing the transcription can focus her or his attention on what is on the tape, rather than on reaching out to control the tape-recorder.) External noise and interruptions are a primary source of inaccurate transcription, and quite small errors can have significant consequences later on (see Box 1).

Box 1: How a tiny transcription error spoiled a study

Steve[1] had been working on a project that looked at the organisation of a surgical outpatient unit in a local hospital. Central to this was the role of the clinical director's relationships with a number of senior nurses. In the course of transcribing an interview with one of his key informants, Steve typed the following:

'frankly, I think this guy's a bit too concerned about his own impotence when he's dealing with the charge nurses.'

Not unnaturally Steve drew a set of conclusions from this that focused his attention on the limits of the clinical director's authority. But the nurse had said something quite different:

'frankly, I think this guy's a bit too concerned about his own importance when he's dealing with the charge nurses.'

---

[1]'Steve' is a pseudonym. I am grateful to him for letting me use material gathered as part of his MSc dissertation in this chapter. All the names and some other details in the exemplars drawn from his work have been changed to ensure the anonymity of his respondents.

Accuracy is more important than speed, and transcribing is painstaking work that needs to be taken seriously. A 60-minute interview may take between 4 and 10 hours to transcribe accurately, so ensure that you build time for this into the design of a research project.

- **Work in an environment where you can concentrate without interruption.**
- **Transcribe in short sessions, stop to read what you have transcribed and look for errors.**
- **Check your transcripts against the tape regularly.**

Editing transcripts for formal analysis

A transcript is, in research terms, a formal document on which interpretative procedures are going to be carried out, so a key question is the extent to which the everyday infelicities of speech are edited out. In everyday encounters, any piece of conversation is littered with ungrammatical utterances, false starts and interruptions. This means that it can be quite hard to make sense of it when it is transcribed verbatim. In Box 2 I have included some verbatim transcription from Steve's project in a surgical outpatients department. It is not always easy to follow and parts of it are really not very informative.

Box 2: Verbatim transcript

Steve: So, uh what do uh you think of the way things have turned out with uh, oh uh this new appointments system?

Helen: Well, you know, it's uh difficult to tell but the truth is that oh, you know, it's Jackie Chan the clinical director. Well, uh how can I put it, it's uh well it's ah difficult, you know, because I think that ahhh, how can I put it, frankly, I think this guy's well uh, a bit too concerned about his own importance when he's dealing with the charge nurses, d'you know what I mean? You know in the case where Mrs Jones made that complaint 'cos her husband died, uh and it was uh, well our fault . . .

In this case, editing for understanding is a matter of removing utterances that spoil the line of the account. But it is important to do this in a way that does not alter its sense or meaning. In addition to editing for understanding, it may be necessary to excise individuals' or institutions' names on ethical grounds, to protect the anonymity of interviewees and their colleagues and patients (a simple set of code numbers or letters can be used in their place). In Box 3, we can see how Steve edited this item of text in a way that retained the sense of uncertainty in the interviewee's account while removing both conversational hesitations and individual names. In practice, this kind of editing can be done while the tape is being transcribed, but there are circumstances in which it is not desirable to do so, especially if the interviewee's account is complex or difficult to understand. The maxim here ought to be: if in doubt do not edit out.

Box 3: Edited transcript

Steve: So, what do you think of the way things have turned out with this new appointments system?

XR3: Well, you know, it's difficult to tell, but the truth is that, you know, it's [name] the clinical director. Well, how can I put it, it's – well it's difficult, you know, because I think that – how can I put it – frankly, I think this guy's well, a bit too concerned about his own importance when he's dealing with the charge nurses, d'you know what I mean? You know in the case where [name] made that complaint 'cos [the patient died], and it was – well our fault . . .

There are no hard-and-fast rules about the editing of transcripts: if a project relies on reporting an interviewee's account as it is spoken – as in some kinds of discourse analysis – then it clearly makes no sense to 'clean' the transcript in this way, and there are special rules of notation that enable discrete speech acts to be rendered textually (see Silverman, 1993). However, the principal rules of editing transcripts are:

- **Edit out the minimum necessary to make an interviewee's account comprehensible.**
- **Edit out the names of individuals and institutions whose anonymity you have promised to protect.**
- **Clearly indicate that a transcript has been edited, and where names have been removed or other material altered.**

Setting out the transcript for formal analysis

Once an interview or set of interviews have been transcribed, the transcripts need to be organised in a way that makes them easy to use. Word-processing software such as Word or Wordperfect makes this easy because margins and line spacing can be automatically set, as can font sizes. (This is especially important if you intend to use a software package like QSR NUDIST, which can – at the time of writing – only cope with the unreadably small Courier 10 point font). Even more usefully, most word-processing packages permit paragraphs and individual lines to be automatically numbered, as well as having cross-referencing and indexing functions.

- **Using a standard layout for transcripts means that they can be easily processed and interpreted in groups.**
- **Line and paragraph numbering allows the indexing of text, so that points of interest can be clearly identified and easily located.**
- **Headers and footers can be used to make sure every page of a transcript can be clearly related to a specific interview.**

So what should the final copy of a transcript look like? In Box 4 I have included part of a page from Steve's interview data. We can now see the transcript set up in a way that will make subsequent work easy.

Keeping organised

Even quite small qualitative studies can generate considerable amounts of paper. How this paperwork is kept and organised contributes crucially to the success of any project. Of course most data will be on disk, and thus be retrievable at a moment's notice (assuming that you have made back up disks – and remember that if you have not, your PC will crash). Even so, you will need paper copies to read and make notes on. Filing – and keeping them safe – is a boring but necessary part of organising your data. Never leave paper copies of interview transcripts lying around where others may read them: if you have promised confidentiality to your respondents it is unethical to do so.

Text as data: categories, codes and memos

The object of preparing interview transcripts in the way that I have described is to make them easy to use when you come to the serious business of formal data analysis. How you go about formal analysis of qualitative data will depend on a number of things: the discipline in which your study is set; the theoretical approach that you have adopted; and the kind of interviews that you have conducted. Each of these will structure your approach to the 'data'. What is important to note here is that what is commonly called analysis in qualitative research is a highly focused and selective kind of reading – it is an act of interpretation rather than a set of mechanical procedures.

Box 4: Interview XR. 27 April 1995

Page 11 of 32

S[teve] 33: So, what do you think of the way things have turned out with this new appointments system?

XR34: Well, you know, it's difficult to tell, but the truth is that, you know, it's [name] the clinical director. Well, how can I put it, it's – well it's difficult, you know, because I think that - how can I put it – frankly, I think this guy's well, a bit too concerned about his own importance when he's dealing with the charge nurses, d'you know what I mean? You know in the case where Mrs [name] made that complaint 'cos [the patient died], and it was – well our fault . . .
S35: What happened there?

XR36: Well basically, he just walked all over us, we tried to insist that the complaint was dealt with quickly and openly, because we figured that if we showed willing and were properly apologetic that would be good enough. And I think we were right, all she really wanted was an explanation – it was an accident after all – but he just stonewalled. The system clammed shut. So the next thing was that the lawyers were involved, just so she could get at the truth. Once that happened then it was going to be about damages. It dragged on and on, but he just wouldn't show any sympathy or be open at all. The Trust settled before it got to court for £200,000, but if he'd just been open at the beginning of everything it wouldn't have cost the Trust a penny, and we could all have avoided a lot of stress.

Staying organised

One of the sub-texts of this chapter is the importance of maintaining a purchase on what is actually going on during the research process. I have already observed that the boundaries between different components of the research process – data collection, transcription and interpretation – are blurred, and that each involves critical engagement with the 'data', whatever form the latter take. I have suggested that keeping a research journal is an important part of this process. At the stage of interpreting and analysing data, however, organising the paperwork becomes even more important. The key point here is to keep to a system of dealing with the transcripts. We will see how important this is when we come, in a moment, to the process of identifying categories and coding.

- **Keep transcripts safe and use a consistent method of filing them.**
- **Use a research journal throughout the process of data analysis to keep track of your ideas about what the data mean.**

Categories of data

At its most basic, the business of analysing interview transcripts is about finding the common features of events and accounts across a number of cases. Although much research using the kinds of approach discussed in this, and in related chapters, emphasises the extent to which interviewees bring their own subjective and reflexive accounts into the interview, it is worth stressing that these do not suddenly just 'appear'. The whole purpose of the interview is to construct accounts that relate to particular topics. When reading transcripts analytically (and critically) the objective of the researcher is to define common features of those accounts, and to seek what Sayer (1984) calls 'relations of similarity'. In seeking categories of data, it is these relations of similarity that are important, and the process of categorisation involves identifying thematic elements across the general body of data collected. To take an example: in the process of analysing data that was collected in the course of my own PhD – which was about the ways in which nurses on wards defined and organised their relationships with terminally ill patients (May, 1991) – respondents' accounts seemed to be organised around three general categories of data. The first of these related to the obstacles that the organisation of nursing work seemed to place in the way of developing a meaningful relationship with the patient; and the second related to the activities that were involved in constructing such a relationship. These two categories of data – about the pragmatic negotiation of work and interaction with patients – were linked by a more general and diffuse thematic element, which related to the ways that they conceived of these relationships as being a morally important component of their work, structured by ideas about what 'good' nursing might be defined by. Ragin (1994:

81–103) provides a useful discussion of the process of identifying 'categories' and 'themes' within qualitative data. A more detailed discussion is to be found in Strauss (1987).

Categories or 'themes' can be defined as the general features of a set of interview transcripts. They are 'first order' constructs of the kind that I noted earlier in the chapter. They are distributed relatively uniformly across most or all of the body of data that is under scrutiny, and they may be identified during the process of fieldwork itself. This was certainly the case with the first two thematic elements of my own study, described above. The third, however, which acted to link them, only emerged after a careful reading of the transcripts. Identifying categories, or thematic elements, is not always an easy task. Where interviews have been gathered from a heterogeneous group of respondents, it may sometimes be very difficult to define the common features of their accounts. As a general guide, however, my own study showed three kinds of thematic elements and these have emerged in several subsequent studies of professional–patient interaction, although they are by no means exhaustive – every study will engender its own set of categories or themes. These three elements are structure, agency and discourse.

Structure: *thematic elements that pertain to the environment or conditions in which actors are located.* In particular, this relates to the ways that external factors provide a kind of framework in which individuals and groups are set and promote or limit certain paths of action. In my research on nurse–patient relationships in terminal care settings, several kinds of structural elements were in play at any one time: for example, the physical layout of the hospital ward, the division of labour between different groups of health care professionals and the management organisation of their work and time, and the 'career' or 'trajectory' of the terminally ill patient, all acted to define a general set of conditions in which relationships between patients and nurses came into being.

- **Structure is about where people are located and about the resources that they can draw on to perform specific kinds of role.**

Agency: *thematic elements that pertain to the activities that individuals and groups undertake within the structural conditions that frame them.* These might refer to very precise kinds of interaction – how nurses talk or act with patients, how patients respond to this, or how nurses negotiate the boundaries of their work with managers or doctors – or to more general considerations about what they aspire to and can achieve.

While structure provides a framework for action, agency is about the ways in which individuals and groups operate within that framework, and about how it is reproduced and transformed by their activities.

- **Agency is about how people respond to events and interactions within specific structural frameworks; it relates to the kinds of interactional talk and behaviours that they perform within it.**

Discourse: *How interviewees characterise the structural conditions and activities in which they are involved, or the ways in which they define and conceptualise attributions of self or group identity, is itself a key thematic element of any study.* The key here is the way in which interviewees draw on sets of ideas about the topic of study. For example, in my study of terminal care nursing, many of the respondents drew on a set of ideas about caring for the 'whole person' that reflected not simply their own grounded experiences but wider ideological imperatives in the professional rhetoric of nursing. Interview-based research is about the language that people use to describe their experiences and thoughts, and it pays to attend closely to this, but it is also important not to assume that a set of verbal constructs has a direct correspondence with 'real' events. Accounts are often highly idealised descriptions of events, and are frequently 'edited' in the telling to present events in a particular light.

- **Discourse is the strategic language that individuals and groups use to characterise their perspective on interactions and relationships.**

Developing a set of ideas about categories or themes within a qualitative data set involves not only identifying the general features of interviewees' accounts, but also thinking about the conceptual linkages between them. In grounded theory research, it is at this stage that basic theoretical constructs come to the fore, but in other models of research – for example those with a constructionist basis, this is the point at which theory and data come together to begin to form a perspective on the data.

Coding

If categories or thematic elements are the general features of a body of qualitative data, then coding is the procedure by which these are systematically broken down into their constituent parts for formal analysis. A code is a means by which individual items of data are defined and indexed on the transcript, in the research journal and in other recording procedures. At its simplest, it is a label that identifies specific kinds of data as components of a subset of a general category. In Box 5, I show how one of the general categories of data that was developed in my study of nurses' relationships broke down into a set of codes that represented different aspects of a category.

Box 5: Coding from categories

Interviews with 22 staff nurses on general medical and surgical wards in a Scottish general hospital about their relationships with terminally ill patients led to the development of three major categories of data. One of these related to ideas about what a 'good' nurse–patient relationship meant in terms of the practical activities with which nurses were involved. Within this the following subsets, or codes, were defined:

1.   ENSURING COMFORT (physical)
1.1   Physical care
1.2   Pain control
1.3   Food and drink
1.4   Noise and interruption

2.   ENSURING COMFORT (psychological/emotional)
2.1   Building open relationships
2.2   'Talking and listening'
2.2.1   Listening to 'hopes for the future'
2.2.2   Identifying concerns and fears
2.2.3   Making time to 'be there'
2.2.4   Listening 'to relatives too'
2.3   Dealing with anxiety
2.4   Building bridges between staff and relatives
2.5   Being involved
2.5.1   Being close to the patient
2.5.2   Maintaining boundaries
2.5.3   Avoiding over-involvement
2.5.4   Making difficult decisions

The codes described in Box 5 arose out of a line-by-line scrutiny of an initial group of five transcripts. Then, across the whole body of transcripts, every identifiable meaningful statement was assigned a code and indexed, using the paragraph and line numbers added during transcription. Of course, some statements defy coding for they may relate to things that lie outside of the remit of the study. Other segments of the transcript might easily be interpreted as 'fitting' within more than one code, in which case they were assigned the code that seemed to fit most closely in the context of the general line that the nurse seemed to be taking in her or his account. Software packages for qualitative analysis usually enable the identification of particular patterns of words and enable coding to be done quickly and efficiently, but simple coding on relatively small data sets can be done easily on the transcript itself with a set of coloured marker pens. Statements that accord to a particular code, or label, can simply be identified with a different colour highlight. Software packages such as QSR NUDIST and Hypersoft have internal procedures for coding data. The former is also able to generate diagrams that show the 'layout' of categories and codes.

Rigorous coding is an important part of analysing interview transcripts, but it is important to understand that it is not a mechanical activity. Instead it is part of a process of reflexively reading and re-reading the transcripts and actively interpreting what the respondent seems to be saying. This is a subjective process that is about trying to engage with the world in which interviewees live. It is easy to be overburdened with a complex system of coding and indexing that means that the researcher concentrates on what the codes are, rather than what the interviewee is saying. The essence of qualitative research is trying to understand the respondent and the experience that a transcript represents. This is why it is so much fun: but over-coding and unreasonably complex coding strategies inhibit the process of data analysis – they do not promote it.

- **Read and re-read the transcripts; get to know them well.**
- **Use the simplest coding strategy that you can.**
- **Index coded statements using software or a research journal.**

Detailed and helpful discussions of types of coding strategy and technique may be found in Strauss (1987) and Strauss and Corbin (1990). The latter provides one of the most explicit and researcher friendly accounts of coding and places it in the context of grounded theory research.

Recording codes with lists and grids

The danger with complex coding strategies is that they end up treating qualitative data as though they could be reduced to a set of numbers. All the time the qualitative researcher has to strike a balance between going through the transcripts thoroughly and rigorously, labelling and indexing data as they appear to be relevant to the task in hand, and working to grasp the meaning of what the interviewees have said. Interpreting what the data mean is the principal objective in this kind of work. On the other hand, however, it can be useful to be able to demonstrate that categories and codes really are common features across the data. The simplest way to go about this is to use a grid as an instrument to record the location of particular codes across a body of interview transcripts. Box 6 shows a grid drawn up as part of a study (Sirur, 1997: 38) that explored the reasons why some general practitioners are attracted to the use of homeopathic remedies rather than orthodox medicines. An important theme or category that arose from this study concerned the factors that inhibited interviewees' use of homeopathy. The study was small, and the researcher chose to label specific kinds of data with an alphabetic rather than numeric code. He defined these as follows:

NUE: No exposure to homeopathy during undergraduate medical training.
NAC: Negative attitudes to homeopathy amongst professional colleagues.
PPR: Problems of professional regulation.
LSP: Lack of scientific proof that homeopathy works.

He was then able to draw up a grid that showed how these were distributed across 10 interviews, using paragraph numbers to show their location in each interview transcript. The grid tells us several things. Most important, it suggests that the problem of peer-disapproval is the obstacle to using homeopathy that interviewees discussed most often. It also suggests that the absence of conventional scientific proof about the efficacy of homeopathy was talked about much less. Not all qualitative researchers would regard using a grid like this as being in the 'spirit' of this style of research. Others, like Silverman (1993) regard 'simple counting' like this as being of value. I agree with him. It is very valuable at the stage of formal analysis to be able to look at a 'map' of the data, to see how different categories and codes are distributed across the transcripts and thus to be able to demonstrate that respondents in interview-based studies really are discussing particular kinds of issue with greater frequency than others.

Box 6: Distribution of codes across a set of interview transcripts				
Code Interview	NUE	NAC	PPR	LSP
Doctor 1	2	12	22	21
Doctor 2	2	2, 11	16	13
Doctor 3	2	8, 16, 18		26
Doctor 4	3, 35			49
Doctor 5	8	24, 37	35	
Doctor 6	32	23, 25, 37		
Doctor 7		28, 34	26	
Doctor 8			25	
Doctor 9	1	18	36	
Doctor 10		2, 20	27	20

The second benefit of a grid like the one in Box 6 is that it provides an index to the data that is easily accessible to the researcher. Having an index such as this is an important part of keeping organised, and being able to find the items in a particular transcript or group of transcripts that are useful in either the interpretation or presentation of the data. A grid is not a statistical device for defining the quantity of data collected – it simply defines where it is, in individual transcripts and across the body of data collected.

● **Consider using a grid to index your coded data.**

Memoranda

At different points throughout this chapter I have stressed that the principal objective of the qualitative researcher who uses interviews is to explore what a particular practice, process or interaction means to a group of respondents. I have outlined some simple procedures for preparing and organising interview data, but these are of no value at all unless the data are interpreted. Establishing meanings through subjective interpretation simply cannot be achieved through any mechanical process: it is something that takes place inside the researcher's head, or in discussion and exchange between groups of researchers. On the other hand, these interpretations do need to be recorded in some way. Memoranda are a simple means of recording this: they are a written record of the researcher's thinking about a particular item of data, a code or category. They may include an interpretation of a particular statement, thoughts about the nature of a category or theme, ideas about how categories and codes relate to each other, or thoughts about how they relate to work undertaken by others. Writing memoranda is a part of the process of interpreting the data, where ideas are recorded and organised and where the development of those ideas through the course of the study may be recorded.

- **Keep a written record of ideas about what the data mean.**

Strauss and Corbin (1990) provide a detailed account of different ways of using memos to contribute to analysis. Whatever strategy you use, remember to keep it as simple as possible and to be consistent.

Inter-rater testing and interviewee feedback

The process of collecting, coding and interpreting qualitative data is, by its very nature, an individual and subjective task. This sometimes leads to questions about bias in interpretation and coding, especially from agencies that fund research in the health care sector. Inter-rater testing is one way to respond to those kinds of questions, and it involves the independent adjudication of coding by someone unconnected with the study in question. Put simply, it means that the researcher asks the question: 'Do you agree that the data that I have coded in this way actually "fit" the criteria through which codes have been defined?' The inter-rater then examines a sample of transcripts and checks the coding that has been undertaken by the researcher.

Although such a procedure is not really in the 'spirit' of the philosophy of qualitative research, and I think that there are some good epistemological reasons for objecting to it, the fact is that many of the agencies that fund or otherwise sponsor do have anxieties about the formal rigour of a research strategy that is, by its very nature, subjective. Inter-rater checks are one means by which those anxieties can be responded to: they simply offer a measure of agreement about what the data are, but they can only ever offer a partial measure of agreement about what they mean.

A much stronger means of ensuring that the interpretation of data that the researcher achieves really does represent in some way the thoughts and experiences of respondents in such studies may be found in feeding back provisional results and conclusions to members of the study group itself. This can be done individually or in a meeting, and it serves a number of purposes.

First, it can support emerging analyses of the data by checking them against the perspective of those who have been interviewed, and the extent to which respondents agree or disagree with what the researcher has made of their accounts is one kind of 'reality check', but it brings with it some key problems too. It can be a very uncomfortable experience if the results of the project are at variance with interviewees' own views. If the work concerned is theoretical in orientation it may be difficult to convey to respondents what the study reveals in a way that is meaningful to them. It is also important to be aware that commissioned research in the health sector is often undertaken for reasons about which respondents may feel fundamentally opposed (May, 1995).

Second, feeding research back to members of a study group offers an opportunity for them to contribute to the research process not simply through being interviewed, but also by offering alternative interpretations of the data. These can sometimes be extraordinarily valuable. Respondents are, after all, experts in the field of their own experience and views, and their interpretations of these can offer novel ways of understanding and interpreting the data that have been collected in the course of the study. This too can be uncomfortable, for it can reveal the researcher's misunderstandings. In the case of my own PhD, discussed earlier in the chapter, returning to a group of nurses to discuss my provisional findings led to the discovery that I had simply not understood their descriptions of what was undertaken at the 'report' that takes place when shifts change on a ward, and that I had profoundly over-estimated what 'involvement' with patients meant to them. The important point about this was that I was able to return to the data and re-analyse some of it in a way that ultimately made much more sense and led me to a new understanding of the relationship between the nurses' aspirations about providing 'holistic' care for their patients and the pragmatic negotiation of nursing work (May, 1993). Although this kind of feedback is useful for the reasons that I have described above, it is no substitute for the researcher's own critical faculties. Qualitative analysis is just that: it is first and foremost the creative engagement between the researcher and the data.

● **Inter-rater testing and respondent feedback may strengthen the validity of your analysis, but they are not substitutes for it.**

Deviant cases

In every body of interview transcripts there will be individual respondents or descriptions of events that somehow do not 'fit'. Silverman (1993) describes these as 'deviant cases', and they may take a number of forms. It may be that they depart strikingly from the line that other respondents take, or that the events that they describe take an unusual form. There is a temptation to discard these in a model of analysis that focuses on the commonalties that exist within and between data. Studies that focus on relations of similarity can be thrown into doubt by the discovery of something that is fundamentally dissimilar. For instance, in Sirur's (1997) study of general practitioners who use homeopathy there was agreement from nine of the ten doctors that lay homeopaths (i.e. non-medically qualified professional homeopaths) should be permitted to practise and to advertise their services. The tenth bitterly rejected this proposition. In fact, it was his description of why lay homeopathy should not be permitted that threw the other nine into sharp relief by pointing to the extent of medico-legal responsibility for treatment that structures all general practitioners' work. By defining the 'problem' of professional responsibility in law this respondent permitted a much greater degree of clarity in the researcher's examination of other accounts, and it became apparent that they too had significant reservations about lay homeopaths.

Silverman (1993) provides a detailed account of the analysis of 'deviant' cases, stressing their value in assisting in the interpretation of other data, but also pointing to the extent to which they can in themselves produce valuable analytic material.

Presenting conclusions

The use of excerpts from interview transcripts to illustrate reports of interview-based studies is one of their most compelling features. Respondents' own accounts frequently offer powerful descriptions of the problem at hand. How these are selected and presented opens up a number of problems, however.

Ethical problems in the presentation of qualitative data

The first of these concerns the protection of respondents' anonymity and confidentiality. It is standard practice in this kind of work to offer some degree of anonymity to interviewees, and without such an assurance it would be difficult to conduct even quite routine studies. However, it does present problems where extracts from interview transcripts are intended to be presented in the public domain. The use of numbers rather than names to identify respondents will go some way towards meeting this requirement, as will careful editing of their accounts. What people talk about, however, as well as their names, will sometimes give an informed reader an indication of their identity. Great care needs to be taken, therefore, to make sure that anonymity and confidentiality are maintained if they have been promised. Even so, there is a limit to the extent to which it is possible to do this before an account becomes so modified that it is a fiction. In such cases it is better to paraphrase it or leave it out of the report or article altogether.

Are excerpts typical?

The second problem concerns presenting relatively few extracts from a large body of data. This will always raise critical questions about whether they are typical of the data as a whole. Subjective accounts, of course, represent very specific individual perspectives on interactions and events, and because of this they can never be seen as directly comparable or compatible. This undermines the idea of 'representativeness' to some extent, but not entirely. When presenting the results of such studies it is important to avoid fixing on the most striking and exotic examples of a particular analytical category, but rather to focus on those that lie in what one might call the middle range. Where the most striking examples of a kind of account are used, the danger is not only that they will seem implausible to the reader but, more importantly, that they will genuinely not represent the generality of the data pertaining to a category or code. Sometimes, of course, it is useful to use the most extreme and atypical description, and it is also important to present deviant cases. The key here is to make it clear to the reader that this is what is being done and why.

Are excerpts 'in context'?

A similar consideration applies to the question of whether excerpts are being presented in a way that maintains its intended meaning and context. In part this is a function of transcription and editing, but when excerpts are presented in the text of a report it is important to give the reader enough material to make a judgement about the sense of a particular statement. Very short extracts from transcripts simply do not do this and it is often necessary to reproduce quite lengthy items of reported speech to ensure that meaning is represented accurately.

Summary

What I have tried to do in this chapter is to define in relatively simple terms the practical procedures that are involved in preparing and analysing interview data. I have presented this in the form of a 'how to' guide, although the truth is that the nature of such research makes it rather inhospitable to such an approach. The key point here is that it is ultimately vital to demonstrate that a research project has been conducted rigorously and to show that an explicit set of procedures has been used to reach the conclusions that are presented in the final report, dissertation, or article. One of the chief problems for the reader of qualitative research is that so much has to be taken on trust. One can rarely find space to provide a full account of the methods and procedures used in such a study, for no research journal can be edited down to the 300 words or so that most editors will permit in published accounts of qualitative work. What this means is that the audit trail that is available to readers of quantitative research – where an elementary knowledge of sampling and statistical tests enables the reader to draw conclusions about the validity and reliability of a study – is simply not available to those who read and use qualitative studies. There are some general rules, however, which go some way to showing that the study has been conducted with proper attention to rigour and procedure.

- **Identify the method employed and the coding strategy used; indicate how particular categories and codes arose during the research process. It is simply not** enough to say 'a hermeneutic-phenomenological method was used' as one recent author in a nursing journal did.

- Provide typical examples of interviewees' accounts to illustrate the text. (It is tempting to use the most interesting and exotic, but this often makes your analysis appear implausible to the very people you want to read it.)

- Show how the data collected led to particular conclusions and interpretations, and make clear the ways in which your theoretical interests and orientation have contributed to this.

- When including excerpts from interview transcripts in reports of publications always make sure that you do so in a way that protects anonymity and confidentiality if you have promised it, and use interview and paragraph numbers to show that your excerpts are typical of responses across the study group.

- Never, ever, fit excerpts from respondents' accounts into a written report in a way that your analysis and coding do not clearly support. This is research misconduct.

My final point is that whatever theoretical perspective, or specific analytical technique you adopt for your study, the kind of research that I describe here can be extraordinarily interesting and it can be fun too. I can think of no other model of research that provides such privileged access to the lives of others, or which permits the subjects of research to be heard so clearly by policy makers and professionals. Being rigorous and cautious in data preparation and analysis is not simply, therefore, just part of the business of doing research, getting results and writing it up, it is also part of a bargain that the researcher makes with those who agree to give their time to an interview. Have fun!

References

Bernstein R (1976) The Restructuring of Social and Political Theory. London: Methuen.

May C (1991) 'Getting to know them': An Exploratory Study of Nurses' Knowledge and Nursing Work with Terminally Ill Patients on Acute Medical and Surgical Wards. Unpublished PhD thesis, University of Edinburgh.

May C (1993) Subjectivity and culpability in the constitution of nurse–patient relationships. International Journal of Nursing Studies 30: 181–92.

May C (1995) More semi- than structured: some problems with qualitative research methods. Nurse Education Today 16: 289–92.

Ragin, C (1994) Constructing Social Research. London: Pine Forge Press.

Sayer A (1984) Method in Social Science: A Realist Approach. London: Hutchinson.

Silverman D (1993) Interpreting Qualitative Data: Methods for Analysing Talk, Text and Interaction. London: Sage.

Sirur D (1997) Doctors who practise homeopathy: a qualitative study of their motives and influences on their behaviour. Department of General Practice, University of Manchester.

Strauss A (1987) Qualitative Analysis for Social Scientists. Cambridge: Cambridge University Press.

Strauss A, Corbin J (1990) Basics of Qualitative Research: Grounded Theory, Procedures and Practices. London: Sage.

Acknowledgements

Much of what I now practise as a qualitative researcher I first encountered in a seminar on research techniques at the University of Edinburgh, led by Tom McGlew, Fran Wassoff and Kath Melia, who also supervised the PhD thesis which I discuss in this chapter. I am grateful to them, and to the colleagues who have collaborated with me since. My thinking about what this chapter ought to incorporate has been greatly influenced by working with Carolyn Chew, Karen Fairhurst and Deepak Sirur.

Chapter 6
Meta-analyses and systematic reviews of the literature

Fahera Sindhu

Introduction

The literature review has traditionally been the process through which findings from primary studies have been identified and summarised, serving the function of 'taking stock' of what is known about a particular treatment or intervention. This chapter therefore begins with a discussion of the traditional approach to reviewing literature. There then follows a discussion of the potential problems with this form of reviewing. The 1980s saw the development of the science of reviewing literature systematically. Overviews, meta-analyses and systematic reviews are forms of reviewing research evidence systematically and statistically.

The steps involved in a meta-analysis are identified and associated methodological issues are discussed. In particular, issues such as defining *a priori* inclusion criteria and conducting a comprehensive and systematic literature search, to ensure that all relevant studies are identified and included in a meta-analysis, are addressed.

Following a critical discussion of the technique of meta-analysis, the chapter concludes with a list and description of the steps involved in conducting a meta-analysis.

Reviewing the literature

The literature reviewing process is not new and has probably existed as long as research in many fields. Reviews are a very useful and versatile way to take stock of what is known in a particular research area. They are a form of summarising the research that has been undertaken and can highlight what needs clarification or the future questions for newly commissioned research. They are also a means to inform decisions about cost-effectiveness for purchasers and managers.

The reasons for conducting a review fall into two categories. First, individual primary studies may provide insufficient or inconclusive evidence because of poor design. This may be because of an inadequate sample-size. Second, a study may show evidence of effectiveness for only a certain type of patient, leaving the reader to

> 'speculate whether other patients, especially those in their care, will benefit from the intervention under study' (Haynes, 1992: 330).

It is often difficult to ascertain the extent to which findings from one particular study can be applied generally.

Types of reviewing techniques

The review

A summary of the results of a collection of research studies is normally referred to as a review. Sackett et al. (1991: 379) state that a review is 'the general term for all attempts to synthesise the results and conclusions of two or more publications on a topic'.

Traditionally reviews have been conducted in which pertinent studies are read and the evidence is qualitatively reported. However, there is usually no formal reporting of the procedure involved in the identification of pertinent studies. Hence the search cannot be replicated and it is difficult to assess whether such a review has been conducted systematically – in other words, whether all studies that have been conducted have been included in the review.

The last decade has shown an exponential increase in primary research, even in specialist literature such as that assessing the effectiveness of non-pharmacological nursing interventions in the management of acute pain in adults. This has made it difficult to identify all the relevant studies. The process of identifying all the relevant studies and reading each and every one is often difficult in practice. The development of electronic databases and indices, in the 1980s, has meant that a larger amount of literature is more easily and rapidly accessible. However, this is only beneficial if the user is equipped with the necessary skills to conduct comprehensive searches. The procedure involved in conducting searches on such databases requires a certain level of training in order to ensure that a comprehensive search is conducted (Closs and Cheater, 1994).

Further, no two researchers conduct exactly the same search or retrieve more than a portion of the same articles, even if they are experts at searching (Haynes et al., 1990). Electronic searching is not as straightforward as it may seem and particular concerns about this type of searching medium are discussed later in the chapter.

Even if a traditional review is based on a systematic search of the literature, it can still be biased by the very fact that it relies, typically, only on published studies. This is commonly referred to as publication bias. This bias highlights the tendency that exists in journals to accept only statistically significant findings and to not even report (let alone discuss) the direction of non-significant effects (Dickersin, 1990). (This issue is addressed later in the chapter.) The selective and unsystematic identification of literature, in a traditional review, may also mean that the review incorporates only those studies that confirm a reviewer's own beliefs or those carried out by acquaintances and/or colleagues. Hence the research and opinion of a sub-sample of the researchers may dominate research in an area.

In terms of someone reading a traditional review and/or attempting to replicate it, there is usually no documented systematic form in the process of reviewing research. Hence a reader may be unable to judge whether such a review is reliable and accurate or whether it has been carried out comprehensively. This problem was highlighted by Mulrow (1987), who surveyed 50 reviews published in four major medical journals in 1985 and 1986. She found that only one of these reviews had specified the methods employed in identifying studies for inclusion. It is apparent, then, that although researchers conduct rigorous primary studies, this rigour is lacking in the reviews conducted by the same researchers.

A further concern is that not all evidence is formally statistically combined. Most reviews report qualitatively on the general conclusions of individual studies and, at most, on the direction of any findings.

The overview

In recent years, many authors have acknowledged the problems associated with traditional reviews outlined above. The technique of overviews has been developed to address these problems. An overview systematically identifies primary studies. Sackett et al. (1991: 379) state:

> when a review strives to comprehensively identify and track down all the literature on a topic, we call it an overview.

Systematically searching for relevant literature will increase reliability and representativeness, and hence generalisability, of any review. Overviews, however, do not statistically accumulate findings from primary research studies. Overviews, like reviews, typically ignore information about the magnitude of findings (Light and Smith, 1971). Simple 'vote counts' are made (Cooper, 1989) of the frequency with which hypotheses are and are not significant. This is conservative as those results that are not significant (maybe due to low power) will be counted as 'failures' even if the relationship is in fact positive. So there still remained the problem of statistically pooling available study findings with respect to both magnitude and direction. A quantitative statistical technique, called meta-analysis, was developed to address this issue.

The meta-analysis

Background

Meta-analysis is a quantitative statistical reviewing method. It is a set of techniques for reviewing research in which data from several primary studies are statistically combined (Cooper, 1979; Cook and Leviton, 1980; Cooper and Arkin, 1981; and Cook and Leviton, 1981).

A meta-analysis, like an overview, comprehensively identifies all the literature on a topic, but incorporates a specific statistical strategy for accumulating the results of several studies into a single estimate (Sackett et al., 1991).

Nomenclature

Meta is derived from the Greek word *meta* meaning 'after'. Medical and social scientists use the term meta-analysis most frequently, although research integration and research synthesis are also used. Physical scientists use the terms *critical reviews* and *critical evaluations*. Many of these terms are used interchangeably. In this chapter, the term meta-analysis will be used to denote the statistical accumulation of reported results from a number of primary research studies identified through a systematic literature search.

Evolution

Although meta-analysis has its origins in educational research (Glass et al., 1981) the term meta-analysis can be traced back to the work of

Tippet (1931), Fisher (1932), Pearson (1933) and Cochran (1937). This early work combined findings from agricultural studies and had two different objectives. One objective involved testing the statistical significance of the combined results across primary research studies, while the other involved the estimation of the magnitude of the experimental effect (treatment) across these studies. The former have become known as combined significance tests and the latter approach refers to methods of effect size.

Meta-analyses can sometimes have a substantial life cost. This was demonstrated by Antman et al. (1992) who found that the majority of experts did not recommend the use of thrombolytic therapy until six years after the publication of a quantitative review of the area despite the fact that a quantitative review would have indicated a 25 per cent reduction in heart attack death rate as a result of using thrombolytic therapy.

A further objective of meta-analysis is to describe existing knowledge (which is ever-increasing) in a concise manner, to indicate weaknesses or gaps requiring further investigation. Strube and Hartmann (1982) suggest that a major indirect value of meta-analysis is its contribution to the quality of studies in that area and identifying areas requiring further study, and those areas that are saturated in terms of having already been extensively researched. A traditional review does achieve this latter objective to a limited extent, but a meta-analysis attempts to do this in a systematic and scientific manner.

Use of meta-analysis

The meta-analytical approach has been advocated to enhance the effective and efficient use of research findings in health services in general (Chalmers et al., 1992) and specifically in nursing practice (Smith, 1988; Closs and Cheater, 1994).

Meta-analysis is now widely used internationally and across disciplines, demonstrating its applicability. Rosenthal (1976) used a meta-analysis to test the influence of interpersonal expectations on behaviour. Glass (1976) cites a meta-analysis relating to teaching methods, television instruction, and socio-economic status as they relate to IQ, and an example of meta-analysis in the medical field is given by Yusuf et al. (1985) investigating the use of beta-blockers in myocardial infarction. A 1995 MEDLINE search of clinical research using the keyword 'meta-analysis' alone identified 223 citations from over 20 countries.

Meta-analysis was first used in nursing research in 1982 (O'Flynn, 1982) to assess the effect of behavioural interventions on weight loss in the obese. This was followed by a meta-analysis by Turley (1985) evaluating the effectiveness of maternal-infant interactions, and Devine and Cook (1986) looking at the effects of a psycho-educational intervention with surgical patients. In 1986, Hathaway assessed the effect of pre-operative information on post-operative outcomes. Other meta-analyses in nursing include studies of the effectiveness of pain interventions with children (Schwartz, 1987, Brown, 1988; Heater et al., 1988; Broome, et al., 1989). More recently, Wilkie et al., (1989) looked at the use of the McGill Pain Questionnaire, McCain and Lynn (1990) conducted a meta-analysis of a narrative review and Sindhu (1994, 1996a) conducted a meta-analysis of the literature assessing the effectiveness of non-pharmacological nursing interventions in the management of acute pain.

The systematic review

Although a meta-analysis may use tabular data supplied directly by triallists, it usually relies on statistics reported in a study's manuscript. They may not, however, be reported in a form to facilitate the 'best' statistical accumulation of the evidence. To address such problems systematic reviews were developed. These involve the accumulation of the raw data from individual primary studies. The development of such reviewing techniques arose out of concern over the quality of data reported in study manuscripts. These concerns can only be addressed with access to raw data (Clarke et al., 1992). Systematic reviews involve close collaboration with the study authors. This is often not feasible in practice and may be time consuming. However, the fact that the validity of individual study results may be checked outweighs the time and effort spent in retrieving individual raw data and involves a number of methodological issues.

Methodological issues in meta-analysis

Most of the methodological issues relevant to a meta-analysis are common to a systematic review. For simplicity, these issues will be discussed within the context of a meta-analysis.

Many of the methodological issues important in conducting primary research studies are also relevant in conducting a meta-analysis. These include:

- the need to specify the research question;
- the selection and representativeness of the sample;
- the need to take account of confounding variables;
- use of appropriate statistical techniques;
- considerations of data quality and independence in the studies reviewed (a primary study may be published in two different forms and may inadvertently be included in a meta-analysis twice).

It is apparent, then, that a meta-analysis is not too dissimilar from a primary research study in its design and methodology.

In contrast to primary research, however, the study is the unit of analysis in a meta-analysis (as opposed, for example, to each individual in a primary research study). The findings and study characteristics of each study are what form the data set for a meta-analysis, the measure of effect defined by the independent and dependent variables forms the 'effect'. In addition it is sometimes useful to consider other factors, such as methodological issues (e.g. sample size) and patient type, or form of intervention from each study, as possible explanatory variables.

Inclusion criteria

Definition of inclusion criteria

In carrying out a meta-analysis, the meta-analyst must decide which studies to include and which to exclude. For instance, are only experimental studies to be included, or observational studies too? Are all relevant studies that have been identified to be included?

The problem of inclusion criteria has caused considerable debate. The definition of inclusion criteria is one of the subjective decisions in a meta-analysis and may involve a range of different types of criteria, for instance either clinical criteria such as specific patient groups or methodological criteria such as only randomised controlled trial (RCT) based research. The former will depend upon research interests, whilst the latter involves theoretical and methodological considerations.

Study design

The RCT has become widely accepted as the methodological 'gold standard' for comparing alternative forms of care (Chalmers et al., 1989). For this reason, many meta-analyses include only those studies with an RCT design. The majority of meta-analyses in health care research have assessed the effectiveness of therapies in RCTs designs only, but a few have assessed aetiological issues by accumulating evidence from observational studies such as the examination of the relationship between alcohol and breast cancer (Longnecker et al., 1988).

According to Sacks et al. (1987), Whither (1987) and Bulpitt (1988), only RCTs should be accumulated in a meta-analysis. Although meta-analytical techniques have been applied to data from non-randomised studies (Goldsmith and Beecher, 1984; Schneider, 1986; Eddy, 1987), Thompson and Pocock (1991: 1128) recommend that 'as the value of any meta-analysis is totally dependent on the lack of bias in its component studies' only RCTs should be reviewed in a meta-analysis. This is because RCTs reduce systematic bias, which is especially important in intervention studies or studies in which attribution of effect to one particular source (such as one specific health care professional) is difficult to make. But what if RCTs are unethical or inappropriate in a particular clinical context? Does this mean that no meta-analysis should be conducted? There are advantages to an overview in which a systematic search for pertinent studies is conducted irrespective of whether the studies are RCTs or not. Areas of research in which RCT designed studies are rare or do not exist could still be 'overviewed' if not 'meta-analysed'.

Having defined the inclusion criteria, the next stage in a meta-analysis involves the collection (search) of pertinent primary studies. As the generalisability of any findings from a meta-analysis is contingent upon the inclusiveness of all relevant studies, the meta-analysis should be preceded by a search for all relevant studies in the literature. A systematic search for both published and unpublished RCTs should therefore be conducted. Electronic and manual searching of databases and indices needs to be supplemented with attempts to identify and retrieve (primarily unpublished) studies from experts in the area being reviewed.

Should all pertinent studies be incorporated in a meta-analysis, or only those of high quality?

The methodological quality of each primary research study should also be assessed. The judgement of how to measure the quality of a study is unresolved and this is reflected in the fact that no definitive rating scheme currently exists. The methodological quality of a research study is important in assessing the level of confidence that can be placed in its findings. This is also important in a meta-analysis in which findings from a number of studies are to be accumulated. Opinions about how to measure quality of individual primary studies in a meta-analysis vary and these are discussed by Chalmers et al. (1981) and Sindhu (1996b). Assuming it can be assessed, how should the quality of a study be incorporated in a meta-analysis? Detskey et al. (1992) suggest ways in which quality can be incorporated into a meta-analysis:

- The simplest approach is to use quality rating as a way to decide whether a specific study should be excluded from the meta-analysis. For instance to include only those trials rated above a specific quality threshold (either the average or some other standard).
- The quality scores may be used as weights, akin to weighting analyses for sample-size (Klein et al., 1986). In this case studies of 'better' quality are given larger weights.
- The association between study quality and effect size may be examined graphically by plotting effect size against quality score and/or using statistical modelling techniques to investigate the relationship and to conduct subgroup analyses if necessary.
- A sequential combination of trial results based on quality scores can also be used (Detskey et al., 1992). They tentatively suggest a new method of incorporating quality into a meta-analysis, whereby they construct a set of overall pooled confidence intervals for the estimate of effect size using logistical regression procedures (see Chapter 10), starting with the highest quality study and then sequentially adding the next highest quality study and so on. It is a form of sensitivity analysis.

Criticisms of meta-analysis

Although meta-analysis has advantages over the traditional qualitative reviewing techniques *vis-à-vis* the systematic identification of studies and the statistical accumulation of results, it has been criticised. The criticisms can be grouped into four categories:

- *Meta-analysis combines too diverse a group of studies using different measuring techniques and different types of subjects.* This is commonly referred to as the 'apples and oranges' problem: in other words not comparing like with like (Eysenck, 1978). This is one of the more common criticisms of meta-analysis: that it mixes apples and oranges. It is not a general criticism but a warning of the potential danger of conducting too broad a meta-analysis. However, a properly conducted meta-analysis should be conducted with the same methodological constraints as any primary research, and hypotheses should be specific rather than broad. A meta-analysis allows the analysis of 'apples' and 'oranges' separately if heterogeneity is extensive, in which case only individual homogeneous groups are reviewed. In fact, the majority of meta-analyses accumulate studies in which similar therapies or interventions are being evaluated (in similarly designed studies) in an attempt to address exactly this problem.

- The meta-analysis research accepts the findings from studies that are poorly designed or are otherwise of low quality (Wilson and Rachman, 1983). Although there may be consensus on some general criteria in assessing the quality of research, there is no standard. A meta-analysis can address this issue either by applying stringent inclusion criteria or through a rating system that can then be used to weight analyses. (The issue of whether or not studies of 'poor' quality should be excluded in a meta-analysis is discussed elsewhere in Sindhu, 1996b. Suffice it to say here that a meta-analysis can address this issue.)

- A meta-analysis relies on published studies whereas the evidence suggests that such studies are biased (Dickersin, 1990). A meta-analytical review is likely to be more representative and rigorous in its procedures than a traditional qualitative review. A well-conducted meta-analysis (like an overview) should use and report objective rules for identifying and retrieving studies through a systematic and comprehensive search strategy whereas the qualitative review often uses undocumented subjective decisions. Further, meta-analysis protocols promote the searching for unpublished studies unlike a traditional review which may not necessarily do this.

- The meta-analysis can be invalidated by a lack of independence between hypothesis tests arising in a variety of ways (Cooper, 1979). For example multiple results are derived from the same study in which more than one outcome is used. This means that the data are not independent and can lead to unreliable results. Care in reading primary studies before accumulating findings from individual studies should ensure that only one finding from each study is accumulated.

Searching the literature

Data collection involves the process of identifying pertinent studies through a systematic and comprehensive literature search of all available and relevant sources to form a collection, or register, of studies to be reviewed. These sources should include as many available relevant sources that it is possible to search within the financial and time-constraints of the meta-analysis. Hence, journals, books, dissertations, theses, indices, reports from conferences and meetings and unpublished research retrieved through both formal and informal contacts should be used. This searching stage is important since the studies identified form the sample (as patients do in a primary study) and the representativeness of this sample defines the extent of generalisations and the level of confidence that can be placed in any conclusions reached. Thus, ideally, all available accessible relevant sources should be searched using electronic and print sources.

Conducting reviews in some areas may require searching across semi-related sources, which may make establishing a complete list of pertinent studies difficult. Although the advent of electronic databases over recent years has made it easier and faster to access a large body of published literature, as discussed earlier, placing reliance on these alone is ill-advised.

Limitations of conducting literature searches using solely electronic sources

Electronic searches, although fast and convenient, have been shown to identify only between 20 and 50% of the eligible studies (Bernstein, 1988; Gotzsche and Lange, 1991; Chalmers et al., 1992). However, Jadad and McQuay (1993) found that one such database, namely MEDLINE, identified 87% of the eligible studies assessing the effectiveness of pharmacological pain therapies, whilst Silagy (1993), reviewing RCTs in primary care, found that 63% of the eligible studies were identified by MEDLINE alone. Sindhu (1994), reviewing RCTs assessing the effectiveness of non-pharmacological nursing therapies in pain, found that MEDLINE identified 51% of the eligible studies. These figures suggest that the degree of completeness offered by electronic searches will not necessarily be the same in different research areas.

Electronic databases are available on-line or as CD-ROM versions. Generally, the on-line versions provide access to a larger body of literature than do the CD-ROM versions. Evidence shows that with MEDLINE, which is probably one of the most frequently used electronic databases by researchers in health-related disciplines, no two researchers conduct exactly the same search or retrieve more than a portion of the same articles, even if they are experts at searching (Haynes et al., 1990). This may be due to the indexing or due to the search strategy employed by searchers. Whatever the reason(s), this evidence supports the need for an iteratively refined search strategy to identify the optimum number of pertinent studies.

Further difficulties in the identification of relevant studies

There are several further difficulties with the identification of relevant studies. First, relevant studies may fail to be identified if for instance:

- after completion, a study is submitted only to a 'minor' (obscure) journal where there is a problem of small readership and the journal is probably not indexed in a database like MEDLINE;
- after completion, the study is submitted and accepted by a journal such as the *British Medical Journal (BMJ)*, but is indexed under 'spurious' keywords, not used by the searcher;
- after completion, the study is submitted to a major journal, such as the *BMJ*, but is rejected. Will this study be 'lost' forever? The study will either be left unpublished (and so 'lost') or submitted to a minor journal with a chance (albeit small) of possible identification and retrieval.
- there are delays in publication. There is evidence that textbook chapters and articles accepted for publication may lag behind due to publication delays which may exceed one year (Teagarden, 1991), again leading to publication bias. Of course, if a meta-analysis is 'updated' at a later date, then such studies would probably be identified, retrieved and incorporated.
- they remain unpublished. Studies that lie unpublished in people's filing cabinets will not be easily accessible. Rosenthal (1979) points out that these unpublished studies might well refute findings from published studies. Again this emphasises the need to contact researchers in an attempt to identify relevant unpublished studies. This problem could be reduced with the use of registers/directories in which all primary studies are registered at their inception. It would then be easier to identify all research in a particular area regardless of whether it had been published or completed.

As a result of publication bias, and the problems of non-identification and non-retrieval discussed above, a meta-analysis (even after attempts have been made to identify and retrieve unpublished studies) is likely to suffer from bias toward significant positive rather than negative studies. Numerical formulae exist which estimate the number of unidentified studies that would need to exist in order to refute the meta-analysis findings (Rosenthal, 1979). Although such estimates are helpful, they do not address the problem of sample bias as its calculation is based on a sample which may not really be representative of the population of studies that exist anyway. Hetherington et al. (1989), after an analysis of retrospective and prospective searches, concluded that it is not possible to estimate the size of publication bias by attempting to identify unpublished trials retrospectively. But is there evidence to suggest that placing reliance on published studies could lead to bias in the conclusions of a meta-analysis?

Publication bias

Publication bias is the bias that results when the decision to publish a study is based on the direction or significance of the findings (Dickersin, 1990). Usually only those studies that appear in published sources are included in a review. This is probably due to the ease with which these are identified. Cooper (1979) suggests that such studies are thought to be more methodologically sound than unpublished research. And Chalmers et al. (1987: 317), say that

> informal and personalised methods of obtaining data are probably more liable to error and bias than employing only published data.

They refer to two conflicting meta-analyses (Conn and Blitzer, 1976 and Messer et al., 1983) in which each analyst contacted the same RCT investigator and obtained opposite answers to the same question. Chalmers et al. (1987: 317) say: 'we are convinced that we should emphasise data in print which the investigator has indicated a willingness to stand behind in public.' Further, Chalmers et al. (1987) report that different meta-analyses of the same subject, differing in the number of studies included (so not all studies are included), usually reach similar conclusions, suggesting that publication bias may not be a serious concern.

Nevertheless, publication bias may arise in several different ways and much evidence has been accumulated to support its existence. The impact of such bias depends on how many important unpublished papers remain inaccessible to the reviewer and whether these are representative of all studies conducted. In a survey of 58 investigators who had conducted, in total, 921 RCTs, of which 96 were unpublished, Chann (1982) found that positive RCTs were significantly more likely to be published than negative trials, suggesting that publication policy is biased toward those studies showing significant findings. Further, Mahoney (1977) submitted articles to different referees, varying the results without altering the methods. He found that the articles from 'respected' institutions and showing positive results were more readily accepted.

Assessing bias in publication policy further, Peters and Ceci (1982), resubmitted 12 already-published research articles to the journals in which they had initially appeared. The articles were unaltered except that the names and institution of the authors were changed from 'high status' to 'low status'. Only three of the twelve articles were recognised as being resubmissions by editors. Of the remaining nine articles, eight were not accepted for publication. This suggests that publication policy may further be biased toward the prestige of authors and/or their institutions.

In a review of 246 published trials of treatment for cancer, Berlin et al., (1989) and Begg and Berlin (1989) found a strong association between sample size and treatment effect. Studies with smaller sample sizes had larger treatment effects, which suggests that small trials with large effects were more likely to be published, while large trials were likely to be published regardless of their findings. This may be due to the assumption that larger trials are more rigorous. It has also been suggested that published sources tend to contain studies that 'worked' and that 'fit' into current scientific thought (Glass et al., 1981), so that any studies not confirming established practice will either not be accepted for publication or might deter the author from submitting for publication altogether.

The evidence thus suggests that the publication process is not entirely free from bias: positive, significant large studies from 'well-known' authors in prestigious institutions confirming traditional theories are more likely to be published. Publication bias has serious implications for the validity of meta-analysis (and indeed for any other reviewing process). It is crucial to ensure that all studies that have been conducted, both published and unpublished, are identified and included in the meta-analysis to minimise possible publication bias in a meta-analysis (Cooper, 1987). Even if a systematic, rigorous search is conducted, a reviewer may still find it difficult to identify and retrieve all relevant studies and may never know if all have been found. Attempting to identify all relevant studies (both published and unpublished) is practically impossible. However, it is possible to attempt to assess the extent of publication bias retrospectively after the search has been completed. The methods used to do this are either graphical (Light and Pillemer, 1984) or numerical (Rosenthal, 1979).

Reducing publication bias

The validity of a meta-analysis is contingent upon minimising the level of publication bias. This can be reduced by taking steps to identify unpublished studies, such as searching conference proceedings, writing and making contact with experts and/or requesting unpublished studies from editors of relevant journals. As discussed earlier, a comprehensive literature search akin to that outlined above is needed.

Thus far the issues of representativeness and inclusiveness of all relevant studies have been discussed. The problem of the quality of the data reported in the study manuscript needs to be addressed after the identification and retrieval of the relevant studies to be reviewed as these form the data for the meta-analysis.

Abstracting data

Problems with data from published studies

Examination of data quality, criteria for study inclusion, and how study information should be coded, represent several of the more subjective decision points in a meta-analysis. The reporting of each step helps to systemise the process and allows anyone reading the meta-analysis to scrutinise the selection and classification procedures.

Data quality

Normally, a meta-analysis relies upon information abstracted from individual studies, so the data can only be as accurate as the data that have been reported in the study manuscript. This reliance on reported information is one of the reasons for the development of systematic overviews.

A meta-analysis may be incomplete if the reported data are incomplete, although in some cases the necessary statistical information can be reconstructed (Glass, 1980) and, if possible, clarification may be sought from the author to facilitate analyses. Many editors impose a word limit on articles submitted for publication, again restricting the amount of information that is reported. Some authors suggest that further details are available from them and give addresses for correspondence.

Reliability and validity

In a primary study the reliability and validity are important. Strictly speaking, reliability refers to consistency of measurement. Measurement in meta-analysis refers to the coding of the characteristics and findings of studies based on the written reports. The principal source of measurement unreliability in meta-analysis, therefore, arises from this coding. So inter-study reliability is assessed as inter-coder and intra-rater reliability.

Validity of outcome measurement depends on the adequacy of the measurement tools used. This refers to the meaning of a coded or measured characteristic and includes such things as clarity of definitions and the adequacy of the reported information. Some problems of validity can be corrected by greater care in reading and coding studies. Other problems of validity cannot easily be corrected; one might have to infer that in a particular study the assignment of subjects to experimental conditions was non-random because random assignment was not specified (although again clarification may be sought from the author, if possible).

The need for systematic overviews

Problems due to the quality of reported data in a study manuscript mean that attempts should be made to request raw data from the study author(s) and systematic overviews should therefore be conducted wherever possible.

Statistical accumulation

The traditional procedure of accumulating evidence consisted of the so-called 'vote-counting' method (Cooper, 1989) whereby the numbers of positive and negative significant results were counted. Relying on significant findings only, however, was recognised to be overly conservative as it does not take into account the magnitude of effect – it considers only the direction. As a consequence, meta-analytical statistical reviewing techniques have been developed and Rosenthal (1984) and Bangert-Drowns (1986) provide comprehensive descriptions of these. The method of combining effect sizes is important.

Two types of models are normally fitted to a set of studies in a meta-analysis. The first of these is referred to as a *fixed-effects model* and assumes that the true treatment effect in all the studies is the same, or that it is zero. This model allows for systematic differences between individual studies. By contrast, a *random-effects* model assumes that the study effect sizes are a random sample from a population of effect sizes and allows for random variations between studies (Hedges and Olkin, 1985). There is a fundamental difference between the fixed-effects model and the random-effects model: the former leads to inferences about the particular studies reviewed whereas, in theory, the latter leads to inferences about all studies in a hypothetical population of studies. There are problems with both the models and the reader is referred to Thompson and Pocock (1991) and to a meta-analyst for advice.

Heterogeneity in the group of studies in a meta-analysis is usually assessed using the Homogeneity test (Hunter and Schmidt, 1990). This test assumes that under the null hypothesis (see Chapters 7 and 10), the studies in the meta-analysis share a common, but unknown, effect size. The alternative hypothesis suggests that at least one of the studies' effect sizes differ. This test has low power and if for instance the test implies that the null-hypothesis stands, it would be quite dangerous to infer that heterogeneity does not exist. The common approach then is to stratify the studies into 'logical' subgroups with the aim of obtaining more homogeneous subgroups. No meta-analysis is complete without an estimate of the heterogeneity.

In conclusion, the steps involved in performing a meta-analysis are presented here and these are summarised in Figure 6.1 in the form of a flowchart.

STEP 1 Problem formulation: This step involves the specification of the aims for a meta-analysis. Although a meta-analysis involves the accumulation of findings from a number of primary individual studies, it is still a research study in its own right. Hence, as in a primary study, specific *a priori* aims should be set out and a protocol set up for the research.

STEP 2 Data collection: This involves the search for all possible pertinent studies which will form the data set of this meta-analysis and will be referred to as the meta-analysis register: a listing of all the studies to be reviewed in this meta-analysis. Before conducting a search, *a priori* inclusion criteria need to be defined.

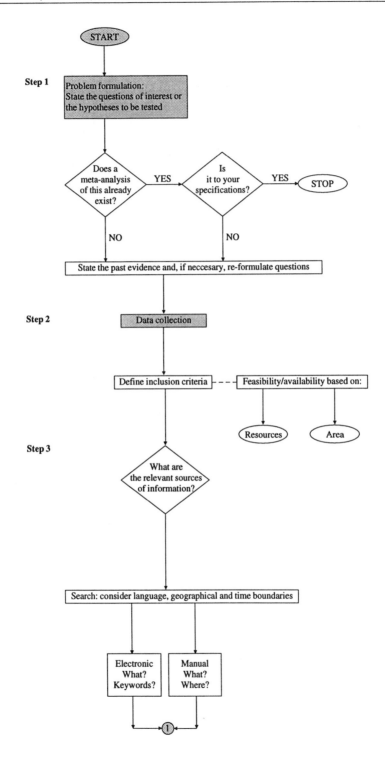

Figure 6.1: Steps involved in a meta-analysis – a flowchart representation.

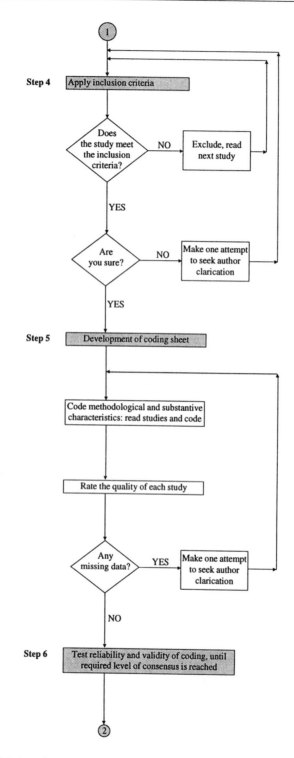

Figure 6.1: (contd)

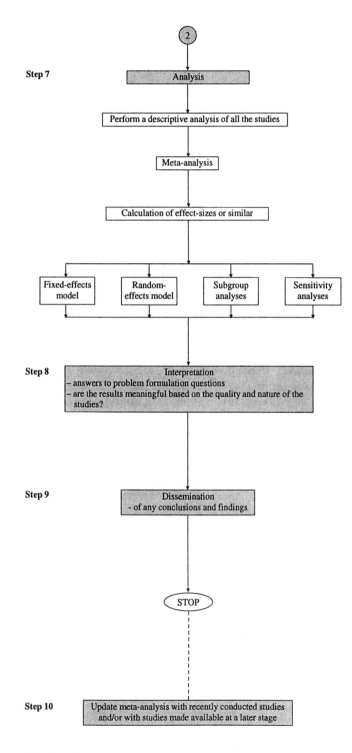

Figure 6.1: (contd)

STEP 3 What are the potentially relevant sources of retrieval?

STEP 4 Selection of studies for inclusion: Having identified and retrieved the studies in the meta-analysis, each identified study should be read to ascertain whether it satisfies the inclusion criteria, and author clarification should be sought if there is uncertainty. In cases where this is not forthcoming, the study should be given the benefit of the doubt: for instance if the study manuscript stated that randomisation had been conducted, but no further details were given, it should be included. Nevertheless, the primary author(s) of each study should be contacted to:

- ascertain if conclusions/findings have altered since publication of their research;
- ask whether they wish to amend their report in any other way; and
- request a copy of the raw data to facilitate analyses.

STEP 5 Coding and quality rating of the studies: Methodological study characteristics (such as sample-size) and substantive characteristics (such as intervention type) should be abstracted from the study manuscripts and entered on to a coding sheet for analysis. Where study manuscripts do not report sufficient information, clarification should be sought from the author(s).

STEP 6 Inter-coder reliability testing of the coding: Having rated and coded the studies, the inter-coder reliability of the coding and of the quality rating, need to be assessed. More succinctly, the aim of Step 6 is to ascertain whether the coding form is reliable in the sense that inter-rater reliability between independent raters is 'high' (Bland and Altman, 1986).

STEP 7 Analysis: This involves the analysis of the full set of studies in the meta-analysis register and subgroup and subsidiary analyses. The methodology involved in each of these techniques is now described, with statistical details given in Hedges and Olkin (1985).

Analysis should begin with key descriptive summary statistics of the studies in the meta-analysis as well as the calculation of effect size estimates for each study. An effect size is defined here as the standardised difference between the control and experimental groups regarding the measure of interest (for instance a pain score) in each study. The difference between the two groups is standardised by dividing this difference by the pooled standard deviation of the two groups. When the necessary information is not available, the effect size can be calculated from selected statistics (such as t-statistics) (Glass et al., 1981) or further information can be sought from the author(s) of the study. If this is not forthcoming, the studies should be assigned a zero effect size and analyses carried out excluding these studies because they might increase the magnitude of the average effect due to the tendency for minimally reported findings to be non-significant and relatively small in general. This is one of the problems faced when relying on only the information reported in a study manuscript. Calculation of effect size estimates and their confidence intervals relies upon the assumption that observations within individual studies are normally distributed. However this assumption is not always realistic. Non-parametric, distribution-free methods to calculate effect size estimates exist. However, estimates such as those provided by Kraemer and Andrews (1982) and Hedges and Olkin (1985) require access to the raw data (such as actual ranges and median scores) from individual studies for an effect size to be calculated, which is difficult in practice. Without access to the raw data, it is impossible to ascertain whether the distributions of observations within a study violate the assumption of normality and, as it would be too optimistic to assume that primary authors had investigated normality, caution is needed in any interpretation of the results. Once effect sizes have been calculated, meta-analysis can be conducted.

STEP 8 Discussion and interpretation of the results of the meta-analysis: Relating findings back to questions posed at the Problem Formulation stage.

STEP 9 Dissemination of the conclusions of the meta-analysis: This involves conference presentations and publications.

STEP 10 Updating the meta-analysis at regular intervals: This depends on if and when relevant studies are completed and/or become accessible. Updating a meta-analysis is a continuous process and specialist review groups already exist to monitor literature for pertinent studies and to update reviews at regular intervals or when the need arises (under the auspices of The UK Cochrane Centre NHS R and D Programme, Summertown Pavilion, Middle Way, Oxford OX2 7LG which, as part of the 1992 National Health Service Research and Development Strategy, is summarising research-based healthcare evidence for practitioners).

Summary

Literature reviews help to summarise literature and determine the current status of a research area. Literature reviews are not new, but traditionally have tended to be qualitative in nature. Unless a review is comprehensive and conducted systematically, the reader may be left with biased conclusions that could have implications for patient care.

Overviews systematically identify relevant research studies and meta-analysis and systematic reviews go on to accumulate quantitatively findings from individual studies, thus facilitating the collation of a larger number of studies than traditional reviewing techniques. The fundamental difference between the procedure involved in a meta-analysis and that of a primary study is 'the unit of analysis, and should not be the scientific principles that apply' (Oxman and Guyatt, 1988: 697). This emphasises the objectivity and rigour of a meta-analysis (Pocock, 1993).

In order to perform a meta-analysis, certain assumptions have to be made, one of which is that all studies that have been performed in the area of interest are included and that these satisfy the stated inclusion criteria. This means that if certain studies were not published because of either publication policy or due to reasons such as non-submittance, the results could be biased, a phenomenon known as publication bias. Hence the need for a comprehensive literature search, which will at least reduce publication bias to some extent.

There are potential hazards with meta-analytical procedures and these require careful attention. Before drawing any conclusions from a meta-analysis, care should be taken to scrutinise the defined identification, retrieval, inclusion, and coding strategies employed. Guidelines for reading and assessing the evidence from reviews exist (Oxman and Guyatt, 1988) and the procedure (and its comprehensive reporting) should follow set guidelines so that if a reader notes faults or limitations then the meta-analysis can be repeated, enhancing the procedures appropriately or treating conclusions with caution. This needs to be reflected in the form in which meta-analyses, reviews and overviews, are reported.

In conclusion, a meta-analysis involves a series of complex, sometimes subjective decisions on the part of the reviewer. Nevertheless, a carefully conducted meta-analysis can inform a healthcare professional by:

- summarising the current knowledge base;

- systematically and quantitatively assessing the effectiveness of intervention(s); and
- highlighting deficiencies in current methodologies and suggesting directions for future research.

Research and researchers have much to benefit from systematic literature reviews. This is reflected in the increased use of these reviewing techniques and the evolution of organisations such as The Cochrane Collaboration (international with UK base in Oxford), and the NHS Centre for Reviews and Dissemination in York. Researchers, practitioners, managers and purchasers will at some stage need to use findings from a review and may even need to conduct a review themselves. The critical appraisal of research should, after all, be an integral part of any research study. For busy clinicians it may well be better and easier to spend time reading a thorough, rigorous meta-analysis than to read a handful of selective, hence potentially biased, primary studies. A carefully conducted, comprehensive review will certainly summarise more evidence in a research area than an individual primary study. The reader can then go on to scrutinise the references of such a review to identify primary studies of particular interest.

References

Antman EM, Lau J, Kupelnick B, Mosteller F, Chalmers TC (1992) A comparison of results of meta-analyses of randomised controlled trials and recommendations of clinical experts. Treatments for myocardial infarction. Journal of the American Medical Association 268: 240–8.

Bangert-Drowns RL (1986) Review of development in meta-analysis methods. Psychological Bulletin 99: 388–99.

Begg CB, Berlin JA (1989) Publication bias and dissemination of clinical research. JNCI 81: 107–15.

Berlin JA, Laird NM, Sacks HS, Chalmers TC (1989) An assessment of publication bias using a sample of published clinical trials. Journal of the American Statistical Association 84: 381–92.

Bernstein F (1988) The retrieval of random clinical trials in liver disease from medical literature: manual versus MEDLARS searches. Controlled Clinical Trials 9(1): 23–31.

Bland JM, Altman DG (1986) Statistical methods for assessing agreement between two methods of clinical measurement. The Lancet 2: 307–10.

Broome ME, Lillis PP, Smith MC (1989) Pain interventions with children: a meta-analysis of research. Nursing Research 38: 154–8.

Brown S (1988) Effects of educational intervention in diabetes care: a meta-analysis of findings. Nursing Research 37: 223–30.

Bulpitt CJ (1988) Meta-analysis. The Lancet 2: 93-4.

Chalmers I, Dickersin K, Chalmers TC (1992) Getting to grips with Archie Cochrane's agenda. British Medical Journal 305: 386–8.

Chalmers I, Hetherington J, Elbourne D, Kierse M (1989) Materials and methods used to evaluate the effects of care during pregnancy and childbirth. In Chalmers I, Enkin M, Keirse MJ (Eds) Effective Care in Pregnancy and Childbirth. Oxford: Oxford University Press. pp 39–65.

Chalmers TC, Smith H, Blackburn B (1981) A method for assessing the quality of a randomised control trial. Controlled Clinical Trials 2: 31–49.

Chalmers TC, Smith H, Blackburn B (1987) Meta-analysis of clinical trials as a scientific discipline. I: Control of bias and comparison with large co-operative trials. Statistics in Medicine 6: 315–25.

Chann SS (1982) The epidemiology of unpublished randomised control trials. Clinical Research 30: 234A.

Clarke M, Gray R, Dunn J, MacLennan I (1992) Combination chemotherapy for myelomatosis. The Lancet 340: 433.

Closs SJ, Cheater FM (1994) Utilization of nursing research: culture, interest and support. Journal of Advanced Nursing 19: 762–73.

Cochran WG (1937) Problems arising in the analysis of a series of similar experiments. Journal of the Royal Statistical Society 4 (Suppl): 102–18.

Conn HO, Blitzer BL (1976) Non-association of adrenocorticosteroid therapy and peptic ulcer. New England Journal of Medicine 294: 473–9.

Cook TD, Leviton LC (1980) Reviewing the literature: A comparison of traditional methods and meta-analysis. Journal of Personality 48(4): 449–72.

Cook TD, Leviton LC (1981) What differentiates meta-analysis from other forms of review? Journal of Personality 49: 231–6.

Cooper H (1979) Statistically combining independent studies: a meta-analysis of sex differences in conformity research. Journal of Personality and Social Psychology 37: 131–46.

Cooper H (1987) Literature searching strategies of integrative research reviews: a first survey. Knowledge 8: 372–83.

Cooper H (1989) Integrating Research: A Guide for Literature Reviews. 2nd edn. London: Sage.

Cooper H, Arkin RM (1981) On quantitative reviewing. Journal of Personality 49: 225–30.

Detskey A, Naylor CD, O'Rourke K, McGeer AJ, L'Abbe KA (1992) Incorporating variations in the quality of individual randomised trials into meta-analysis. Journal of Clinical Epidemiology 45: 255–65.

Devine EC, Cook TD (1986) Effects of psychoeducational interventions with surgical patients: a meta-analysis of 102 studies. Nursing Research 35: 124.

Dickersin K (1990) The existence of publication bias and risk factors for its occurrence. Journal of the American Medical Association 263: 1385–9.

Eddy DM (1987) The use of confidence profiles to assess tissue-type plasma activator. In Califf RM, Wagner GS (Eds) Acute Coronary Care. Boston: Martinus Nijhoff Publishing Company. Ch 7.

Eysenck HJ (1978) An exercise in mega-silliness. American Psychologist 33: 517.

Fisher RA (1932) Statistical Methods for Research Workers. 4th edn. London: Oliver & Boyd.

Glass GV (1976) Primary, secondary and meta-analysis of research. Educational Researcher 5: 3–8.

Glass GV (1980) Summarising effect sizes. In Rosenthal R (Ed) New Directions for Methodology of Social and Behavioural Science: Quantitative Assessment of Research Domains. San Francisco: Jossey-Bass.

Glass GV, McGaw B, Smith ML (1981) Meta-analysis in Social Research. Newbury Park, CA: Sage Publications.

Goldsmith JR, Beecher S (1984) Strategies for pooling data in occupational epidemiological studies. Annals of Academic Medicine of Singapore 13 (suppl. 2): 297–307.

Gotzsche PC, Lange B (1991) Comparison of search strategies for recalling double-blind trials from MEDLINE. Danish Medical Bulletin 38: 476–8.

Hathaway D (1986) The effect of pre-operative instruction on post-operative outcomes: a meta-analysis. Nursing Research 35: 269–76.

Haynes KB (1992) Clinical review articles. British Medical Journal 304: 330–1.

Haynes RB, McKibbon KA, Walker CJ (1990) On-line access to MEDLINE in clinical settings, a study of the use and usefulness. Annals of Internal Medicine 112: 78–84.

Heater BS, Becker AM, Olson RK (1988) Nursing interventions and patient outcomes: a meta-analysis of studies. Nursing Research 37: 303–7.

Hedges LV, Olkin I (1985) Statistical Methods for Meta-Analysis. New York: Academic Press Inc.

Hetherington J, Dickersin K, Chalmers I, Meinert CL (1989) Retrospective and prospective identification of unpublished controlled trials. Paediatrics 84: 374–80.

Hunter JE, Schmidt FL (1990) Methods of Meta-analysis. Newbury Park, CA: Sage Publications.

Jadad AR, McQuay HJ (1993) A high yield strategy to identify randomised controlled trials for systematic reviews. On-line Journal of Current Clinical Trials (27 February): Document number 33.

Klein S, Simes J, Blackburn GL (1986) Total parenteral nutrition and cancer clinical trials. Cancer 58: 1378–86.

Kraemer HC, Andrews G (1982). A non-parametric technique for meta-analysis effect sizes calculation. Psychological Bulletin 91: 404–12.

Light RJ, Pillemer DB (1984) Summing Up: The Science of Reviewing Research. Cambridge, MA: Harvard University Press.

Light RJ, Smith PV (1971) Accumulating evidence: Procedures for resolving contradictions among different research studies. Harvard Educational Review 41: 429–71.

Longnecker B, Berlin J, Orza M, Chalmers T (1988) A meta-analysis of alcohol consumption in relation to the risk of breast cancer. Journal of the American Medical Association 260: 652–6.

McCain N, Lynn O (1990) Meta-analysis of a narrative review. Western Journal of Nursing Research 12(3): 347–58.

Mahoney MJ (1977) Publication prejudices: an experimental study of confirmatory bias in the peer review system. Cognitive Therapy Research 1: 161–75.

Messer J, Reitman D, Sacks HS, Smith H Jnr, Chalmers TC (1983) Association of adrenocorticosteroid therapy and peptic ulcer disease. New England Journal of Medicine 309: 21–4.

Mulrow CD (1987) The medical review article: state of the science. Annals of Internal Medicine 106: 485–8.

O'Flynn AI (1982) Meta-analysis of behavioural intervention effects on weight loss in the obese. Unpublished doctoral thesis, University of Connecticut.

Oxman AD, Guyatt GH (1988) Guidelines for reading literature reviews. Canadian Medical Journal 138: 697–703.

Pearson K (1933) On a method of determining whether a sample size n supposed to have been drawn from a parent population having a known probability integral has probably been drawn at random. Biometrica 25: 379–410.

Peters D, Ceci S (1982) Peer-review practices of psychological journals. The fate of published articles, submitted again. Behavioural and Brain Sciences 5: 187–255.

Pocock SJ (1993) Editorial. Statistical Methods in Medical Research 2: 117–19.

Rosenthal R (1976) Experimenter Effects in Behavioural Research. New York: Irvington.

Rosenthal R (1979) The file drawer problem and tolerance for null results. Psychological Bulletin 86(3): 638–41.

Rosenthal R (1984) Meta-analytic Procedures for Social Research. Beverly Hills, CA: Sage.

Sackett DL, Haynes RB, Guyatt GH, Tugwell P (1991) Clinical Epidemiology – A Basic Science for Clinical Medicine. 2nd edn. Boston/Toronto/London: Little, Brown & Co.

Sacks HS, Berrier J, Reitman D, Ancona-Berk VA, Chalmers TC (1987) Meta-analyses of randomised control trials. New England Journal of Medicine 316: 450–55.

Schwartz R (1987) A meta-analysis of critical outcome variables in nonnutritive sucking in preterm infants. Nursing Research 36: 292–95.

Schneider AP (1986) Breast milk jaundice in the new born: a real entity. Journal of the American Medical Association 255: 3270–4.

Silagy C (1993) Developing a register for randomised controlled trials in primary care. British Medical Journal 306: 897–900.

Sindhu F (1994) Are non-pharmacological nursing interventions in the management of pain effective? A meta-analysis. Doctoral thesis, Faculty of Clinical Medicine, University of Oxford.

Sindhu F (1996a) Are non-pharmacological nursing interventions for the management of pain effective? A meta-analysis. Journal of Advanced Nursing 24(6): 1152–9.

Sindhu F (1996b) Development of a tool to rate the quality assessment of randomised controlled trials using a Delphi technique. Journal of Advanced Nursing 25: 1262–8.

Smith MC (1988) Meta-analysis of Nursing Intervention Research. Birmingham, AL: Birmingham Printing and Publishing Company.

Strube MJ, Hartmann DP (1982) A critical appraisal of meta-analyses. British Journal of Clinical Psychology 21: 129–140.

Teagarden JR (1991) Meta-analysis: whither narrative review? Pharmacotherapy 9: 274–84.

Thompson SG, Pocock SJ (1991) Can meta-analyses be trusted? The Lancet 338: 1127–30.

Tippet LHC (1931) The Methods of Statistics. London: Williams & Norgate.

Turley MA (1985) A meta-analysis of informing mothers concerning the sensory and perceptual capabilities of their effects on maternal-infant interaction. Maternal Child Nursing 14: 183–97.

Whither A (1987) Meta-analysis. The Lancet 1: 897–8.

Wilkie DJ, Savedra M, Holzemer W, Lynn O (1989) Use of the McGill questionnaire to measure pain: a meta-analysis. Nursing Research 39: 36–41.

Wilson GT, Rachman SJ (1983) Meta-analysis and the evaluation of psychotherapy outcome: limitations and liabilities. Journal of Consulting and Clinical Psychology 51: 54–64.

Yusuf S, Collins R, Peto R et al. (1985) Intravenous and intracoronary fibrinolytic therapy in acute myocardial infarction. European Heart Journal 6: 556–85.

Note

The views expressed in this chapter are those of the author and not necessarily those of the National Audit Office.

Chapter 7
Quantitative research designs

Kathryn Getliffe

Introduction

Quantitative research is characterised by the measurement of qualities or variables present in populations by assigning numerical data to them in accord with some rule. The reason for measuring these qualities is usually to identify and establish relationships between variables or to detect changes that may occur either spontaneously or as a result of an intervention. The likelihood of such data occurring by chance, or in response to an identifiable cause, can be calculated by using statistical analysis. Quantitative research designs commonly attempt to control extraneous variables that could cause bias by contributing to the observations measured or by masking existing relationships.

The quantitative research approach employs a formal process that is rigorous, systematic and objective. The philosophy and principles underpinning this approach are centred on the logical analysis of observations and the aim to explain nature through the testing of hypotheses and development of theories. Experimental designs are credited as the most effective way of determining relationships between variables, enabling understanding, prediction and control (Munhall, 1982). Such designs play an important role in attempts to identify cause-and-effect relationships, which are essential for nursing science because of their relevance to clinical practice (Schumacher and Gortner, 1992). There is a need to establish an evidence base for practices performed and to be able to predict the likely consequences of certain events and interventions under given conditions. This is important not only with respect to patient care but also to inform policy, planning and allocation of resources.

Although statistical analysis can be used to inform decision making it must be remembered that tests of significance allow relationships between variables to be expressed according to a specified level of probability and do not provide information about the clinical significance or practical importance of study results. Statistical significance does not necessarily equate with clinical significance and clinical implications are subject to interpretation by the researcher.

However, not all quantitative studies are designed to test hypotheses and research designs may be classified into two broad groups (Figure 7.1).

Experimental research

         _____ true experiments

         _____ quasi-experiments

Non-experimental research

         _____ descriptive surveys

         _____ correlational surveys

Figure 7.1: Quantitative research designs.

The main purpose of survey designs is to describe and document the variables of interest in a given population, situation or setting. In a purely descriptive survey it may not be possible to make any inferences regarding relationships between variables although descriptive statistics can be applied to quantify frequencies of variables and central tendencies (see Chapter 10). This type of research may provide preliminary data for future studies but can also lead to practical applications based on increased awareness of variables. For example, a survey designed to identify the prevalence of smoking amongst teenagers will not necessarily contribute to understanding why teenagers smoke but will provide data on the percentage of smokers in the teenage population and may inform decision making about future anti-smoking policies and campaigns. By contrast, a correlational survey is designed to identify and test the strength of relationships between variables by statistical analysis. Using the example above, questions to teenage smokers might be designed to elicit information about how or why they started smoking and why they continue.

Quantitative designs (particularly experiments and quasi-experiments) are criticised at times for their focus on specific variables, sometimes in comparative isolation from the whole, for example examination of the effects of compression bandaging on the healing of venous leg ulcers without including inquiry into patient characteristics such as comfort and satisfaction. Whereas the holistic view commonly taken in qualitative designs is clearly important in providing data which can be recognised as describing the 'real' world, it must be remembered that the purpose of quantitative research is different to that of qualitative approaches. Research designs should be selected according to their appropriateness and ability to provide answers to the research question identified, and may include both quantitative and qualitative techniques.

This chapter begins by addressing the principles of quantitative research design, highlighting both strengths and potential limitations, and then focuses on three main types of quantitative design:

- quasi-experimental designs
- true experimental designs
- non-experimental designs – surveys.

A consideration of ethical issues that might arise in quantitative research is included within appropriate sections and the chapter concludes with a summary of the key points. Greater details of methodologies and techniques commonly employed in the designs discussed are provided in the following chapter.

Principles of quantitative research design

Quantitative research usually follows a clearly defined process (Figure 7.2), which begins with the identification of a research problem or area of concern for a particular population.

Developmental stage

The precise aims of the study may be defined from a review of existing literature that identifies 'gaps' in current knowledge, or from a combination of questions arising from experience and examination of the literature to confirm that the required answers are not already in existence. Even where previous work has been conducted in the same problem area a critical review is required to establish whether adequate knowledge exists to make changes in practice or whether additional work is needed.

Developmental stage
research problem and purpose
- literature review
- theoretical framework
- research objectives, questions, hypotheses
- study variables – operational definitions

Research design, methodology and data collection
- research design
- population and sample
- ethical issues
- methods of measurement – pilot studies, reliability, validity and sensitivity
- data collection

Data analysis and interpretation
- data analysis
- research outcomes and dissemination

Figure 7.2: Steps in the quantitative research process.

A theoretical framework provides the logic on which the study is based. It attempts to explain why it is thought that certain variables may be linked and provides a basis for the interpretation of the data collected. Often the framework used is founded on a well-tested, well-developed theory that has been used as a framework for many studies but, alternatively, if little previous work in the area has been undertaken, the framework may represent a newly developed theory to be tested. It is common in published research for the theoretical base to be implicit rather than explicitly defined. In studies using physiological measurements, for example, this may be partly because the science underpinning such studies is well-established and often considered to be fact rather than theory. It may also be partly because the concepts used, such as blood pressure, wound healing, cardiac output and so forth are less abstract than many of those used in behavioural studies.

Research objectives, questions and hypotheses focus the research purpose and provide precise criteria against which the outcomes of the research can be measured. In descriptive studies a research purpose may be sufficient to guide the study but when the aim of the study is to identify and establish relationships between variables, specific questions and/or hypotheses need to be formulated. A hypothesis can be defined as a formal statement of the expected relationship(s) between two or more variables in the study population. As a statement that explains or predicts the outcome of the study being performed, the hypothesis can be tested against the results of the research and either accepted as true for that population or rejected. However, the extent to which the conclusions drawn may be applied to alternative populations is a very different question and will be addressed later in the chapter when issues of validity are considered. In quantitative research, which will be subject to statistical analysis, the research hypothesis is commonly expressed as a null hypothesis (see Chapter 10). In this case, instead of predicting the outcome of the research and the expected relationship between variables, the null hypothesis states that no relationship will exist between the defined variables. For example:

> Research hypothesis (sometimes referred to as the alternative hypothesis H_A): 'the incidence of sleep problems in infants will be reduced by providing parents with information and advice in the early post-natal months'.
> Null hypothesis (sometimes referred to as the statistical hypothesis H_o): 'the incidence of sleep problems in infants will not be affected by providing parents with information and advice in the early post-natal months'.
> (Kerr et al., 1996)

Mention has already been made of the importance of measurement in quantitative research. Clearly, it is important that 'what is being measured' is precisely defined, not only to assist the interpretation of results obtained but also to allow comparisons with results from other studies. Definitions of variables may be characterised in two ways:

- conceptual definitions: which explain the meaning of a given concept or idea;
- operational definitions: which define the variable in a way which can be measured.

For example, in a study of the prevalence of urinary incontinence in a nursing home population the following definitions might be used:

- **Conceptual definition of urinary incontinence:** the uncontrolled loss of urine in an unacceptable place at an unacceptable time.
- **Operational definition of urinary incontinence:** the uncontrolled loss of urine measured by the presence of a wet pad on two or more occasions in one week.

Often further operational definitions may be required, for example what is meant by a wet pad and how wet should it be to be included?

In this case the pad might be weighed and a certain increase in weight defined as the minimum required to accept the pad as being 'wet'.

In studies designed to examine associations or cause-and-effect relationships, variables are often classed as independent and dependent. The independent variable is the characteristic thought to exert an influence on the dependent variable, i.e. the characteristic being measured. In experimental designs where some intervention or manipulation is introduced by the researcher, the variable that is manipulated is the independent variable and its effect on the dependent variable is measured. For example, in the study of infant sleep disturbances referred to above, the independent variable is the information and advice given to parents whilst infant sleep is the dependent variable.

Research design, methodology and data collection

Except for purely descriptive studies most quantitative research aims to examine the nature of relationships between phenomena – for example, whether a certain nursing intervention produces a decrease in patient anxiety. The research design directs the way in which the study is conducted and attempts to maximise control of factors that could influence the study outcome and its purpose. For example, it attempts to control the influence of other factors, such as noise or lack of information, which might increase (or reduce) patient anxiety while the nursing intervention is taking place. The strength of the true experimental design (discussed later in this chapter) is that the experimenter can achieve greater confidence in the genuineness of relationships because they are observed under carefully controlled conditions. The research design also aims to minimise the risk of making two types of error when deciding if the null hypothesis should be accepted or rejected (see Chapter 10).

The risk of rejecting the null hypothesis when it is actually true is termed a Type I error. For example, in a study of the effectiveness of a new and expensive mattress in reducing the incidence of pressure sores, the risk of a Type I error is the risk of introducing the mattress when it is not effective (and therefore wasting limited resources). The acceptable level of risk of a Type I error is chosen by the researcher and is generally the same as the level of statistical significance selected. This is most commonly 0.05 or 0.01 which means that the researcher is prepared to take a 5% or a 1% chance of being wrong. The risk of a Type II error is the risk of accepting the null hypothesis when it is false – that is, not detecting changes that exist. In this example, the risk of a Type II error is the risk of not identifying that the new mattress is effective when actually it is. Type II errors are often caused by faults in the study design where sample sizes are too small to be able to detect changes with statistical certainty or where measurement instruments are insufficiently sensitive to detect small changes.

The sample must be carefully selected from the target population, using a randomisation procedure if at all possible, because of the need to maximise control over variables that could cause bias in the study. The target population refers to all the individuals (or objects and so forth) who meet certain criteria for inclusion in the study. This is the population about which the researcher would like to be able to draw some conclusions. For example, in the study of infant sleep disturbance the target population might be all parents in the UK with a child of less than six months. Since it would be impossible to include all parents in the UK with a child of less than six months in the study, a smaller sample must be selected that is representative of the target population. If the sample accurately reflects the range of characteristics present in the target population there is a greater possibility of being able to generalise the results obtained from the study to the target population. Sampling techniques are discussed further in Chapter 10, but randomisation is the best technique available to obtain a representative sample.

Ethical issues

In any study involving human subjects there are ethical issues that must be considered, particularly in experimental and quasi-experimental designs where some intervention occurs that will affect at least some of the subjects. This will be discussed further in relation to specific research designs but in all studies involving patients the approval of the local ethics committee must be granted before any data collection takes place. Some of the key points that must be addressed are presented here:

- potential subjects must be informed of the study protocol and the extent of their own involvement. They must be fully aware of any possible risks to themselves and they must be free to withdraw from the study at any time should they choose to do so;
- subjects must be assured that they will not be disadvantaged in

any way either by choosing to take part in the study or by refusing to take part;
- subjects' anonymity must be maintained;
- subjects' informed consent must be obtained before data collection commences. The issue of informed consent is extremely important and the procedures employed in obtaining consent should be described in the research report.

Pilot study

Prior to commencing the main research data collection it is usual to conduct a small-scale pilot study to test the elements of the study design. This can save costly and time-consuming mistakes by demonstrating that the research design is appropriate and that the methodology and measurement techniques are capable of producing the results expected. If faults in the design or measurement instruments are detected these can be corrected before the full-scale data collection begins. The pilot sample comprises a small number of subjects drawn from the same population as the main study sample. The results gained from the pilot work are normally excluded from the analysis of data from the main study because of methodological or other changes occurring between the pilot and the main study.

The quality of any quantitative research study depends to a large extent on the quality of the measurement techniques used to collect the data. A critique of a method of measurement requires examination of three key characteristics:

- reliability
- validity
- sensitivity.

These characteristics will be considered further in relation to the different types of quantitative designs but the differences between them can be illustrated by the example of a set of scales. The reliability of a measurement technique or instrument refers to its ability to provide consistent measurements every time it is used. For example, if a set of scales is used repeatedly to weigh an individual whose weight has not changed, if the scales are reliable they will consistently record the same weight. However, if the scales record the individual's weight consistently as 60 kg when the true weight is 62 kg, they are reliable but they are not providing a valid measurement because they are not measuring what they are supposed to be measuring, namely the individual's true weight. If this particular set of scales was actually designed to weigh heavy equipment rather than people it may be that the scales are only capable of weighing to the nearest 5 kg, in which case they would not be sufficiently sensitive to record the difference between 60 kg and 62 kg. The sensitivity of an instrument is an important design feature in avoiding Type II errors.

In studies which require repeated measurements by researchers or in which more than one researcher collects data, issues of intra-rater and inter-rater reliability arise. Intra-rater reliability can be assessed by the test–retest method in which measurements of the same variable are repeated twice by the same researcher/rater under the same conditions within a prescribed period of time, and the results compared. Similarly inter-rater reliability can be assessed by comparing scores obtained by different raters for the same variable under the same conditions.

Data analysis and interpretation

The process of organising and extracting meaning from the data collected occurs during the data analysis stage. It includes the use of both descriptive and inferential statistics usually by computerised statistical techniques. However, there are two points that are worth considering here. The first is associated with data protection and the need to install procedures to ensure that the data collected remain confidential. The second point is that sometimes the use of computers can detract from the researcher's own understanding of the data gathered. Whereas it may be impractical in large scale studies with very large datasets, in smaller studies simply 'looking' at the data to see what they suggest can be very helpful. Further statistical analysis can then be used to test possible unexpected relationships.

The final stage of the research process is the identification of the research outcomes, and the conclusions drawn, together with recognition of the limitations of the study. Implications for practice and further research should be acknowledged and the report of the study prepared and disseminated appropriately.

Experimental and quasi-experimental designs

Experimental and quasi-experimental research designs aim to provide evidence to support or refute issues of causality. The key characteristic that distinguishes them from non-experiments is that the researcher introduces some intervention, in order to observe or measure its effect on the subjects in the study or on the variables of interest. A true experiment is a scientific study characterised by the following three attributes:

- manipulation
- control
- randomisation

(Polit and Hungler, 1991).

Manipulation involves some intervention on the part of the researcher. This may involve actually doing something to one group of subjects (the experimental group) and withholding it from others (the control group), or selecting two or more groups of subjects on the basis of characteristics which they already possess. For example, in the introduction of a new type of dressing over an intravenous cannulation site to examine its effect on the incidence of bacteraemia, the experimental group receive the new dressing whilst the control group receive the usual dressing. The intervention, i.e. the new dressing, is referred to as the independent variable whilst the factor which may be influenced by it, i.e. the incidence of bacteraemia, is the dependent variable. In another experiment to compare the effects of a particular teaching approach on young student nurses and on older students entering nursing later in life, the independent variable is not the teaching approach, because it is the same for both groups, but rather it is the age group of the students. The dependent variable is the outcome of the teaching.

Control involves designing the study in order to minimise the effects of variables other than those that form the focus of the study. This is usually performed using a control group. For example, in a study to examine the effectiveness of different methods of learning pelvic floor exercises on stress incontinence, patients may be assigned to one of three groups. After an initial consultation and examination Group I receive a written handout explaining how to do the exercises and how often. Group II also receives the handout but this group is invited for monthly review visits to the clinic to monitor its progress. Group III receives the same treatment as Group II but at the monthly follow-up visits they use a biofeedback technique that allows them to visualise the strength of their pelvic floor contractions. In order to be confident that after six months any changes in pelvic floor strength are related to the learning programme and not to individual variations amongst group members it is important that extraneous variables such as age, motivation, and initial weakness of the pelvic floor muscles are controlled as far as possible. All groups should therefore be composed of patients with similar characteristics where those characteristics are thought to have the potential to influence the research outcomes. Other elements of control are also important. For example, if a number of different practitioners are involved in providing initial and follow-up consultations, the content of the consultations must be defined and controlled to avoid some subjects receiving more information or greater support and encouragement than others.

Randomisation involves assigning subjects to experimental and control groups in such a way that every subject has an equal chance of being assigned to either group. This sampling technique is also a form of control in that it tries to ensure that there is no systematic bias within groups with respect to attributes that may influence the dependent variable under investigation. However, although randomisation is the best technique available to minimise risks of sampling bias, equality of groups cannot be guaranteed, particularly where sample sizes are small. For example, if there were only 20 women taking part in the above study there is a possibility that the five women with the least motivation to perform pelvic floor exercises might all be assigned to the same group. This risk is reduced as the number of subjects increases. Other sampling methods designed to avoid bias are considered in Chapter 10.

The following section provides examples of different designs and utilises a short-hand notation to map the designs, where:

X = the independent variable or intervention (sometimes written as T for treatment, but this can lead to some confusion where 'T' or 't' is also used to denote time).

O = the dependent variable or observation.

R = randomisation.

Experimental designs

Simple true experiment

Group 1	R	O_1	X	O_2
Group 2	R	O_1		O_2

In this design subjects are randomly assigned to Group 1 or Group 2. Pre-test measurements (O_1) of the independent variable are made for each group. Group 1 then receives the experimental intervention (X) whilst Group 2 acts as a control and receives no intervention. Both groups then undergo the post-test measurements (O_2). Statistical comparisons of the data from the two groups allow the researcher to state the confidence with which they may predict the relationship between the independent and dependent variables.

Randomised clinical trials (RCTs) are a particular example of the simple true experiment and are characterised by the following features:

- they involve the testing of clinical treatment;
- there is random assignment of subjects to experimental or control conditions;
- collection of information on treatment outcomes from all groups;
- they generally use a large and heterogeneous sample of subjects, frequently selected from multiple, geographically dispersed sites to ensure results are not unique to a single setting;
- the required sample size is usually calculated from equations that include a measure of the power of the study – i.e. the ability of the study to detect existing relationships among variables.

The RCT is first thought to have been used in conjunction with human subjects in 1946, in the determination of the effectiveness of streptomycin (Poole and Jones, 1996). This design has been widely endorsed within medicine as a rigorous means of establishing clinical benefits – particularly of pharmaceutical interventions. The Cochrane databases of research evidence underpinning practice are principally compiled from RCTs (The Cochrane Library, 1996).

Experimental research designs can present ethical difficulties if there are potential risks to the subject in either receiving or not receiving an intervention. This is readily illustrated in trials of new medications. It will be difficult to gain approval from an ethics committee to conduct a study if there is evidence of severe side effects caused by the drug. Alternatively, if during the progress of a drug trial it becomes evident that the new drug has the potential to save life, for example in patients with AIDS, it may become ethically unacceptable to continue the trial and to withhold the drug from patients in a control group. Another ethical issue associated with RCTs relates to possible effects on the practitioner/client relationship where patients may be unduly influenced to consent to take part in trials.

Solomon four group design

When data are collected before and after an intervention, the pre-test measure itself can sometimes influence the post-test measure even in the absence of the experimental intervention. For example, in a study to examine the effect of a workshop to improve nurses attitudes towards elderly patients with dementia, a pre-test measure of attitudes may affect subjects' responses to the workshop. The Solomon four group design has the potential to overcome this distortion of the study results since there are two control groups (who, in the given example, do not take part in the workshop) and two experimental groups (who do). One control group and one experimental group undergo the pre-test, and the other groups do not.

| | | | Data collection | | |
			Before	Interverntion	After
Group 1	Experimental – with pre-test	R	O_1	X	O_2
Group 2	Experimental – without pre-test	R		X	O_2
Group 3	Control – with pre-test	R	O_1		O_2
Group 4	Control – without pre-test	R			O_2

Figure 7.3: Example of a Solomon four group design to examine the effects of a workshop to improve nurses' attitudes towards older patients with dementia.

The main limitation of this design is that it requires a larger sample size than simple experimental designs. This is also true of the factorial design.

Factorial design

Using a factorial design it is possible to manipulate two or more independent variables simultaneously within a single study and to collect data on the interaction between those variables. In a 2 x 2 factorial design two independent variables or 'factors' are involved. Each factor is manipulated at two different levels, for example presence or absence of the factors or the presence of the factor at two different levels of intensity (Figure 7.4).

Groups B and C allow examination of the effects of each relaxation technique separately while Group D acts as a control because these subjects are not taught either technique. Group A allows examination of the interaction between the two techniques and provides information that cannot be gained by other experimental research designs. Equivalent numbers of subjects are necessary in each of the four groups and because a large sample size is required this may necessitate the use of several data collectors, giving rise to issues of inter-rater reliability.

Independent variables:	1 – progressive muscle relaxation technique	
	2 – controlled deep breathing technique	

	Muscle relaxation	No muscle relaxation
Controlled breathing	A	B
No controlled breathing	C	D

Figure 7.4: Example of a 2 x2 factorial design to examine the effect of two strategies (independent variables) for promoting relaxation in hypertensive patients.

Quasi-experimental designs

Quasi-experimental research is similar to experimental research in that there is manipulation of an independent variable, but differs in that randomisation and/or control is lacking. These designs are used more frequently than true experiments in health care research because of inherent difficulties in designing true experiments with human subjects. For example, true experimental designs assume all relevant variables are known and can be controlled or manipulated and that randomisation can be used. Often it is impossible to meet these criteria and so quasi-experimental designs must be used. However, they are weaker designs since they are less capable of identifying cause-and-effect relationships with the same degree of confidence as experimental designs.

One-shot case study–X O

(Also known as the *after only* or *post-test design* – X O.) This is the simplest of designs where data are collected only once – after the intervention. An example of the use of this design occurs in educational studies when new curricula are introduced and so their effects cannot have been measured before. The design is weak because no data with which to compare results are collected prior to the intervention and there is no control of other variables that may have influenced the results, such as changes in entry requirements. It is impossible to infer a cause-and-effect relationship with an intervention tested using this research design.

One group pre-test – post-test – O X O

A slightly more complex design includes measures at two points in time – a baseline measure or pre-test (for example, measurement of pain perception by chronic back pain sufferers before commencement of a new analgesic treatment regime, and a post-test measure or outcome measure). This is still a weak design as there is no control and factors other than the independent variable may have influenced the outcome, including the placebo effect or a concurrent reduction in stress levels. The one group pre-test – post-test design is often used when the researcher does not have access to an equivalent group (for example, a similar group of back pain sufferers not receiving medication). A time series design can help to overcome some of these problems. For example, other extraneous variables influencing pain may fluctuate over time and their effects can be recognised.

Time series design

Group 1 $\quad$ O_1 $\quad$ O_2 $\quad$ O_3 $\quad$ X $\quad$ O_4 $\quad$ O_5 $\quad$ O_6

The consistency of baseline observations O_{1-3}, which occur at time 1, time 2, time 3 etc, followed by a change in observations O_{4-6} at times 4, 5 and 6 after the intervention strengthens the probability that X has influenced the observed results.

Static group comparison

$$\frac{X \quad O}{O}$$

This is a stronger design because there is some control through the use of a control group which has not been subject to the intervention. However, in the absence of randomised allocation of subjects to the two groups it cannot be assumed that the subjects in the two groups were similar prior to the intervention and therefore there may be other reasons for observed differences between groups.

Non-equivalent control group pre-test – post-test design

Group 1	O_1	X	O_2
Group 2	O_1		O_2

This design is very similar to the true experiment with the one exception that the subjects are not randomly allocated to the groups and the researcher must assume that they are similar in the first place. However, this assumption can be tested statistically by comparing the data gathered at the pre-test.

Advantages and disadvantages of experimental designs

The strength of experimental designs is undoubtedly in the investigation of causal relationships. However, there are a number of difficulties in undertaking experimental research with human subjects, particularly in clinical settings.

Practical difficulties include:

- Limited availability of subjects who meet the research sample inclusion criteria.
- Inability to control some variables which may influence the experimental results. Examples of such variables include gender, intelligence, the weather, occurrence of disease.
- Some variables could be controlled in theory but ethical considerations prevent such manipulation, for example intervening unnecessarily during the normal delivery of a baby, or studying the effects of drugs with severe side effects.

Threats to internal validity

As considered earlier, the validity of a research instrument or research design refers to its ability to measure what it claims to be measuring. Threats to internal validity are caused by factors that limit the degree to which it can be inferred that the experimental treatment (independent variable), rather than uncontrolled extraneous variables, is responsible for the observed effects (Polit and Hungler, 1991). Such threats may arise because of:

- inability to impose and/or monitor control of variables – for example, in a community based study it would be very difficult to impose and monitor a controlled diet for more than a few days;
- effect of previous experience/extraneous influences, for example the influence of a concurrent television programme on the evaluation of a local anti-smoking campaign;
- maturational effects where the passage of time influences the observed results or affects one group of subjects more than another;
- influence of pre-testing – see the discussion of the Solomon four group design above;
- errors of instrumentation which could include both mechanical and/or human problems;
- selection bias where randomisation or other sampling techniques cannot be applied and samples of convenience are used;
- loss of a proportion of the sample population through 'drop-out' (mortality). This may be difficult to control within the research design, but the loss of subjects can influence the internal validity of the study, particularly if the drop-out rate is greater from one study group than another;
- the Hawthorne effect. This describes the effect on the dependent variable caused by subjects' awareness that they are being studied. It may be possible to 'blind' the subjects, for example by use of a placebo in drug trials but in other situations it may be more difficult. In a double-blind experimental design neither subjects nor data collectors know which subjects are in which group.

In a true experiment attempts are made to control all recognised sources of threats to internal validity. In a clinical environment this may not be possible or it may be considered that extensive control produces an artificial environment which is unrepresentative of 'real life'. In this respect maximising control can present a threat to external validity – i.e. the ability to generalise the results to populations or settings other than the ones studied. It may be necessary to reach a compromise between the two, or to ensure that studies are replicated in new settings and with different subjects. In general, greater confidence can be placed on results if they can be replicated in different environments.

Non-experimental research – survey designs

Surveys are the most common type of non-experimental quantitative research design and do not involve the manipulation of an independent variable. Whilst experimental studies usually look at only a few variables at a time, surveys provide an efficient and effective means of collecting a large amount of data about a population. Such data may be purely descriptive, for example regarding prevalence and distribution of the data within populations, or they may be examined for correlations between variables. For example, a survey of the health histories and dietary habits of a large number of people might be used to identify correlations between dietary habits and certain health problems. When a correlation exists a change in one variable corresponds to a change in other variables. However, it should be remembered that correlation does not necessarily indicate causation and further studies would be required to establish a causative relationship.

Survey designs are sometimes attractive to inexperienced researchers because of the relative ease with which they can be launched and because asking questions is a familiar process that is an everyday part of life. However, poorly constructed surveys can result in a mass of facts, figures, questionnaire schedules and/or interview transcripts that may lack validity and reliability, and are difficult to analyse and make sense of. A well-planned survey is an extensive and potentially costly undertaking for which there should be clearly identified goals.

One of the potential strengths of survey designs is their external validity, but this depends on the use of appropriate sampling techniques. It is usually impossible to collect data from every member of the population of interest and therefore a representative sample must be selected from the target population. Probability sampling uses a randomised method of selecting participants, such that each subject has an equal and independent chance of being included in the study. Sampling techniques are discussed in detail in Chapter 10 but include:

- simple random sampling;
- stratified random sampling;

- cluster sampling;
- systematic random sampling.

By contrast, non-probability sampling uses conveniently accessible subjects who meet the selection criteria. However, there is a clear potential for selection bias in a convenience sample and this severely limits the external validity of results obtained. In most surveys the demographic characteristics of the population are collected. These may enable the researcher to compare characteristics of the sample with those of the target population. For example, if it is found that the target population comprises 50% men and 50% women, but that the sample population contains 85% women, the survey conclusions may not be appropriate for the general population.

Although surveys do not include manipulation or intervention there are other ethical issues which may arise. For example, to approach severely ill patients or their relatives to take part in a survey may be considered unethical unless adequate justification for the need to collect the proposed data can be presented. Alternatively the data to be collected may be of a sensitive nature which may leave subjects feeling distressed and/or unsure where to turn for help even if they are willing to participate.

There are two main methods of collecting survey data:

- questionnaires
- interviews.

In general, questionnaires are most useful in obtaining quantitative data and the practicalities of questionnaire design are considered in the next chapter. Some of the advantages and disadvantages of questionnaires, compared with interviews, are indicated in Figure 7.5.

Types of survey design

The greatest advantages of survey research are its flexibility and broadness of scope. It can be applied to many populations, can focus on a wide range of topics and its information can be used for many purposes. Some alternative survey designs are considered below, but in general surveys may be classified as descriptive or correlational.

Advantages

- generally less expensive and time consuming than personal or telephone interviews
- can be administered to large numbers of subjects simultaneously
- require less skill to administer than interviews
- provide a structured format which enhances the uniformity of measurement from one subject/situation to another, and facilitates computer-assisted data analysis
- provides anonymity which may enable subjects to respond more freely or honestly

Disadvantages

- low response rates are common. A 50% response rate is considered good for a postal questionnaire
- questions may be misunderstood or ambiguous. This risk can be reduced by careful design and piloting
- may be inappropriate where sensitive information is requested. Subjects may be unwilling to answer or may be distressed by the questionnaire material
- accuracy of responses can only be assumed
- information collected tends to be relatively superficial
- no opportunity for follow-up if respondents are anonymous

Figure 7.5: Advantages and disadvantages of questionnaires.

Descriptive surveys

Descriptive surveys may be simple or comparative. In a simple descriptive survey the goal of the survey is to provide as complete a description of the sample as possible, with identification of variables of interest and the frequency of their occurrence. By contrast, in a comparative survey design a comparison is made between two or more groups by statistical analysis of information collected from each group. It is important for the study samples to be as similar as possible in all variables except those under study and therefore random sampling techniques should be used.

Longitudinal designs

Longitudinal studies may be used when the researcher is interested in how variables have changed over time and may follow one of several alternative design approaches:

- trend studies – the researcher selects samples from the general population at specified time intervals, and at each interval new subjects are chosen. This design provides information about the amount of change that has occurred over a specific period of time, for example, smoking in the general population;

- cohort studies – different subjects are also selected at specified intervals but they are drawn from the previously identified groups within the population. This design allows sections of the population to be followed over time, e.g. to investigate the development of a disease such as coronary heart disease in a group of men all born in the same year. This type of design offers an element of control over at least some variables, such as age and changing attitudes within society;
- panel studies – repeated measurements are made of the same subjects at specified time intervals. This design might be used in the follow up of patients treated for a particular condition.

Although longitudinal studies can provide valuable information that may not be identifiable through cross-sectional designs where data are collected at one point in time only, they can be lengthy and expensive. In addition, there is an increasing risk that subjects will be lost to the study over time. Furthermore, they may provide little information on which factors have contributed to the changes observed over time.

Correlational studies

In correlational surveys the aim is to describe existing relationships between variables and to determine whether there is a correlation between them. Variables of interest are identified and the researcher then determines the most appropriate way to measure them, usually through questionnaire or interview. Alternatively the design may be retrospective, in which case the researcher starts with an observed effect, for example a particular disease condition, and then collects data to try to determine what factors occurring in the past may have been associated with the effect. Data may be collected from individuals or from archival records. Retrospective studies are particularly useful when investigating relatively rare conditions when it would be difficult to obtain a large enough sample size using other sampling techniques. The retrospective approach may also be quicker and less expensive than prospective designs because it uses existing data. However, there are certain disadvantages that must be considered. Where subjects are questioned there may be problems of poor recall of events that can create threats to validity. There may also be an element of recall bias causing either over-reporting or under-reporting. Over-reporting can occur when subjects are very aware of their personal histories and may over emphasise events, whilst under-reporting may exist when sensitive or socially undesirable outcomes are under investigation. Difficulties can also arise when archival records are used as a source of data. Access to records may sometimes be difficult to obtain and the records themselves may be incomplete or missing.

Summary

Research designs should be selected on the basis of their ability to achieve the purpose of the proposed research. Quantitative designs can be employed in a number of different ways:

- descriptive – identifying variables;
- explanatory – looking for relationships and correlations;
- predictive – estimation of the probability of a specific outcome;
- intervention – involving some manipulation of variables to test the outcome

(Burns and Grove, 1995).

Quantitative designs provide the strongest designs for investigation of inter-relationships between variables and issues of causality. They are characterised by the assignment of numerical data to the measurement of variables but also by efforts to enhance objectivity in the measurement process.

References

Burns N, Grove S (1995) Understanding Nursing Research. London: Saunders.

The Cochrane library (1996) Issue 2 Database on disk and CD-Rom. London:BMJ Publishing

Kerr SM, Jowett SA, Smith L (1996) Preventing sleep problems in infants: a randomized controlled trial. Journal of Advanced Nursing 24: 938–42.

Munhall P (1982) Nursing philosophy and nursing research; in apposition or opposition? Nursing Research 31(3): 176–81.

Poole K, Jones A (1996) A re-examination of the experimental design for nursing research. Journal of Advanced Nursing 24: 108–14.

Polit D, Hungler B (1991) Nursing Research: Principles and Methods. Philadelphia: Lippincott.

Schumacher KL, Gortner SR (1992) (Mis)Conceptions and reconceptions about traditional science. Advances in Nursing Science 14(4): 1–11.

Chapter 8
Methods of data collection for quantitative research

Anne Mulhall

Introduction

This chapter concerns the ways in which data are collected for quantitative research in clinical nursing practice. Before proceeding, however, we must define two terms – *methodology* and *methods* – which appear frequently in this chapter. Research methodology has been defined in a number of ways but, for the purposes of this chapter, it refers to the approach to a research topic that is taken within a specific paradigm. A paradigm is a worldview based on the particular assumptions and values shared by a research community – see Chapter 2. Examples of research methodologies include experimental research, survey research and ethnography. Research methods refer to the ways in which data are collected when undertaking research, for example by asking questions or observing situations or individuals.

How does research look from practice?

For new and experienced practitioners, and indeed nurse educators, the pursuit of research-based practice has caused a sense of unease as they attempt to unravel how they should achieve this objective. This dilemma has produced two responses. On the one hand many nurses report that they lack the skills to undertake, or even critique, research (Pearcey, 1995; Veeramah, 1995). Others contend that since they spend much of their working life observing, assessing, implementing and evaluating, then they are 'doing research'. Either way there is a problem for, in reality, like nursing itself, research is a complex activity that requires many years of training and experience to master. Furthermore, unlike medicine, which has been reluctant to examine different ways of undertaking research, nursing has embraced a range of research methodologies and methods. Gaining knowledge about these presents both neophyte researchers, and those who aim to critique such work, with an uphill task. Such is the gradient, that for many the sheer bulk of information that they are required to understand is a sufficient block to their pursuing such a course. In addition, research methods have frequently been taught in isolation, and often by teachers who have little research experience themselves. This has led to a situation where research remains unintegrated with the main body of nursing knowledge, an appendage which is somehow separate from the activity of clinical nursing.

The problem about research methods, then, is one of overload of information and, let's face it, boredom. Some aspects of thinking and learning about research are stimulating and enjoyable. Trying to define questions from practice in a researchable format, exploring the different routes through which questions might be tackled as discussed in Chapter 2, more easily fall into this category. Actually trying to decide how to collect the data to answer these questions is more taxing, and often rather frustrating. Furthermore, many of the problems inherent in particular methods do not make themselves apparent until well into the data collection phase. Such difficulties are well known only to those who have the opportunity to undertake research

Although recent studies suggest that research is viewed positively by many practitioners (Lacey, 1994; Veeramah, 1995), the challenge in terms of promoting a better understanding of methods remains. It remains because in general those who teach research methods are embedded in the world of research/education, and this world is fundamentally different from the world of practice (Mulhall, 1997). Thus the forces that drive and motivate these two groups do not coincide. Practitioners are, at the bottom line, interested in the answers to questions that arise as they care for patients and clients and they are concerned with nursing practice. In contrast, although some researchers at least attempt to gear their work to providing these answers, much of their energies are focused on research practice. This raises two important questions fundamental to this chapter, and indeed this book:

- Why should clinical nurses concern themselves with research methods?

●   If a knowledge of methods is important how may practitioners be more optimally engaged in acquiring this understanding?

The importance of research methods to clinical nursing

To conform to the standard of professional practice in the 1990s nurses will require a knowledge of research methods. However, although statutory requirements and professional pressure are essential in shaping an ideology of research in nursing, in the battle of the hearts and mind they only address the latter. Research-based practice will not become a sustainable reality until the purveyors of practice are convinced of its intrinsic and fundamental importance to the care of their patients and their own abilities to deliver that care. Once converted on this point, the importance and relevance of a knowledge of research methods will be all too apparent.

Part of the problem related to research methods concerns the different foci of practitioners and researchers and the general mystique surrounding research and researchers. It is not difficult to engage researchers in a heated debate about methodologies or methods, whereas such discussions leave most practitioners stone cold. How can research methods be perceived as essential to excellent practice? Perhaps the central task with regard to methods is, first, to demonstrate their crucial importance in underpinning research-based practice, and second, to attempt to convey some of the excitement and rewards, both personal and professional, that a closer engagement with methods brings.

Getting excited about methods!

The discussion so far has begun to indicate why clinical nurses need to acquire an adequate knowledge of research methods. It is important, however, to also consider why quantitative methods in particular are important to nursing. Early forays into nursing research, not surprisingly, were modelled on the approaches and methods that prevailed in other relevant disciplines, in particular medicine. Research was therefore designed and conceived under the auspices of the scientific model (see Chapter 2). However, in the last decade there has been a growing movement of nurse researchers who contend that investigation of the social world of health care is not amenable to the methods of natural science (Melia, 1982; Duffy, 1985). This movement has gained such a foothold in both social science and nursing that Hammersley (1995: 1) notes:

No one today, or hardly anyone, refers to themselves or their own work as
positivist.

Within nursing this movement towards more naturalistic methodologies has particular attractions. First, such approaches are eminently
suitable vehicles for the exploration of much nursing practice. Second,
the ideology of nursing celebrating, as it does, a holistic approach to
care and the importance of the individual, fits comfortably into the
naturalistic framework. Third, the adoption of another research paradigm different from that of medicine has acted as a professional strategy for emphasising the difference between these two domains.
However, there are a multitude of questions in clinical nursing that are
more appropriately tackled through quantitative research. In the
remaining sections of this chapter the three main methods of collecting quantitative data will be described and, alongside them, examples
will be provided of where such methods have made an impact in clinical nursing. Illustrating methods in this way is crucial to underwriting
their importance for clinical nursing. If a convincing case can be made
that quantitative results have much to offer clinical nursing it is but a
short step to capturing the interest of practitioners in the quantitative
methods that made those results possible.

Although the practical significance of quantitative methods in
producing useful information for nursing practice is important there
is another reason which may explain researchers' genuine interest in
methods. It is the question of methodologies and the philosophies
that underpin them that was first discussed in Chapter 2, and it
involves the relationship between researchers and their research.
These ideas will be explored in the final part of this introduction.

Researchers and their research

Thomas Kuhn (1970) challenged the conception of science as a
process whereby increasingly correct descriptions of the physical
world were discovered. Nielsen (1990: 13) neatly summarises Kuhn's
arguments thus:

> . . . data or observations are theory laden (that is the scientist only sees data
> in terms of their relevance to theory); . . . theories are paradigm laden
> (explanations are grounded in world views); and . . . paradigms are culture
> laden (worldviews, including ideas about human nature, vary historically
> and across cultures).

In essence this says that the way we go about research, and the explanations that we draw from it are, to a certain extent, grounded in
who we are, where we have come from and where we find ourselves.

Or, putting it another way, research methodologies, and therefore methods, may be socially constructed. Although this idea may be new, it brings the issue of methodologies and methods alive. It indicates that the perception of a research problem, and also the way in which research questions are asked, may be influenced by the philosophies that underlie the different research perspectives. At a personal level therefore it is very important to reflect carefully on the ways in which you perceive potential research topics, the questions that you frame in order to explore these topics, and the methodology and thence methods that you consider appropriate to address these questions. Seen in this light, discussions about methodologies and their attendant methods take on a deeper meaning. With a knowledge of paradigms and a recognition of your own preferences and why you hold them, then the debate about why a particular methodology and method were selected, and whether they were appropriate (either when considering your own research, or appraising that of others) becomes much more significant, potentially contentious, and therefore hopefully exciting! As Guba and Lincoln (1994: 116) conclude:

> Paradigm issues are crucial; no inquirer, we maintain, ought to go about the business of inquiry without being clear about just what paradigm informs or guides his or her approach.

Quantitative research

The remainder of this chapter will describe some of the methods used for collecting data for quantitative research, but what do we mean by this term? There is some confusion, and indeed controversy, in the literature as to what exactly the terms qualitative and quantitative research refer. Many nurse researchers reserve these terms to describe the methods of data collection, rather than the underlying approaches or methodologies involved. However, Bryman (1988:3) in his well known discussion of these two approaches to research suggests that these terms have come to

> ... signify much more than ways of gathering data; they come to denote the divergent assumptions about the nature and purpose of research in the social sciences.

This view of the terms quantitative and qualitative goes beyond method to methodology, and eventually to paradigms and their underlying philosophies. It reflects a more widespread view within the research community, and this interpretation is adopted here. It takes the definition of quantitative research beyond the presence of numerical data alone to include a consideration of where, in terms of a worldview, this type of research emanates from.

The worldview or paradigm underlying quantitative research is underpinned by the practices of natural science, and the philosophies of positivism and empiricism (see Chapter 2). The logic and procedures of the natural science paradigm are therefore the 'epistemological yardsticks' against which quantitative research is judged (Bryman, 1988: 3), and social scientific knowledge is distinguishable from other ways of knowing through its foundation in rigorous natural science methodology. Positivists assume that there is an objective (i.e. independent of the knower) world to be known and that by applying the methods of natural science it is possible to discover it. There is, for them, a fundamental difference between facts and values, the former being produced by scientific methods (Hughes, 1990). Two of the hallmarks of natural science are a desire for generalisability and replicability. This is manifested in a quest for law-like findings, which may be universally applied, and a general unease with values intruding on the collection or interpretation of data.

The main research approaches or methodologies in quantitative research are surveys and experiments (see Chapter 7), but secondary analysis of data sets and content analysis (the quantitative analysis of documents) may also fall within its remit. Data which are collected within these approaches are used to describe whatever is being surveyed – for example, the distribution of hospital-acquired infections in a hospital, or to test hypotheses and analyse the relationships between variables, for example whether poor nutrition might predispose hospitalised patients to infection. However, whatever methodology is chosen, because of its philosophical underpinnings in natural science, the results of quantitative research are based on the researcher's interpretation of the observed phenomena.

This discussion of the paradigms and methodologies that underpin quantitative research has been necessary because the rigour of these methods is based on the extent to which they meet the criteria for natural science. In other words, as quantitative researchers design and apply certain data-collecting instruments, they are striving to conform to the values and assumptions that underlie the paradigm of natural science. Thus they believe that:

- natural science methods can be applied in the social world (the fact that humans think, communicate, and are individuals, is not an obstacle);

- only observable phenomena may be admitted as sources of valid knowledge;
- scientific knowledge is established through objective, systematic and controlled methods.

In the sections that follow we will explore how researchers have attempted to ensure that these criteria are met.

Methods of collecting data

In both quantitative and qualitative research there are only a limited number of ways in which data may be collected. These include:

- undertaking observations;
- asking questions;
- taking measurements;
- retrieving and reconstructing data from evidence collected for another purpose.

Although some or all of these methods can be used across quantitative and qualitative approaches, the way in which the method is undertaken is driven by the methodology within which it is being applied. For example, a behavioural psychologist might undertake a series of highly structured observations of the ways in which nurses and patients interacted during the provision of 'intimate' care. A list of possible behaviours would be predetermined and then trained observers would check when, and how often, these behaviours occurred. In contrast, anthropologists might observe the same interaction, but instead of having a checklist they would describe everything about the encounter including the context in which it occurred and the participants who were involved.

The sections that follow will explain how the first three data collection methods listed above are used to best effect to collect data for quantitative research. For a discussion of their use for qualitative research, refer to Chapter 4. The specific hallmarks of each technique will be outlined and examples provided of where such methods have been used to good effect in clinical nursing research. The retrieval and reconstruction of data from information collected for other purposes is beyond the remit of this chapter. A discussion of the use of the secondary analysis of data in nursing research may be found in Adams et al. (1994).

Observation

Observational research has a long history in health care and includes many well know studies such as Piaget's work on child development (1936), and the Masters and Johnson (1966) laboratory-based research that explored the physiological and psychological response to sexual stimulation. Many researchers have also used the technique of observation to collect data, and some of these studies will be discussed later. In relation to quantitative research, one of the hallmarks of positivism is the contention that valid knowledge may only be derived from empirical observations. Thus acceptable knowledge only comes from the objective measurement of observable phenomena. Observation is therefore central to the philosophy of research in the natural science paradigm and it is a key method of collecting data for quantitative research in the social sciences and nursing. Methods for observation fall into two categories – structured and unstructured. The latter is generally used to collect qualitative data within a naturalistic paradigm (see Chapter 4). Structured observation is associated with the natural science paradigm and aims to provide measurable and quantifiable data that are valid and reliable.

The characteristics of structured observation

As mentioned earlier some practitioners contend that since they use 'observation' in caring for patients, they are doing research, and, of course, observing others is part of everyday life. However, observation as a research method

> signifies a particular systematic approach to the business of quantifying behaviour (Bakeman and Gottman, 1987: 818).

Observational research may be conducted in natural settings such as a clinic, or in contrived settings such as the laboratory that Masters and Johnson used for their work. Studies proceed through the use of checklists that record the presence or absence of particular behaviours. The researcher predetermines these behaviours before the process of data collection begins, and other behaviours that might occur during the period of data collection are ignored. The aim of structured observation is to:

- record in a systematic way the behaviours of interest;
- record them accurately and reliably;
- avoid subjectivity.

Several observers can be trained to collect data simultaneously so the method is relatively cost and time effective and may be used for large scale studies (Pretzlik, 1994).

The process of collecting data

Before collecting data it is necessary to determine that observational methods will be suitable for gathering information about the phenomenon of interest. In other words the method of data collection must be suitable to both the research question posed and the paradigm in which it is framed. Furthermore, it must be possible to observe and record the phenomenon. Sometimes this is straightforward – for example, an infection control nurse might use observation in a survey which aimed to record the frequency of hand washing. On other occasions the phenomena may not be 'visible' or so easily defined – for example, the way in which patients anticipate surgery. Observation, whether structured or unstructured, must be guided by a framework or schedule that uses a formal recording technique (Cormack, 1984).

The main steps in collecting data using observational techniques are as follows:

- What is to be observed and measured must be defined. For example, if the project was concerned with studying nurse/patient communication then it would clearly be important to define exactly what was meant by 'communication', 'nurse' and 'patient' and to work out how communication could actually be observed and recorded.
- To achieve this it is necessary to determine the vocal or motor responses that might occur naturally in relation to this phenomenon, and define them in a taxonomy. Behavioural taxonomies are systems of responses to particular situations (Sackett et al., 1978). They are generated by the investigator by reviewing the literature for the type of responses that might be expected to occur in relation to the phenomenon, and/or by directly observing people as they participate in the phenomenon.
- The behaviours need to be defined and categorised either singly or in groups which encompass a number of behaviours. In the example above behaviours such as gaze aversion would need to be defined, say, as 'movement of the head such that eye contact is avoided for at least 5 seconds'. This might be combined together with behaviours such as body stiffening,

and non-verbal response to direct questions to form a more generic category of 'resistance to communication'.

- The validity of the taxonomy must be established.
- Investigators must decide how the data will be collected, either by live observation or on videotape. The former will capture the context of an observed phenomenon and is more economical when the phenomenon can be observed in a single event. However, once the event has passed it is lost and there is no possibility of rechecking. Observers must therefore be carefully trained.
- Videotaping can be undertaken in the absence of data collectors and it is essential for continuous observations. Checklists for recording either from live or videotaped observations must be developed with great care and need thorough piloting (Hinde, 1973). An example of a structured recording sheet is provided by Ashworth (1980). Hand-held computers are now available to record data electronically.
- A sampling strategy must be developed. This may be intermittent or continuous and the data collected may be time- or event-based. In the former, intervals during which observations will take place are selected systematically or at random. In event-based sampling, behaviours or prespecified events, such as mealtimes or nursing handovers, are selected for sampling. In this case the data collector must have knowledge of the occurrence of events. The research question being posed, and the phenomena being observed will determine the sampling strategy adopted.
- Intra- and inter-rater reliability must be determined.

This outline indicates the essential steps which need to be considered when collecting data by observational methods. More details are provided in a useful volume of *Nurse Researcher* (1994, volume 2), which includes articles on drawing up a schedule for observations (Barlow, 1994); objectivity in observations (Endacott, 1994); and validity (Redfern and Norman, 1994). The main concerns related to data collection using observation are discussed by Lobo (1992) who illustrates her arguments with examples of research involving children.

Examples of clinical nursing research which uses observation to collect data

We have already noted that observational methods of collecting data originated in the early work of child psychologists. Interestingly, many nursing studies using these methods have also focused on babies or children. This illustrates that although research methodologies and methods can be used across disciplines and clinical specialities, certain trends or preferences may develop that are more related to the social nature of research work. As O'Connell Davidson and Layder (1994: 51) note,

> social researchers are members of society as well as scientists. They are formed and informed by the very things which they study.

Some recent examples of observational research involving children include a study of the ways in which nurses and parents interact in their care of children in hospital (Cleary, 1992); Horgan's (1995) comparative observations of pain in new-born babies who had or had not undergone surgery; and an investigation of paediatric nursing interventions that tested the hypothesis that 'there is no difference in the quality of nursing care provided for sick children by nurses who are qualified RSCNs and those who are RGNs' (Barlow, 1996). These studies provide evidence concerning not only individual micro-level encounters between nurses and patients, but also more managerial issues that might have implications for the ways in which nursing care is organised and delivered. Communication is another area of nursing care that has been extensively studied using observational techniques. An early example is Ashworth's (1980) study of care and communication. Other researchers have focused on touch in the care of older people (Le May and Redfern, 1989).

These are just a few examples of research that has involved observational data collection techniques. They illustrate how this method can provide systematic information about a wide range of nursing activities, and across a range of specialities. Research that uses structured observation can inform clinical nursing both by providing an unbiased picture of what may be happening in certain environments or interactions, and by examining hypotheses that might be related to these events. Sometimes observations are relatively simple, for example a study by Crow, et al. (1988) recorded the number of times closed urinary drainage systems were broken by observing an indelible mark on the catheter/drainage tube junction for misalignment. Alternatively, observations may involve a sophisticated process of developing behavioural taxonomies and defining sampling and data collecting strategies that will identify and accurately record the phenomenon of interest, for example empathy between a midwife and a mother in labour. The level of sophistication associated with the data collecting instrument will depend on the phenomenon of interest and the original research question. Observational techniques can provide clinical nursing with valuable quantitative data, which may be used to develop the quality of care and to make the case for improvements in organisation – for example by suggesting the necessity for increased staffing levels.

Asking questions

The second way of collecting data for quantitative research involves asking questions. Questions may be asked either through the use of written questionnaires or by interviewing. Although these techniques differ, it is important to realise that both methods are about the same thing – asking questions. You might like to consider here how the information collected by asking questions might differ from that obtained by observation. From a strictly practical point of view it is easy to recognise that asking questions is the simplest and most economical way to obtain data about samples or populations. For example, it would be time consuming and almost impossible to attempt to assess the ages, clinical experience and grades of a group of ward staff through observation. The simple option would be to ask them to fill in a questionnaire. At a more theoretical level, structured observations cannot provide us with information about the meaning which, say, nurses give to a 'communication' with a patient, or their motivations and intentions.

In some circumstances meaning may be construed from data collected through structured observation. For example, Lobo (1992) suggests that a child's response to a health care procedure may be quantified in terms of co-operation by looking for behaviours which indicate this state, such as lying quietly or assisting in the procedure. However, it is important to note that this is the researcher's interpretation of the meaning of what has been observed. To collect certain types of factual data, and information that people hold in their heads, methods such as questionnaires and interviews are more useful than observations. Although both questionnaires and interviews ask questions, they will be discussed separately.

Characteristics of questionnaires

Jacobsen and Meininger (1985), in a review of research journals between 1956 and 1983, reported that questionnaires were the commonest data collecting instrument used. All of us, whether researchers or not, will have encountered questionnaires, and many will have attempted to design one. Unfortunately it is this apparent familiarity with questionnaires, and the pressures under which practitioners are often placed to evaluate practice, which results in the production of instruments that are badly constructed and inappropriately applied. It is deceptively easy to dash off a list of questions and put them together to undertake a survey of, say, patient satisfaction. However, as this section will illustrate, questionnaire design and use is technically demanding and requires considerable knowledge.

Advantages and limitations of questionnaires

The strengths and limitations of questionnaires are discussed by Parahoo (1993) and Mulhall (1994). Summarising these, the advantages include:

- Savings of time (both researcher's and respondent's) and money.
- Anonymity – useful when sensitive topics are being explored such as sexual practices, working conditions.
- Avoidance of interviewer bias where the interviewer affects the answers to questions by the manner in which they conduct an interview.
- Uniform delivery of the same questions to each respondent.
- More relaxing and less intimidating than interviews. May be completed at time of respondent's choosing.
- Rapid analysis using computerised statistical packages.

The limitations include:

- Reliance on accurate reporting of behaviour or events. There is a gap between intentions and subsequent behaviour (Mechanic, 1989).
- Bias introduced through the desire to give socially acceptable answers.
- Limited responses in that people may have contradictory views on the same topic, their response often being conditional on the context in which an event or situation may occur.
- The answers to earlier questions may be biased if the whole questionnaire is read before it is completed.
- Poor response rates and thus lack of confidence in the data and more particularly in their generalisability.

Collecting data using questionnaires

There are two types of questionnaire: those with standardised and predetermined questions, and those with questions that may be expanded on (Parahoo, 1993). In this section we will discuss the former, the latter being described in the section on interviews. The standardised questionnaire assumes that the respondent is completing the answers without assistance. Often such questionnaires are used in postal surveys but they may be used in the presence of the researcher (who takes no part in the exercise). Questionnaires may be used to collect data for qualitative research but their use in this respect is limited (see Chapter 4). Essentially, questionnaires emanate from the positivist paradigm and usually collect quantitative data. As with structured observations, the categories of information about which questions will be asked are predetermined by the researcher. Similarly the range of responses will be pre-set, there is no room for the respondent to expand on the answers, or to answer questions that are not posed.

A questionnaire is simply a list of questions that respondents are requested to answer. However, there are a number of methodological pitfalls that await the inexperienced researcher and these will be described here. A very useful practical guide is *Designing and Analysing Questionnaires* by Youngman (1987).

Steps in producing the standardised questionnaire

Production of the instrument:

1.   The questionnaire structure must, from the beginning, include the apparatus and format necessary for a successful analysis. Although this seems rather like putting the cart before the horse, it is essential that the coding for the analysis takes place as questions are developed. This avoids the situation where some responses cannot be coded, and cannot therefore be included in the analysis. However, particularly if closed questions are used, this mandates that the researcher must have a good grasp of the possible responses that might be anticipated. In addition, the strategy for dealing with non responses, obvious incongruency, and missed pages should be defined in advance. An example of a data collection sheet used in a study of catheter associated bacteriuria is shown in Table 8.1.

2.   Concepts used within the questionnaire must be operationalised – i.e. they need to be defined in terms of specific observable characteristics. For example, a study which explored the effect of stress on overeating would need to define what was meant by 'overeating' and 'stress' in advance.

3.   There must be a theoretical basis for including questions, although in a more general sense the content of questions will be determined by the researcher's empirical or theoretical agenda (O'Connell Davidson and Layder, 1994). The concepts to be addressed in the questionnaire need to be operationalised by specific questions.

4.   The format of questions must be considered: closed or forced questions are easy to code and analyse but disallow any qualification by respondents. On the other hand, answers to open questions are notoriously difficult to code, although Youngman (1987) contends that their inclusion, especially at the end of sections, may act as a safety valve for respondents who do not feel the questions are doing justice to their views. However, inserting open questions merely to increase compliance would be considered by many researchers as exploitation of the respondent.

5.   Question wording should be short, clear, unambiguous and bereft of jargon. The way in which questions are phrased will also affect responses. For example a nurse might be reluctant to answer 'Yes' to a question which asked 'Have you ever endangered you patients because you felt stressed?' A more general question such as 'In what ways does stress affect your ability to provide care?' is more suitable. Similarly, it would be better to ask people exactly what they ate on certain days than to ask if they under- or over-ate, as one person's gluttony is another's normal healthy appetite! Finally, respondents must understand any terms that are used. This is particularly relevant to clinical research, and the structure of the questionnaire must not be so complex that it defeats completion.

6.   Questions must relate to the concepts pertinent to the study and should not stray into other areas, particularly those of a personal nature. If such data are to be collected, researchers must be forthright about their purpose in investigating such areas.

Many of the problems identified above can be eliminated during the pilot phase.

Administering the questionnaire

The administrative work involved in producing and distributing a questionnaire should not be underestimated. It is essential to keep

Table 8.1: Example of a pre-coded data collection sheet

FORM D   Catheter Associated Bacteriuria Study – Original Equipment Details

Study No. ....

Catheter Details		Drainage Bag	
Name		Name	
....		....	

1	MANUFACTURER		8	MANUFACTURER	
	Warne Franklin	1		Bard	1
	Eurosil	2		Wallace	2
	Bard	3		Universal	3
	Simpla	4		Simpla	4
	Rusch	5		Other	5
	Dow-Corning	6		Not known	9
	Argyle	7			
	Other	8	9	TYPE	
	Not known	9			
				Uriplan	1
2	TYPE			Urimeter	2
				Cystocare unit	3
3	NUMBER OF OUTLETS			S4	4
				Trident	5
	2-way	2		Leg bag	6
	3-way	3		Other	7
	Other			Not known	9
	Not known	9			
			10	Non-return valve	
4	LENGTH		11	Drip chamber	
	Male	1	12	SUSPENSION	
	Female	2		None	0
	Not known	9		Floor stand	1
				Bed hanger	2
5	Balloon size			Cot sides	3
				Bed side	4
6	Gauge			Chair	5
				Patient's leg	6
7	MATERIAL			Other	7
				Not known	9
	P.V.C.	1			
	Siliconised latex	2			
	Silicone/teflon coated latex	3			
	Solid silicone	4			
	Other	5			
	Not known	9			

good records and, where appropriate, to ensure the anonymity of respondents (but ensure that a master list which identifies code numbers with respondents' names is kept in a secure place). Poor response rates are a problem, particularly with postal questionnaires. There is a golden rule here – know your customers and treat them as you would wish to be treated yourself.

1.   A covering letter, which explains the purpose of the study and ensures that respondents are clear about what they are committing themselves to, should always be sent with the questionnaire. This letter should also explain how the results of the study are to be disseminated. Unless the cost is prohibitive it is reasonable that all respondents should receive some written feedback concerning the results of the study and the implications that it has for clinical practice where applicable.

2.   The appearance of the questionnaire is extremely important: a professional looking document is sure to further your request

Table 8.2: Characteristics of interviews versus questionnaires in collecting data for quantitative research

Characteristic	Structured interview	Standardised questionnaire
Cost	High	Low
Opportunity to explain questions	Some	Little
Opportunity to confirm understanding of interviewer/ interviewee	Some	No
'Everyday' language	Yes	No
Uniform delivery of questions	Yes	Yes
Anonymity maintained	No	Yes
Inclusion of sensitive material possible	Sometimes	Yes
Completion rates	High	Low
Large samples possible	No	Yes
Literacy of respondent necessary	No	Yes
Over complicated or academic jargon used	Usually not	Sometimes
Number of questions	Small	Large
Pressure to participate	High	Low

Adapted from Mulhall (1994).

and increase the response rate. Youngman (1987) suggests the
following tips:

- Liberal spacing makes for easier reading.
- Reduction by photocopying produces more space without reducing content.
- Consistent positioning of response boxes is helpful.
- Use of different typefaces for instructions and questions.

3. The instructions for completing the questionnaire must be
   clear and unambiguous. There are usually some general
   instructions at the beginning and end, and more specific
   instructions throughout the text.

4. The order of questions may affect whether the respondent
   completes the questionnaire. The first section is critical; it is
   important to quickly engage the respondent's interest and
   provide questions that are not too taxing to answer (often these
   are biographical). However, beware: some people are sensitive
   about their age and qualifications!

5. Finally, respondents should be thanked for completing the
   questionnaire and always provided with a stamped addressed
   envelope for return. A cut-off date for the return of the questionnaire must be stated (both in the covering letter and at the
   end of the questions).

6. A reminder letter will usually need to be sent to some participants and the timing for this should be considered when
   designing the study.

Finally, it is worth remembering the concept of researcher validity
(Mulhall, 1994). Your respondents are people and their reaction to
your questionnaire will inevitably rest on both their opinion of the
topic and the data collecting instrument, but also on you. It is vital,
therefore, that investigators establish their credentials as competent
researchers. It is worth noting that researchers with nursing qualifications, especially in the speciality being investigated, will have an
advantage here since they will be perceived as 'like' professionals
with 'clinical credibility' by the respondents.

Characteristics of interviews

There are three types of interview methods – structured, semi-
structured, and unstructured. Unstructured interviews are used to

collect qualitative data. The nature of each method differs because different researchers consider the interview process in different ways according to their paradigm preferences (Cohen and Manion, 1989). Research texts may elaborate in more detail concerning what is meant by these terms but research articles are often more vague. In addition, although researchers may include in their publications some of the questions used, without being present at the interview it is almost impossible to ascertain how the process occurred. This contrasts with structured questionnaires where one has a clearer picture (provided the questionnaire is published).

Structured interviews are most commonly used in collecting data for quantitative research. The interview here is strictly a means of transfer of information from interviewee to interviewer. This reflects a natural science perspective and, as with the other methods discussed in this chapter, the concern is with maintaining objectivity, control of bias, and measurement. Positivist research aims to identify, classify and measure human behaviours or attributes across populations. Thus the same information must be gained from each interviewee in the same way and it must not be affected by the opinions or biases of the interviewer. To achieve this the researcher must be in control of the interview and retain a detached and formal position. Categories of information that will inform the analysis are chosen before the interview. Most of the questions are closed, the interview will be standardised and a schedule will be used to guide the researcher and enable him or her to ensure the validity and reliability of the process and thus the subsequent data. These concepts will be examined in more detail below.

This approach to interviewing rests on three assumptions (Nay-Brock, 1984):

- respondents and interviewers share a similar vocabulary, phraseology, dialect and so forth, so that each question means the same thing to each person;
- the words used in exploring the topic will have a uniform meaning to all respondents;
- the order in which the questions are posed will provide the same stimulus to respondents.

Some researchers argue that semi-structured interviews which use both open and closed questions fall within the confines of qualitative research. However, usually the questions are quite specific and their order is pre-determined by the researcher. Many researchers would thus disagree that qualitative data may be collected using this type of interview. In reality data collected using this method cause problems, for semi-structured interviews seldom have sufficient structure for data to be analysed statistically, nor are they 'sufficiently flexible and responsive enough to allow exploration of anything beyond surface meanings' (King, 1994: 15).

For an insight into the different ways in which semi-structured interviews are used you might like to compare Barriball and While (1994) with Conway, et al. (1995).

The advantages and limitations of interviews

Table 8.2 compares the characteristics of interviews and question-naires. The relative importance of the factors mentioned will be affected by several circumstances including the study population (its accessibility; level of education; language); the topic of the study (is it sensitive?); the sample (how large does it need to be and where is it situated geographically?); the amount of funding for the project; the time available to complete the research; and the skills of the researcher.

Collecting data by interview

When collecting data for quantitative research through question-naires or interviews the aim is to develop neutral instruments that can measure an objective reality which natural scientists contend exists separate from the individual. This goal is rather easier to achieve when data are collected through the use of questionnaires than when they are collected by interviewing. This is because an interview is a series of social interactions between the respondent and the researcher. Both parties are conscious, purposive actors who bring to the interview their particular beliefs, values and expectations and these could obscure or distort the 'truth' that emerges. Structured interviews used for quantitative research attempt to deal with this central problem through standardisation and control.

Steps in structured interviewing

1.   As with questionnaires the concepts used within the interview must be operationalised and there must be a theoretical basis for including questions.
2.   The categories for analysis are chosen before the interview, and this leads to the production of specific, closed, fixed alter-native questions (Brink and Wood, 1994).

3.   Since the interviewer/interviewee interaction is a prime source of bias, it is argued that the relationship between the two should remain formal and interviewers should never proffer opinions or advice. At the same time it is suggested that interviewers need to establish a rapport with respondents.

4.   For the same reason the researcher should control the interview, asking the questions that the respondent answers.

5.   Interviews are standardised, i.e. the same information is collected in the same way from each interviewee. The introduction to, and explanation of, the interview are similarly standardised. Questions must be posed in a neutral way, avoiding verbal intonation, facial expression or other overt body language.

6.   An interview schedule is used. Interview schedules instruct the interviewer in the precise wording of questions, their order, and the probes that may be used. Probes are used to clarify answers and in the case of the standardised interview these must use neutral language or pregiven phrases such as 'Is there anything else?'

7.   Closed questions are presented in the same format, as discussed for questionnaires – i.e. with a limited selection of responses for ticking or perhaps as a Likert scale.

8.   The responses to the questions are recorded by the interviewer. If pre-coded questions are used then respondents are given a limited choice of replies. Sometimes the question is asked in an open format and the interviewer chooses which of the pre-coded response boxes should be ticked.

9.   As with questionnaires, respondents should be thanked for their time and provided with information as to how they will be informed of the results of the study.

From a practical standpoint, the expense and time involved in interviewing suggests that all arrangements should be confirmed in writing and double checked the day beforehand. A quiet and comfortable room away from the respondent's immediate workplace, telephone and bleep will greatly enhance the encounter. Finally it needs to be appreciated that interviewing is a complex activity that requires skills and knowledge of a different nature from those used in 'interviews' with patients that occur in the course of clinical nursing. Furthermore, practitioners should be aware that if the respondents in interviews are drawn from their own clinical 'caseload', then problems with identity might ensue. Subtle changes with the relationship may occur as the nurse is presented first as a 'carer' and then as a 'researcher'. These roles have fundamentally different goals and often incompatible agendas (Mulhall, 1995). This difference in persona will be particularly marked in the case of structured interviews, which follow the precepts for rigour as listed above.

Examples of clinical nursing research that uses questionnaires and interviews to collect data

Questionnaires are used extensively in nursing and other social research because, if properly constructed, they provide an inexpensive vehicle for obtaining data from a large number of respondents who may be located in a wide geographical area. They find their greatest use in descriptive surveys (see Chapter 7) which aim to describe a population or collect data about opinions. For example, Stone (1996) used a structured questionnaire to assess the amount of pain experienced by patients who had undergone tonsillectomy and had been discharged from hospital. She then related this to the amount of information regarding pain control they had received before discharge and the actual analgesia taken. From this she was able to make concrete recommendations for practice concerning the need for more detailed pain information and further staff training in analgesia.

Questionnaires may also be used in experimental research to collect information on outcome that cannot be recorded by physiological measurements. Such data might include information on symptom control, patient satisfaction, or knowledge. Nurse educators also make extensive use of questionnaires to gather information concerning students' experiences and knowledge (see for example Courtney, 1991), whereas managers use this technique for collecting data for policy and planning purposes. Clark and Cullum's (1992) survey of pressure sores and pressure relieving equipment in one District Health Authority, and a similar study of the availability of urethral catheters in the same district (Mulhall et al., 1992), are examples where questionnaires were used by researchers to collect data that aided in the formulation of purchasing policy. Finally, questionnaires are also used in the evaluation of nursing practice, in which case they often consist entirely, or substantially of recognised measurement scales (see Chapter 15).

Structured interviews are used to a lesser extent than questionnaires in nursing research, but some examples do exist. In the field of education Harrison and Novak (1988) used interviews in a quasi-experimental research design to evaluate the effect of a gerontological training programme on practice. A representative sample of patients was interviewed before and after the introduction of the training programme for nurses. The outcome measures used were patient satisfaction with, and perceptions of, their care. However, the potential expense and complexity of interviewing undoubtedly deters novice researchers, or those who have little research funding. This is illustrated by a study conducted in the USA of how different ethnic groups and mental health professionals perceived problematic behaviour (Flaskerud, 1984). It involved 12 nurse researchers in different parts of the country conducting structured interviews with 68 mental health professionals and 159 minority group members. In the broader arena of public health and epidemiological research, structured interviews are used in large surveys that require substantial funding, often provided through governmental agencies. The data collected through studies that use interviews may be put to all the uses described above in the case of questionnaires.

Taking measurements

The previous two sections have described three familiar and often-used methods of data collection for quantitative research – observation, questionnaires, and interviews. As these methods were explored it became apparent that they were often concerned with attempting to measure, in a valid and reliable way, particular phenomena. Indeed at the beginning of this chapter it was stressed that one of the central characteristics of quantitative research concerned the objective measurement of phenomena. This is in contrast to qualitative approaches where researchers are concerned to understand, explain, or describe phenomena. Measurement has been defined as the assignment of numbers to represent properties (Campbell, 1952). In other words a property is measured when it is assigned a number or a category label (for example, male/female or mild/moderate/severe pain) to represent it. The principles of measurement are more fully described in Chapters 9 and 10, but two aspects will be covered in this chapter. Firstly, although their use will not be discussed extensively, it is helpful to examine here the differences between measurement scales and questionnaires. Secondly, the topic of physiological measurement in nursing research will be briefly explored.

Questionnaires and measurement scales

Parahoo (1993) states that questionnaires are used to collect data about different aspects of a particular topic for example, the attitudes of staff nurses towards patient self medication. In contrast, measurement scales aim to identify the dimensions underlying a particular concept and then to develop subscales for those dimensions. The scale is then used to determine to what extent an individual exhibits the particular attribute. Measurement scales have been developed for subjective phenomena such as mental states, anxiety, pain, and observable activities such as mobility, sleeping, eating etc. In addition many complex indices have been developed to measure the outcome of nursing care. These may be used when attempting to evaluate the impact of care. Thus functional ability can be measured by the Index of Activities of Daily Living (Katz et al., 1963), perceived health status by the Nottingham Health Profile (Hunt et al., 1986) and psychological well being by the Hospital Anxiety and Depression Scale (Zigmond and Snaith, 1983). Bowling (1991) and McDowell and Newell (1987) provide comprehensive reviews of such rating scales.

Measurement scales are always used from a natural science perspective, and produce quantifiable data that may be used to measure certain phenomena in individuals and groups, explore differences between groups, or demonstrate causality. There is, however, much controversy over the use of scales to measure psychological aspects of human behaviour. This revolves around the argument that, in accepting that attributes such as anxiety are real and that people may possess these 'things', we are 'reifying' such ideas. In other words abstract concepts are made concrete by the assumption that they can be measured objectively, and then people are labelled as having such attributes. It is very important to examine all such scales and consider in what ways they have been overladen by the values of both the researchers who produced them, and the society in which they are used.

Physiological measures

Polit and Hungler (1993) define physiological measures rather grandly as 'those physiological and biological variables that require specialised technical instruments and equipment for their measurement'. Such measures are, of course, commonly performed during clinical practice. For example, the measurement of blood pressure and body temperature form a cornerstone of monitoring a patient's condition in hospital. However, this definition, by specifying the use of specialised technical instruments excludes, say, the measurement of urine output, fluid intake, or volume of wound exudate. In addition, what constitutes a sophisticated technical instrument varies according to one's perspective: the thermometers used to take oral temperature would hardly justify this label. The important issue with regard to physiological measurements is that they are undertaken accurately and reliably. These two concepts will be explored in detail in the next section. Ensuring that measures are valid and reliable is more difficult to achieve when using human judgement rather than machines. Vomiting 'several times', 'copious' wound exudate, 'moderate' amounts of pain are all expressions that may be interpreted differently by different nurses. They are not valid and reliable expressions of measurement. Simply specifying the use of technical instruments detracts from the principle that all measures and observations should strive to be accurate and reliable.

Physiological measures may be undertaken *in vivo*, literally in life, on or within a person. Examples include measuring blood pressure using an intra-arterial catheter, determining respiratory parameters using a spirometer, monitoring foetal heart rate using an ECG. Other measurements are made *in vitro* (in glass): these encompass the very many microbiological, biochemical and histological 'tests' that are available to measure certain variables. Relevant examples are the measurement of rubella antibodies in pregnant women, serum potassium and sodium estimations, and cytological examination of tissues for malignant cells.

Physiological measures are frequently used when collecting data for quantitative research. Most familiar is their use in determining base line data and outcome in clinical trials, but they may also be used in studies of prevalence and incidence; surveys, and instrument development. Many 'research' posts for nurses involve them in undertaking such physiological measures for trials of drugs or other new treatments.

Some examples of research where physiological measurements have been central to the collection of data include: a series of studies on the factors which predispose to the development of pressure sores (Cullum and Clark, 1992); an exploration of the factors related to the encrustation and blockage of urethral catheters (Getliffe, 1992); a survey of the prevalence of bacteriuria in catheterised patients (Crow et al., 1988) and a large health and lifestyle survey that measured fitness alongside health-related behaviour, attitudes and beliefs (Blaxter, 1990). Further information about the use of physiological measures in nursing research and practice may be found in Oldham (1995). Tierney et al. (1988) provide a useful general article about measurement in nursing research.

Reliability and validity

All the methods of collecting data discussed so far can be used to describe and measure particular phenomena. Where the methods differ is in the process through which this is achieved – by observing, asking questions, or using technical instruments. However, in each case it is essential that the ways in which the data are collected and recorded are valid and reliable. Validity refers to how closely the observed or measured state of affairs aligns with reality. That is, does a scale, a question, an observation, an instrument measure what it purports to measure? Reliability is concerned with consistency and replicability: will the methods being used give the same results over time irrespective of who is administering them? Oppenheim (1984) provides a simple example of these two concepts. If a clock consistently showed the time as ten minutes fast, then it would be reliable, but not valid.

Observation

The validity of a behavioural taxonomy is usually tested through the use of a panel of experts who ensure that what is being observed accurately reflects the phenomenon of interest. Barlow (1994) shows how she sought the advice of senior paediatric nurses during the development of an observational schedule to be used in the study of the quality of nursing care provided for sick children. As with other methods of collecting data for quantitative research it is also crucial to ensure that the process of measurement is unbiased – i.e. it is undertaken objectively. Two sources of potential bias that may occur during observations are:

- The Hawthorne effect, where the presence of the researcher alters the behaviour which they are attempting to observe.
- Prior explanations to those being observed which may distort subsequent data collection.

Endacott (1994) describes these sources of bias in more detail. There are two areas of concern regarding the reliability of observations:

- Instrument reliability.
- Data collector reliability.

For an observation schedule to be reliable it must consistently measure the desired behaviour. It also must be sensitive, without always or never identifying the desired behaviour (Lobo, 1992). Difficulties in interpreting the content of the schedule, or biases in responses where, for example, an observer gives all 'no' or 'yes' answers need to be checked out in the pilot phase of a study (Barlow, 1994). During the pilot phase the agreement between observers may also be checked. Inter-observer reliability can be determined by observers watching and coding the same subjects. This is often expressed as Cohen's Kappa co-efficient of agreement (where K = 1 there is total agreement, where K = 0 there is no agreement other than that which might have occurred by chance). Lobo (1992) provides an excellent description of the ways in which observers influence the reliability of data collection and therefore the considerations that need to be taken into account in training them.

Questionnaires

The validity of a questionnaire relates both to the individual questions within it and the process and format through which it is 'administered'. Concepts to be addressed in the questionnaire may be derived from the literature, experts, or the researcher's own experience. Whatever the source these concepts must be relevant to the phenomenon under investigation. Thus a questionnaire exploring patients' perceptions of the quality of nursing care must include concepts which might reasonably encapsulate quality of care, such as provision of information, physical comfort, time taken to respond to requests, etc. Furthermore, it should be possible to identify the concept that each question is addressing.

The layout, instructions, wording of the questions, and the way in which responses are recorded may all affect both the validity and the reliability of the information that emerges. Again the strategy for ensuring validity and reliability is through the judicious piloting and subsequent modification of the instrument. In this way ambiguous and/or redundant questions can be rephrased or weeded out. Reliability of the information collected may be increased through cross-checking with another method of data collection such as referral to records.

Interviews

Since interviews involve a social interaction it is more difficult to attain the same control and objectivity that may be secured through questionnaires. The steps in collecting data within interviews already outlined in this chapter are all attempts to ensure that reliability and validity are maintained. As with questionnaires, much work is undertaken in developing the interview schedule and training interviewers who must be well versed in the precise questions and the probes that may be used. Objectivity and control must be maintained so that characteristics of the interviewer (such as their age or opinions) do not bias the responses received. Similarly efforts are made to ensure that the respondents do not provide socially or professionally desirable answers.

Physiological measures

Regardless of the scale on which they are made the quality of measurements is encompassed in their validity and reliability. Clinical measurements may take a range of values depending on the circumstances in which they are undertaken. Variation in measurements occurs not only as a result of the actual measuring but also because of biological variability over time and between individuals. Errors in the measurement process are dependent on the performance of both the instrument and the operator. Standard protocols are designed to reduce these errors. Where measures are more reliant on human observations, for example measuring foetal heart rates by auscultation, the potential for variation is more difficult to control. Fletcher et al., (1988) provide further details of measurement and biological variation. Methods of ensuring the validity and reliability of scales used to measure other less objective concepts such as health status, pain, anxiety etc. are discussed in Chapter 9.

Where measurements are made of clinical variables such as serum urea concentrations or blood gases, validity may be attained through ensuring that:

- the method used actually measures the variable of concern;
- samples are correctly collected (Oldham, 1995 provides an example);
- the instruments used have been recently calibrated against known standards.

Within clinical laboratories the issue of quality control is always foremost and thus samples processed through this route should produce reliable and valid data. However, clinical research nurses are often involved in obtaining these specimens and they must therefore ensure correct collection and transport to laboratories. Where physiological measures are made outside of the laboratory it is essential that the instruments used are regularly calibrated and maintained.

Ethics

Ethics pervade all aspects of research and Chapters 2, 3, 4 and 7 have already raised a number of pertinent issues. Eby (1995) also provides a useful overview. Four areas are important in considering ethics and research:

- informed consent
- confidentiality
- deception
- covert research.

Although ethics are commonly discussed in terms of the design and conduct of studies, they also relate to paradigm choices. Thus qualitative researchers in general, and feminist researchers in particular, stress the importance of undertaking research with, rather than on, people. They would thus eschew as fundamentally unethical the controlling and objective nature of much quantitative research. Webb (1990) has described this as 'a smash and grab raid by the researcher.' Ironically, the lack of a common set of rules and the complexity of many qualitative approaches creates particular ethical problems that may be difficult or impossible to solve. For example, if you undertook an ethnography of an antenatal clinic how would you obtain informed consent from everyone whom you observed? Lathlean (1996) provides an excellent discussion of the ethical features pertinent to different methodologies. Accepting the ethical implications of adopting a positivist stance, the ethical dilemmas in survey and experimental research are rather less than for qualitative approaches. However, although the methods of collecting data for quantitative research are more rule bound and overt than qualitative studies, there are many ethical pitfalls involved and these will form the remainder of the discussion in this chapter.

Ethical problems in collecting data for quantitative research

Once a survey or a randomised controlled trial has been designed, and before any data may be collected, informed consent should be obtained. Although requesting consent is now common research practice, the underlying question remains as to how 'informed' such consent is, and when it is obtained (see Chapter 7 and Oakley, 1989). The dilemma for some researchers is their contention that providing information about a potential course of treatment will bias the results and endanger their validity. To avoid biasing the outcome in double-blind trials, both the investigator and the participant remain unaware of which branch of the trial they are in. As Lathlean (1996: 178) states 'People . . . have to take it on trust . . . that they will not be disadvantaged'.

Similarly, participants in surveys should be given sufficient information for them to make an informed choice about participating. However, certain information may be withheld if the researcher considers it may affect the way in which the respondents reply. The implications of this for ethical integrity must be carefully considered. Choice to participate may also be compromised by the relative position of researcher and participant. The position of healthcare professionals within society and the 'situations' in which the sick find themselves may mitigate against such people refusing to participate in research. Where distance and objectivity are the goals, as in quantitative studies, the lack of personal relationship between researchers and participants may make discussions about refusal intimidating. This imbalance in power may also affect the validity of responses:

> Do researchers really believe that questionnaires handed out by uniformed staff to patients lying captive in their nighties in hospital beds on hospital premises, will obtain the same responses as questionnaires filled in after they go home . . .? (Robinson, 1996: 43)

Confidentiality and anonymity are central to the design of many quantitative studies and thus breaches of this ethical canon are not usually a problem. Names and contact addresses are required only where follow up is necessary. Privacy and the right that each person has to live without intrusion causes more concern. It is all too easy to set up ill-conceived surveys that contain questions unrelated to the topic of interest. Ethics must be considered when formulating the content and format of questions for interviews and questionnaires. First, the choice of subject matter is of concern. An unsolicited questionnaire arriving through the post about alcohol dependency, or sexually transmitted diseases may provoke a hostile reaction. Second, the range of responses to closed questions must be sufficient to allow a wide range of replies that go beyond what the researchers or organizations wish to 'hear'. For example, questionnaires often provide no means of distinguishing between different aspects of different individuals' performance. Patients who are trying to be fair will not criticise all staff simply because some did not come up to expectation.

Quantitative studies that purport to measure such attributes as attitudes or personality also have significant ethical problems. How many patients would participate in such research if they understood its true implications? Robinson (1996) discusses four complaints from patients who claimed that they were damaged by pejorative reports that appeared in their records following their participation in psychological research. Psychometric testing, by its covert nature, may also conceal the purpose of research from participants. This is illustrated in a recent report of a training needs assessment (Hicks and Hennessy, 1996: 444), which suggested that since the topic of research-based practice was threatening to nurses, information would be 'better extracted in an indirect way' using an opaque method of assessment that would avoid data distortion introduced by response bias.

Many studies also bypass ethics committees by being labelled audit, rather than research. Consideration must be given as to whether such activities cross the boundaries from audit into covert research.

The final ethical issues to be considered are beneficence (the duty to do good) and non maleficence (the duty not to harm). These principles are enshrined in a central tenet of research, which is that participants should be protected from pain, harm and suffering. Although the situation is not entirely satisfactory, attention is usually given to this issue in designing studies to be undertaken with patients. Hospital ethics committees and professional codes of practice are run and formulated to protect participants. However, many studies involve not patients but staff, and in some organisations approval for such research from the ethics committee is not required. Poorly designed studies may cause considerable psychological damage, loss of self esteem and a breakdown in working relationships amongst staff members. The ethical dimensions of all studies, regardless of whom they target, must therefore receive attention.

Finally, in undertaking research, clinical nurses may encounter situations where they may observe or hear something that puts a patient at risk. In planning and undertaking data collection it is essential that the course of action to be taken in such an event has been thought through in advance. The therapeutic imperative should always override the research imperative (Munhall, 1988). In a more general way, strategies for providing a therapeutic input should always be considered when planning data collection on sensitive topics. Respondents must never be left abandoned to deal with the psychological and emotional trauma that the process of collecting data may have engendered.

Summary

This chapter has included methods of data collection generally used in quantitative studies and has set them in context with the wider issues faced when undertaking research. A comprehensive guide for each of these methods of data collection appertaining to observations, asking questions and taking measurements was presented, and included their principal features, advantages and disadvantages, essential steps that need to be followed and examples of each method used in clinical nursing research. The rigour of each method has been considered by examining key aspects of both validity and reliability, essential requirements for all research endeavour, and, finally, ethical issues often encountered during data collection for quantitative research have been explored.

References

Adams A, Hardey M, Mulhall A (1994) Secondary analysis in nursing research. In Hardey M, Mulhall A (Eds) Nursing Research Theory and Practice. London: Chapman & Hall. pp. 127–44.

Ashworth P (1980) Care to Communicate. London: Scutari Press.

Ashworth P (1994) Analysis of observed data. Nurse Researcher 2: 57–66.

Bakeman R, Gottman JM (1987) Applying observational methods: a systematic view. In Osofsky J (Ed) Handbook of Infant Development. New York: Wiley. pp. 818–54.

Barlow S (1994) Drawing up a schedule for observation. Nurse Researcher 2: 22–9.

Barriball KL, While A (1994) Collecting data using a semi-structured interview: a discussion paper. Journal of Advanced Nursing 19: 328–35.

Blaxter M (1990) Health and Lifestyles. London: Tavistock/Routledge.

Bowling A (1991) Measuring Health: A Review of Quality of Life Measurement Scales. Buckingham: Open University Press.

Brink P, Wood MJ (1994) Basic Steps in Planning Nursing Research. 4th edn. Boston, MA: Jones & Bartlett.

Bryman A (1988) Quantity and Quality in Social Research. London: Unwin.

Campbell N (1952) What is Science? New York: Dover.

Clark M, Cullum N (1992) Matching patient need for pressure sore prevention with the supply of pressure relieving matresses. Journal of Advanced Nursing 17: 310–16.

Cleary J (1992) Caring for Children in Hospital: Parents and Nurses in Partnership. London: Scutari Press.

Cohen L, Manion L (1989) Research Methods in Education. 3rd edn. London: Routledge.

Conway M, Armstrong D, Bickler G (1995) A corporate needs assessment for the purchase of district nursing: a qualitative approach. Public Health 109: 337–45.

Cormack DFS (1984) The Research Process in Nursing. Oxford: Blackwell Scientific Publications.

Courtney M (1991) A study of the teaching and learning of the biological sciences in nurse education. Journal of Advanced Nursing 16: 1110–16.

Crow R, Mulhall A, Chapman R (1988) Indwelling urethral catheterisation and related nursing practice. Journal of Advanced Nursing 13: 489–95.

Cullum N, Clark M (1992) Intrinsic factors associated with pressure sores in elderly people. Journal of Advanced Nursing 17: 427–31.

Department of Health (1993) Report of the Taskforce on the Strategy for Research in Nursing, Midwifery and Health Visiting. London: HMSO.

Duffy M (1985) Designing nursing research: the qualitative–quantitative debate. Journal of Advanced Nursing 10: 225–32.

Eby MA (1995) Ethical issues in nursing research: the wider picture. Nurse Researcher 3: 5–13.

Endacott R (1994) Objectivity in observation. Nurse Researcher 2: 30–40.

Flaskerud JH (1984) A comparison of perceptions of problematic behaviour by six minority groups and mental health care professionals. Nursing Research 33: 190–97.

Fletcher RH, Fletcher SW, Wagner EH (1988) Clinical Epidemiology. Baltimore, MD: Williams & Wilkins.

Franklin B, Osborne H (1971) Research Methods: Issues and Insights. Belmont, NY: Wadsworth Publishing Company Inc.

Getliffe K (1992) Encrustation of Urinary Catheters in Community Patients. Unpublished PhD thesis, University of Surrey, Guildford.

Guba EG, Lincoln YS (1994) Competing paradigms in qualitative research. In Denzin N, Lincoln Y (Eds) Handbook of Qualitative Research. Thousand Oaks CA. Sage. pp 105–17.

Hammersley M (1995) The Politics of Social Research. London: Sage.

Harrison LL, Novak D (1988) Evaluation of a gerontological nursing continuing education programme: effect on nurses' knowledge and patients' perceptions and satisfaction. Journal of Advanced Nursing 13: 684–92.

Hicks C, Hennessy D (1996) Applying psychometric principles to the development of a training needs questionnaire for use with health visitors, district and practice nurses. NT Research 1: 442–54.

Hinde RA (1973) On the design of check sheets. Primates 14: 393–406.

Horgan MF (1995) Application to practice: observational techniques in forming an assessment tool. Research in Paediatric Nursing Society, Liverpool, 28 February.

Hughes J (1990) The Philosophy of Social Research. Harlow: Longman.

Hunt SM, McEwan J, McKenna SP (1986) Measuring Health Status. London: Croom Helm.

Jacobsen BS, Meininger JC (1985) The designs and methods of published nursing research 1956–1983. Nursing Research 34: 306–12.

Katz S, Ford AB, Moskowitz RW (1963) Studies of illness in the aged: the index of ADL – a standardized measure of biologic and psychosocial function. Journal of the American Medical Association 185: 914–19.

King N (1994) The qualitative research interview. In Cassell C, Symon G (Eds) Qualitative Methods in Organizational Research: A Practical Guide. London: Sage. pp. 14–36.

Kuhn T (1970) The Structure of Scientific Revolutions. Chicago: University of Chicago Press.

Lacey EA (1994) Research utilisation in nursing practice. Journal of Advanced Nursing 19: 987–95.

Lathlean J (1996) Ethical issues for nursing research: a methodological focus. NT Research 1: 175–83.

Le May AC, Redfern SJ (1989) Touch in elderly people. In Wilson Barnett J, Robinson S (Eds) Directions in Nursing Research. London: Scutari Press. pp. 11–18.

Lobo ML (1992) Observation: a valuable data collection strategy for research with children. Journal of Paediatric Nursing 7: 320–8.

McDowell I, Newell C (1987) Measuring Health. A Guide to Rating Scales. New York: Oxford University Press.

Masters W, Johnson V (1966) Human Sexual Response. Boston: Little Brown & Co.

Mechanic D (1989) Medical sociology. Some tensions among theory, method and substance. Journal of Health and Social Behaviour 30: 147–60.

Melia K (1982) 'Telling it as it is' – qualitative methodology and nursing research: understanding the student nurse's world. Journal of Advanced Nursing 7: 327–36.

Mulhall A (1992) Nursing research: exploring the options. Nursing Times 7: 35–6.

Mulhall A (1994) Surveys in nursing research. In Hardey M, Mulhall A (Eds) Nursing Research Theory and Practice. London: Chapman & Hall. pp. 77–102.

Mulhall A (1995) Nursing research – what difference does it make? Journal of Advanced Nursing. 21: 576–83.

Mulhall A (1997 in press) Nursing research: our world not theirs? Journal of Advanced Nursing. 25: 969–76.

Mulhall A, Lee K, King S (1992) Improving nursing practice: the provision of equipment. International Journal of Nursing Studies 29: 205–11.

Mulhall A, Le May A, Alexander C (1996) The Utilisation of Research in Nursing: A Phenomenological Study involving Nurses and Managers. London: Foundation of Nursing Studies.

Mulhall A, Alexander C, Le May A (1997) Prescriptive care? Guidelines and protocols. Nursing Standard 11(18): 43–6.

Munhall P (1988) Ethical considerations in qualitative research. Western Journal of Nursing Research 10: 150–62.

Nay-Brock RM (1984) A comparison of the questionnaire and interview techniques in the collection of sociological data. Australian Journal of Advanced Nursing 2: 14–23.

Nielsen JM (1990) Introduction. In Nielsen J (Ed) Feminist Research Methods. Exemplary Readings in the Social Sciences. Boulder, CO. Westview Press. pp. 1–37.

O'Connell Davidson J, Layder D (1994) Methods, Sex and Madness. London: Routledge.

Oakley A (1989) Who's afraid of the randomized controlled trial? Some dilemmas of the scientific method and 'good' research practice. Women and Health 15: 25–59.

Oldham J (1995) Biophysiologic measures in nursing practice and research. Nurse Researcher 2: 38–47.

Oppenheim AN (1984) Questionnaire Design and Attitude Measurement. London: Heinemann.

Parahoo K (1993) Questionnaires: use, value and limitations. Nurse Researcher 1: 4–15.

Pearcey PA (1995) Achieving research-based nursing practice. Journal of Advanced Nursing 22: 33–9.

Piaget J (1936) The Constructions of Reality in the Child (Trans. Cook M). New York: International Press.

Polit DF, Hungler BP (1993) Essentials for Nursing Research – Methods, Appraisal and Utilisation. Philadelphia: JB Lippincott Co.

Pretzlik U (1994) Observational methods and strategies. Nurse Researcher 2: 13–21.

Redfern S, Norman I (1994) Validity through triangulation. Nurse Researcher 2: 41–56.

Robinson J (1996) Its only a questionnaire . . . ethics in social science research. British Journal of Midwifery 4: 41–4.

Sackett GP, Ruppenthal GC, Gluck J (1978) Introduction: an overview of methodological and statistical problems in observational research. In Sackett GP (Ed) Observing Behaviour Vol. II Data Collection and Analysis Methods. Baltimore, MD: University Park Press. pp. 1–14.

Stone C (1996) Post-tonsillectomy pain relief following discharge from hospital. NT Research 1: 57–65.

Tierney A, Closs J, Atkinson I, Anderson J, Murphy-Black T, Macmillan M (1988) On measurement and nursing research. Nursing Times 84: 55–8.

Veeramah V (1995) A study to identify the attitudes and needs of qualified staff concerning the use of research findings in clinical practice within mental health care settings. Journal of Advanced Nursing 22: 855–61.

Webb C (1990) Partners in research. Nursing Times 86: 40–4.

Youngman MB (1987) Designing and Analysing Questionnaires. 2nd edn. Nottingham: University of Nottingham.

Zigmond AS, Snaith RP (1983) The hospital anxiety and depression scale. Acta Psychiatrica Scandinavica 67: 361–70.

Chapter 9
Health status measurement and outcomes

Crispin Jenkinson

Introduction

Recent years have witnessed a growing interest in the measurement of subjective health status and quality of life in the evaluation of health care. The use of patient completed questionnaires has grown with the recognition of the importance of the patient perspective (Spilker, 1996). The purpose of many health care interventions is neither cure nor the prevention of death, but quite simply to improve health status. It is striking, therefore, that systematic attempts to do this have only become part of the mainstream of health assessment in the last few decades. The purpose of this chapter is to provide an introduction to this area of research. The chapter will outline the potential uses of subjective reports of health status, outline the requirements for measures to ensure they are valid and reliable indicators of health status, and discuss the benefits and limitations of this area of research. Quality of life is increasingly recognised as an important aspect of research and the large range of quality of life measures has been comprehensively reviewed by Bowling (1991, 1995).

Patient-based outcomes: the imperative

Health care has historically concentrated on the diagnosis and treatment of physiological and anatomical conditions and evaluation of health interventions has relied upon measures of morbidity and mortality, whereas medical practitioners have based judgements for intervention on traditional clinical, radiological and laboratory measures (Albrecht, 1994). This is anomalous given that clinically assessed outcomes of treatment do not always reflect those of patients (Blazer and Houpt, 1979; Jenkinson, 1994a). However, over the past few decades there has been a gradual shift away from this approach, and increasingly there is incorporation of patient based data into the evaluation of care (Geigle and Jones, 1990; Jenkinson, 1995). The growth in interest in this field has, in part, come about due to the recognition of the limitations of existing clinical and laboratory data. Given the ever increasing demand for health care, and the rising costs of providing it, it is essential that meaningful measures of outcome are developed and applied. For many interventions the only meaningful outcomes are quality of life. Thus, for example, plastic surgery is often regarded as cosmetic and, consequently, of low priority. However, recent studies on the quality of life of women undergoing breast reduction indicate that their subjective health status improves dramatically in a wide variety of areas after surgery (Klassen et al., 1996). Clinicians and policy makers can use data such as these to develop guidelines as to the value of health interventions. The move toward evidence-based health care has provided an impetus to outcomes research. If treatments are to be provided they should be shown to be effective, and if many treatments are designed to improve subjective health status it is important that they are evaluated on these outcomes.

The recognition of the patient's point of view as central to the monitoring and evaluation of health care has brought with it numerous approaches to the measurement of subjective well being. The purpose of such evaluation is to provide more accurate assessments of individuals' or populations' health and the benefits and harms that may result from medical care (Fitzpatrick et al., 1992a). However there are a wide variety of applications of health status measures, and the requirements of measures differ across these applications. To begin with, therefore, this chapter will outline the possible applications of such measures in which data gained directly and systematically from the patient perspective could be of value.

Applications

Subjective accounts of functioning and well being can be used in a variety of ways in the evaluation of health and medical care.

Screening

Health status measures have been advocated as appropriate tools for the screening of patients needing particular care or attention

(Fitzpatrick, 1994). For example, Leigh and Fries (1991) administered the Health Assessment Questionnaire (Fries et al., 1982) to patients with rheumatoid arthritis and found it to be more accurate than traditional measures of health state in predicting long-term morbidity and mortality in this patient group. However, many established health status measures were designed for use at the group level and not the individual level. Thus, scores from many health status measures can be analysed at the aggregate level but not at the level of the individual. Many instruments are simply not reliable enough to be used in this manner (McHorney et al., 1994). The less reliable an instrument (the greater the level of measurement error) the wider the confidence intervals around any individual score. Confidence intervals indicate the likelihood that a given mean score is accurate (see Chapter 10). Thus a mean score of, say 50, with 95% confidence intervals of 40 and 60 would mean that we can be 95% certain that the mean lies between 40 and 60. When confidence intervals are this wide then use of the measure at the individual level for the purposes of screening becomes impracticable. For example the eight dimensions of the Short Form 36 health survey questionnaire (SF-36), which has been the subject of considerable validation (Brazier et al., 1992; Jenkinson et al., 1993; Jenkinson et al., 1996a; Ware and Sherbourne, 1992; Ware et al.,1993), has been found to manifest wide confidence intervals in patient groups and consequently the eight dimension scores cannot be used at the level of the individual.

The clinical interview

Whereas health status measures may be inappropriate for screening patients, it has been suggested that on an individual basis health status data can act as an adjunct to the standard clinical interview and may be useful for informing medical practitioners of the wellbeing of individual patients in their care. This was one of the possible applications suggested by the designers of the Nottingham Health Profile (NHP) (Hunt et al., 1986) although no studies have documented its use in this manner. However, the Dartmouth COOP charts, which contain nine items that measure aspects of functioning and wellbeing, were designed with this purpose in mind (Nelson et al., 1990; Nelson et al., 1996; Wasson et al., 1992). Studies suggest that both patients and clinicians believe the use of the charts has led to improved interaction, and better treatment (Kraus, 1991).

Randomised controlled trials

At the level of group analysis perhaps the most obvious use for standardised health measurement profiles is as outcome measures in randomised controlled trials. Whilst the use of such measures in randomised control trials has been relatively limited their use in this arena of outcomes research is growing (Spilker, 1996). One potential problem with the use of such measures in trials relates to the difficulties in determining meaningful differences on health assessment measures. This problem has probably been one reason for the relatively slow uptake of subjective health outcomes as primary endpoint measures in clinical trials. The relative paucity of trials including such measures has in turn been suggested as one reason why many clinicians have been unwilling to use such measures in clinical practice (Bergner et al., 1992). In many instances clinical trials that have claimed to use quality-of-life instruments have done so with measures that are often limited in the range of dimensions covered, and have not been psychometrically validated (Aaronson, 1989). For results to be meaningful in such studies then it is imperative that psychometrically validated measures covering appropriate domains are used.

Routine outcomes assessment

It has been suggested that routine monitoring of patient groups could be undertaken using health status measures. Such data would give some insight into the effectiveness of treatment regimes and programmes of care. Routine systems to collect outcomes have been successfully demonstrated in England (Bardsley and Coles, 1992) and America (Lansky et al., 1992). Such systems have proved acceptable to clinicians, although widespread use of 'outcomes management' systems has been slow to get off the ground. In part this is due to a lack of a agreement on what standardised measures should be used, and concern as to what, if any, effect such measurement will have upon clinical practice (Wasson et al., 1992).

Cost containment and prioritisation

Perhaps the most emotive use for health status measures is in the arena of cost containment and prioritisation. When used in cost utility studies, measures are required from which a single figure can be derived, which can then be used to rank order treatments, or indeed patients. The most famous attempt that has as yet been made to derive a set of priorities on the basis of a cost–benefit analysis was the Oregon experiment (Oregon Health Services Commission, 1991). It used the Quality of Well-Being Scale (Kaplan and Anderson, 1987) and produced results that were so counterintuitive that informal procedures were used to reorder the resulting list. However, attempts continue to develop methods of evaluating health care that take into account the length of life gained by a treatment, the effect on health status and the cost of treatment. Quality adjusted life years (QALYs) are an attempt to develop an index of quality of life and length (Torrance, 1986; Williams, 1985). Thus one year in perfect health (where perfect health $= 1$) gives the same number of QALYs as 10 years in a health state of 0.1 (which would be relatively poor health). The purpose of QALYs is to determine which treatments give the greatest number of QALYs and to determine which QALYs are the cheapest and which are the most expensive. They can consequently be used in prioritisation and rationing. It is imperative, therefore, that the measures that are used to provide the health status or quality of life component are well validated.

Population monitoring

Health status measures also allow the monitoring of population health, or sub-samples within the population (Ware, 1992). Furthermore, comparisons of the health status of different countries can also be undertaken (Orley and Kuyken, 1994). Thus, there is currently interest in developing measures that can be used across cultures. This is the thrust of the work being undertaken by, for example, the World Health Organisation Quality of Life (WHOQOL) Group (Szabo, 1996) and the International Quality of Life Assessment (IQOLA) Group (Aaronson et al., 1992). The development of such instruments is not without its difficulties. It is certainly not enough to simply translate an instrument from one language to another. Careful checks are required to ensure that the meaning of questions remains the same. This can mean that it is actually necessary to ask somewhat different questions in different cultures to ensure that the same underlying concept is being tapped (Bullinger, 1995). Even more problematic is the possibility that issues of importance in one culture in relation to health are unimportant elsewhere (Hunt, 1995). However, if these problems can be overcome the potential exists of not only comparing the quality of life of different countries, which seems an undertaking of limited value, but, more importantly, also undertaking large multi-centre cross-cultural studies that incorporate self perceived health as a major outcome measure.

Reliability, validity and responsiveness

It would be naive to assume that designing a health-assessment measure or indeed any questionnaire is an easy task (Oppenheim, 1992). A number of issues must be considered when designing a questionnaire. Instruments must be reliable, valid and sensitive to change or 'responsive' (see Chapters 7 and 8).

Reliability

Questionnaires must be reliable over time. Thus, they should produce the same, or very similar, results on two or more administrations to the same respondents, provided, of course, there is good reason to believe that the health status of the patients has not changed. The difficulty with such a method of validating a questionnaire is that it is often uncertain whether results that may indicate a questionnaire is unreliable are in fact no more than a product of real change in health status. Due to the potential difficulties in gaining an accurate picture of reliability in this way, many researchers adopt the Cronbach's alpha statistic (Cronbach, 1951) to determine internal reliability. Internal reliability refers to the extent to which items on a scale are tapping a single underlying construct, and therefore the extent to which there is a high level of inter-item correlation. Assuming that such high levels of inter-item correlation are not a product of chance, it is commonplace to assume that a high alpha statistic indicates the questionnaire is tapping an underlying construct and hence is reliable. There is, however, disagreement as to whether such a method can be viewed as appropriate for assuming a questionnaire is reliable over time (Ruta et al., 1993; Sheldon, 1993).

Validity

Essentially there are four aspects to validity. Face validity, content validity, criterion validity and construct validity.

Face validity refers to whether items on a questionnaire superficially appear to make sense, and can be easily understood. This may seem a simple enough test for a questionnaire to pass, but there are ambiguities on some of the most respected and well-used measures. For example the Sickness Impact Profile (SIP), of which the UK version is called the Functional Limitations Profile (FLP), requests respondents to complete the questionnaire with reference to today. They are thus asked to affirm or reject items on the basis of how they are feeling today. The basis of this judgement should, further, be related to their health. Let us take the example outlined in the SIP/FLP itself. It concerns the ability to drive. The statement given is 'I am not driving my car'. Thus, if a respondent cannot drive a car today, and this is due to a health complaint, then he or she should affirm the question 'I am not driving my car'. If he or she is not driving because they never learnt to do so, then the person concerned must answer this question in the negative. Thus, respondents are asked to make two judgements for each response. It could be argued that in such a long questionnaire (136 items) respondents might well forget or ignore the initial rubric. However, even if this were not the case, some questions do not make any sense on the basis of the rubric. For example, the item 'I have attempted suicide'. Respondents must tick 'Yes' or 'No' to this item. Further, they must not tick 'Yes' if they have attempted suicide today, but did so because their spouse has been killed in a car accident (this is, after all, not a problem with their health). Maybe it would be legitimate to tick 'Yes' if the respondent reasoned that his or her mental health had been adversely affected by a relative's death, and he or she had attempted it today! Problems such as these are by no means unique to the FLP, and must make researchers carefully consider how such questions are interpreted (or re-interpreted) by respondents if results from such instruments are to be of any meaningful use whatsoever.

Content validity refers to the extent to which items on a questionnaire tap all the relevant aspects of the attribute they are intending to measure. In a matter as fundamental as the selection of items a number of approaches are available to the potential designer. Broadly speaking, items can be developed by the researcher, from searches of the literature, from studies of lay or patient surveys, or any combination of these.

Both the NHP and SIP were developed on the basis of surveys of health perceptions of non-medically trained populations, with items weighted by a psychometric scaling technique. Hunt et al., the designers of the NHP, claimed that the scoring and weighting for seriousness of items on many health assessment questionnaires often reflect the values of the clinician and not those of the lay person. As such they claimed that items tapping subjective health status should be generated from studies of lay people (Hunt et al., 1986).

The NHP is a short easily administered questionnaire designed to overcome the potential criticism of many pre-existing instruments that both the domains and the questions contained in them are more a reflection of the assessments of clinicians and academic researchers than of lay people. To overcome this problem Hunt and her colleagues undertook a great deal of research with lay people in order to ascertain what they believed to be the most salient dimensions of health that could be affected by illness. Six distinct dimensions emerged: pain, social isolation, energy, sleep disturbance, mobility, and emotional reactions. Lay people were then asked to generate items that could be incorporated into these dimensions. Large numbers of statements were gained. A small number were then selected and weighted for inclusion in the questionnaire. To undertake this process, Hunt et al.(1986) used a method similar to that which had been used by Bergner and her colleagues in the development of the SIP (Bergner et al., 1976, 1981).

There are 38 questions on the first section of the NHP (designed to assess subjective health state), and each item on the questionnaire carries a specific weight, ascribed to it by the developers, by an attitude scaling technique developed by Thurstone early this century (Thurstone, 1928). Respondents can affirm all or none, or indeed any number, of the statements, as the developers claim they all tap an underlying attribute on any given dimension. It has been suggested that it is misleading to use a scaling technique such as Thurstone's method to attempt to scale statements that are, or could be, viewed as factual (Edwards, 1957). The NHP contains factual statements, or ones that certainly could be viewed in this light (for example, 'I'm unable to walk at all'). It is because of this that the NHP contains illogical groups of (factual) statements. It is possible, for example, to gain higher scores (indicating worse health) for less severe symptoms on the mobility dimension of the NHP. Some of the statements contained in the mobility section of the NHP logically preclude subjects responding to other items. For example an affirmation of the statement 'I'm unable to walk at all' (with a weight value of 21.30) technically precludes positive responses to some other aspects of mobility. For example, if a respondent affirms the statement that they are unable to walk, they should not, logically, be able to affirm the statements 'I can only walk about indoors' (weight 11.54), and 'I have trouble getting up and down stairs and steps' (weight 10.79), which make a total score of 22.33. Thus the score of a respondent with walking difficulties may exceed that of someone who is unable to walk at all. Such an outcome can make the results gained from a questionnaire such as the NHP difficult to interpret (Jenkinson, 1991; Jenkinson, 1994b).

Criterion validity refers to the ability of an instrument to correspond with other measures held up as 'gold standards'. In practice few studies can truly claim to have evaluated criterion validity as gold standards are hard to find in this area of research. Results from questionnaires have been compared with clinical criteria; for example, results from the Arthritis Impact Measurement Scales (AIMS) (Meenan et al., 1980, 1992) were compared with various rheumatological measures; similarly results from the Parkinson's Disease Questionnaire were compared to various clinical assessments of disease progression (Jenkinson et al., 1995; Peto et al., 1995). However, given that subjective health questionnaires are designed to measure different aspects of health than those tapped by traditional measures, such assessments can really only give a very general impression that measures are related. It would be worrying if clinical assessments and subjective health status measures were completely contradictory, but likewise it would be surprising if they correlated perfectly. Questionnaire results on one measure are often compared with those of another. For example the results of the physical and mental health summary scales from the 36-item SF-36 have been compared with results from the 12-item version of the questionnaire and have been found to be almost identical (Ware et al., 1995b; Jenkinson and Layte, 1997). The gold standard in this instance is the longer form measure, and perhaps it is only when comparing longer and shorter forms that proclaim to measure identical phenomena that one could really ever say that one measure truly was a gold standard.

Construct validity refers to the ability of an instrument to confirm expected hypotheses. Thus one would expect those who are ill, who are in lower social classes, and/or who make more frequent visits to their GP to gain scores indicating worse health than those who are well, in higher social classes and rarely visit their GP. Preliminary validation of questionnaires involves ensuring questionnaires can discriminate between such groups (Brazier et al., 1992; Hunt et al., 1985, 1986; Jenkinson et al., 1993a, 1996a; Ware et al., 1993).

Overview of health status measures

Broadly speaking there have emerged two general approaches to the measurement of health status. The first is an attempt to develop instruments that provide a single global score of well-being. These are designed in such a way as to permit all items on a questionnaire to be summed into a single health index. The other method is the development of questionnaires designed to measure a number of dimensions of health status.

Single-index measures of health status

Single-index measures of health status are designed to provide a single figure reflecting overall health status. The Rosser Index (1988) is one of the most famous examples of such an index. This measure, designed initially to place in perspective the magnitude of change achieved in clinical trials, consists of two dimensions, disability and distress, in the form of a matrix. There are eight levels of disability and four levels of distress. For each combination of distress and disability the Rosser Index provides a single figure. The figures in the matrix were developed by Rosser on the basis of a project where 70 subjects, including doctors, nurses, psychiatric patients and healthy volunteers, were asked to rank illness states and estimate relative severity. Whilst this scale gives a single index-figure of health state and, when used in routine clinical practice it takes only a few seconds for those familiar with its use to complete, it has to be borne in mind that the original weighting exercise that produced the matrix was undertaken on a very small sample. The valuations, therefore, are unlikely to reflect those of the population as a whole.

Whilst the Rosser Index was essentially developed for completion by physicians and staff, and not patients, attempts have been made to develop self completion single-index measures. An attempt to gain a single-index value of health from the perspective of the patient is the Quality of Well Being Scale (QWB). The complex method of developing this questionnaire has been described fully elsewhere (Kaplan and Anderson, 1987). The intention of this index is to combine mortality, morbidity and the benefits and side effects of treatment into a single global score. Such a global score can permit the comparison of health states and treatments. Its value in comparing disease states depends, however, on gaining reliable prognoses. Without this latter information it is not possible to calculate potential 'well years' accruing from treatments. Another limitation of this questionnaire is its length. It can take up to 15 minutes to complete, and the developers suggest it is administered by an interviewer, as the self completion version resulted in unreliable data (Anderson et al., 1986). As such, the QWB does not lend itself to easy use in clinical settings, or to routine evaluation of care.

Attempts have been made to devise a questionnaire that is short, easy to complete and a reliable indicator of health state. This has been a venture that has had few successes, although the Health Measurement Questionnaire (HMQ) (Kind and Gudex, 1991), which was derived from the Rosser Index and the EuroQol (EuroQol Group, 1990), have both had their advocates. The HMQ is a relatively brief, easy to complete questionnaire that elicits information on dimensions of mobility, capacity for self care, constraints on usual activities, social relationships and perceived stress. A single-index figure is derived from responses to these domains. More information on this questionnaire is provided in Kind and Gudex (1991). A more widely used measure is the EuroQol EQ-5D (EuroQol Group 1990; Kind, 1996; Rosser and Sintonen, 1993). The EuroQol EQ-5D was developed by a multidisciplinary group of researchers from five European countries (EuroQol Group, 1990). There are five questions covering the areas of mobility, self-care, usual activity, pain/discomfort and anxiety/depression. Each question has three response categories: level 1 – 'no problems', level 2 – 'some problems' and level 3 – 'inability or extreme problems'. Overall health state can ostensibly be calculated from responses to these items. For example the response set '11111' indicates no problems with any of the five areas, and consequently perfect overall health. There are, in total, 243 possible health states (i.e. 3^5), and weighted values have been assigned to each of these on the basis of national and international surveys (Van Agt et al., 1994). A single overall score can also be gained from the EuroQol thermometer, on which respondents mark their overall perceived health from 'worst imaginable health state' to 'best imaginable health state'.

All of these single-index measures are based on questionnaires that include fixed-format items. However, a number of researchers have begun to analyse the possibility of asking patients individually to nominate areas of their life that have been adversely affected by health state, and then to assess the extent of this impact. The results from each of the items selected are then aggregated to form a single-index figure. A variety of methodologies for this approach exist, but in essence they all permit each individual to select and weight their own chosen areas

(McGee et al., 1991; Ruta et al.,1994). Such a procedure has the advantage of not imposing pre-existing definitions of health state on respondents (Ruta and Garratt, 1994; Ruta et al., 1994). Research in this area has been undertaken in a number of groups including patients undergoing orthopaedic surgery, HIV positive patients, arthritis patients and those reporting low back pain (Hickey et al., 1996; McGee et al., 1991; O'Boyle et al.. 1992; Ruta and Garratt, 1994; Ruta et al., 1994; Tugwell et al., 1990). Such methods are, like many research projects attempting to gain single-index figures of health, still in their infancy and hence not widely applied. A number of issues need to be addressed, such as whether respondents should select new dimensions each time they complete the questionnaire in longitudinal studies, whether aggregating potentially unrelated dimensions is an appropriate methodology and whether patients should select dimensions from a list (which perhaps undermines the whole philosophy of this approach) or simply select from any areas they think important. Such issues are at present receiving attention from a number of researchers, and whereas the generalised applicability of this new technique seems a long way off, it is an interesting and potentially worthwhile new approach to the whole field of subjective health measurement.

Health status profiles

Health status profiles are measures that tap a number of dimensions of functioning and well-being. Many instruments that have been developed are illness specific or are aimed at tapping a specific aspect of ill health (such as pain or depression). Generic measures, in contrast, can be used with any community or patient group and cover general aspects of health status, such as emotional well-being, social functioning, pain, energy, mobility, etc. The most frequently reported generic health measures have been the Sickness Impact Profile (Bergner et al., 1976, 1981), the Functional Limitations Profile (Patrick and Peach, 1989), the Nottingham Health Profile (Hunt et al., 1985, 1986), and, more recently, the COOP Charts (Nelson et al., 1996; Wasson et al., 1992), Short-Form 36 (SF-36) (Brazier et al., 1992; Jenkinson et al., 1996a, 1996b; Ware and Sherbourne, 1992; Ware et al., 1993, 1994) and Short-Form 12 (Ware et al., 1995a, 1995b, 1996; Jenkinson and Layte, 1997). These measures cover a wide variety of dimensions of health status and are not primarily designed to give a single index of health status but to provide a profile of scores.

Discussion: benefits and limitations

Single-index figures of health status appeal to those who wish to compare different treatments and interventions. However, whilst such single-index figures give the impression of comparability between illness states and treatments, they may do so unfairly. For example the EuroQol (EuroQol Group, 1990; Kind, 1996) questionnaire does not contain a dimension evaluating sleep disturbance and a treatment aimed primarily at improving this dimension of health may not appear to have been efficacious if assessed by this measure.

Single-index figures gained from patient-generated measures such as the Schedule for the Evaluation of Individual Quality of Life (O'Boyle et al., 1992) and the Patient Generated Index (Ruta and Garratt, 1994) may overcome this criticism. In these measures the dimensions chosen by patients are seen as paramount and so, if a patient is primarily concerned about the impact of illness on his or her sleep patterns, this will be incorporated in the measure. However, difficulties arise here. At initial interview a patient may claim his or her quality of life in five areas is affected. At follow up these areas may have improved, and so if the patient completes the questionnaire using the same dimensions chosen at time one, an improvement in health status will be apparent. However, side effects of drug treatment may have influenced other aspects of the respondent's life, and thus overall quality of life may not have improved at all. When using such a measure it is therefore appropriate also to include a generic instrument so as to ensure as wide as possible coverage of health-related dimensions.

Generic measures, such as the FLP/SIP, the SF-36 Health Survey Questionnaire and the NHP, indicate clearly which dimensions of health status are being measured but the dimensions included may not be appropriate in the assessment of every intervention. For example, the FLP, despite having 12 dimensions, lacks a specific category measuring pain. Results from generic measures can, of course, be compared with data from other populations and illness groups. For example, normative data can be used to compare the health status of a particular patient group with that of the general population (Ware, 1993). However, it is still important that disease-specific measures are used alongside such generic measures, as disease-specific measures are, by their very nature, likely to tap particular aspects of ill health that are unique to particular illnesses.

Many health status measures have been criticised for manifesting so called 'ceiling' and 'floor' effects, which must be considered. For example the NHP has been criticised because it detects only the severe end of ill health, and thus most respondents score zero on many, if not all, of the six dimensions of the questionnaire (Kind and Carr-Hill, 1987). The items on the questionnaire were chosen to represent severe health states, and so individuals who have mild to moderate illness may not be detected with this instrument. In a study of change over time, respondents with minor ailments may improve but if their initial score on dimensions of the NHP was zero, such improvement may not be detected (the floor effect). Similarly respondents may score as maximally ill on a health measurement questionnaire. However, the extent of their illness may still not be fully reflected in the questionnaire. Such severely ill respondents would fall beyond the measurement range. Thus, while these patients may improve over time, it is still possible they may continue to score as maximally ill on the questionnaire (ceiling effect). Such floor and ceiling effects are more likely to be found on instruments with small numbers of items (Bindman et al., 1990). Related to floor and ceiling effects is another important aspect of health status measures: sensitivity to change or 'responsiveness'. For health status measures to be useful in evaluating the impact of health care interventions they must, of course, be sensitive to change. It is thus imperative, when selecting a measure, to determine the exact nature of the questions asked and the time scales used. For example, a questionnaire such as the NHP, designed to tap the extreme end of ill health, is unlikely to be sensitive to small changes in health status among patients with minor illnesses.

Furthermore, in longitudinal studies it is preferable that the mode of administration of questionnaires is, whenever possible, kept consistent. For example, due to the nature of some of the items in the FLP, respondents may gain higher scores in hospital than as out-patients or when at home, and such scores may not actually reflect health state. Items such as 'I stay in bed more' are more likely to be affirmed in hospital, and may not accurately reflect the impact of the illness per se on a person's life (Jenkinson et al., 1993b)

Summary

Subjective health measurement questionnaires are not designed to be used as substitutes for traditional measures of clinical endpoints but are intended to complement existing measures and to provide a fuller picture of health state than can be gained by clinical measures alone. However, such measures must be carefully chosen if they are to be useful. Health status measures can provide a useful adjunct to the data traditionally obtained from mortality and morbidity statistics, or from traditional clinical and laboratory assessments, but careful consideration must be given to the choice of measures. At present it seems reasonable to assume that health status measures may permit scientific questions to be answered fully in the context of clinical trials, and, in time, they may find their way into routine use. In the meantime, however, research is required to determine the appropriateness of measures for various clinical groups and to determine the sensitivity to change and validity of measures across community and patient samples.

References

Aaronson N (1989) Quality of life assessment in clinical trials: methodologic issues. Controlled Clinical Trials 10: 195–208S.

Aaronson NK, Acquadro C, Alonso J, Apolone G, Bucquet D, Bullinger M, Bungay K, Fukuhara S, Gandek B, Keller S, Razavi Sanson-Fisher R, Sullivan M, Wood-Dauphinee S, Wagner A, Ware JE (1992) International Quality of Life Assessment (IQOLA) Project. Quality of Life Research 1: 349–51.

Albrecht G (1994) Subjective health assessment. In Jenkinson C (Ed) Measuring Health and Medical Outcomes. London: UCL Press.

Anderson JP, Bush JW, Berry CC (1986) Classifying function for health outcome and quality of life evaluation. Medical Care 24: 54–69.

Bardsley M, Coles J (1992) Practical experiences in auditing patient outcomes. Quality in Health Care 1: 124–30.

Bergner M, Barry MJ, Bowman MA, Doyle A, Guess HA, Nutting PA (1992) Where do we go from here? Opportunities for applying health status assessment measures in clinical settings. Medical Care 30 (Supplement): MS219–30.

Bergner M, Bobbitt RA, Carter WB, Gilson BS (1981) The sickness impact profile: development and final revision of a health status measure. Medical Care 18: 787–805.

Bergner M, Bobbitt RA, Kressel S, Pollard WE, Gilson BS, Morris JR (1976) The sickness impact profile: conceptual formulation and methodological development of a health status measure. International Journal of Health Services 6: 393–415.

Bindman AB, Keane D, Lurie N (1990) Measuring health changes among severely ill patients: the floor phenomenon. Medical Care 28: 1142–52.

Blazer D, Houpt J (1979) Perception of poor health in the healthy older adult. Journal of the American Geriatrics Society 27: 330–4.

Bowling A (1991) Measuring Health. A Review of Quality of Life Measurement Scales. Buckingham: Open University Press.

Bowling A (1995) Measuring Disease. Buckingham: Open University Press.

Brazier JE, Harper R, Jones NMB, O'Cathain A, Thomas KJ, Usherwood T, Westlake L (1992) Validating the SF-36 health survey questionnaire: new outcome measure for primary care. British Medical Journal 305: 160–4.

Brazier JE, Usherwood T, Harper R, Jones N, Thomas K (1994) Deriving a single index measure from the Short Form 36 health survey (abstract). Journal of Epidemiology and Community Medicine.

Bullinger M (1995) In Guggenmoos-Holzmann I, Bloomfield K, Brenner H, Flick U (Eds) Quality of Life and Health: Concepts, Methods and Applications. Berlin: Blackwell-Wissenschafts.

Cronbach LJ (1951) Coefficient alpha and the internal structure of tests. Psychometrica 16: 297–334.

Edwards A (1957) Techniques of Attitude Scale Construction. Englewood Cliffs, NJ: Prentice-Hall.

EuroQol Group (1990) EuroQol – A new facility for the measurement of health related quality of life. Health Policy 16: 199–208.

Fitzpatrick R (1994) Applications of health status measures. In Jenkinson C (Ed) Measuring Health and Medical Outcomes. London: UCL Press.

Fitzpatrick R, Fletcher A, Gore S, Jones D, Spiegelhalter D, Cox D (1992a) Quality of life measures in health care. I: applications and issues in assessment. British Medical Journal 305: 1074–7.

Fitzpatrick R, Ziebland S, Jenkinson C, Mowat A, Mowat A (1992b) The importance of sensitivity to change as a criterion for selection of health status measures. Quality in Health Care 1: 89–93.

Fitzpatrick R, Ziebland S, Jenkinson C, Mowat A, Mowat A (1993) A comparison of the sensitivity to change of several health status measures in rheumatoid arthritis. Journal of Rheumatology 20: 429–36.

Fries JF, Spitz PW, Kraines RG, Holman HR (1980) Measurement of patient outcome in arthritis. Arthritis and Rheumatism, 23: 137–45.

Fries JF, Spitz PW, Young DY (1982) The dimensions of health outcomes: the health assessment questionnaire, disability and pain scales. Journal of Rheumatology 9: 789–93.

Geigle R, Jones SB (1990) Outcomes measurement: a report from the front. Inquiry 27: 7–13.

Guyatt GH, Berman LB, Townsend M, Pugsley SO, Chambers L (1987a) A measure of quality of life for clinical trials in chronic lung disease. Thorax 42: 773–8.

Guyatt G, Walter S, Norman G (1987b) Measuring change over time: assessing the usefulness of evaluative instruments. Journal of Chronic Diseases 40: 171–8.

Hickey AM, Bury G, O'Boyle C, Bradley F, O'Kelly D, Shannon W (1996) A new short form quality of life measure (SEIQoL-DW): application in a cohort of individuals with HIV/AIDS. British Medical Journal 313: 29–33.

Hunt S (1995) Cross-cultural comparability of quality of life measures. In Guggenmoos-Holzmann I, Bloomfield K, Brenner H, Flick U (Eds) Quality of Life and Health: Concepts, Methods and Applications. Berlin: Blackwell-Wissenschafts.

Hunt S, McEwan J, McKenna S (1985) Measuring health status: a new tool for clinicians and epidemiologists. Journal of the Royal College of General Practitioners 35: 185–8.

Hunt S, McEwan P, McKenna S (1986) Measuring Health Status. London: Croom Helm.

Hunt S, McKenna S (1991) The Nottingham Health Profile User's Manual Revised Edition. Manchester: Galen Research and Consultancy.

Jenkinson C (1991) Why are we weighting? A critical analysis of the use of item weights in a health status measure. Social Science and Medicine 32: 1413–16.

Jenkinson C (1994a) Measuring health and medical outcomes: an overview. In Jenkinson C (Ed) Measuring Health and Medical Outcomes. London: UCL Press.

Jenkinson C (1994b) Weighting for ill health: the Nottingham health profile. In Jenkinson C (Ed) Measuring Health and Medical Outcomes. London: UCL Press.

Jenkinson C (1995) Evaluating the efficacy of medical treatment: possibilities and limitations. Social Science and Medicine 41: 1395–403.

Jenkinson C, Coulter A, Wright L (1993a) Short Form 36 (SF-36) health survey questionnaire. Normative data for adults of working age. British Medical Journal 306: 1437–40.

Jenkinson C, Layte R (1997) Development and testing of the UK SF-12. Journal of Health Services Research and Policy 2: 4–8.

Jenkinson C, Layte R, Wright L, Coulter A (1996a) The UK SF-36: An Analysis and Interpretation Manual. Oxford: Health Services Research Unit, University of Oxford.

Jenkinson C, Layte R, Wright L, Coulter A (1996b) Evidence for the sensitivity of the SF-36 health status measure to inequalities in health. Journal of Epidemiology and Community Health 50: 377–80.

Jenkinson C, Peto R, Fitzpatrick R, Greenhall R, Hyman N (1995) Self reported functioning and well-being in patients with Parkinson's Disease: Comparison of the SF-36 short-form health survey (SF-36) and the Parkinson's Disease Questionnaire (PDQ-39). Age and Ageing 24: 505–9.

Jenkinson C, Ziebland S, Fitzpatrick R, Mowat A, Mowat A (1993b) Hospitalisation and its influence upon results from health status questionnaires. International Journal of Health Sciences 4: 13–18.

Kaplan RM, Anderson JP (1987) The quality of well-being scale: Rationale for a single quality of life index. In Walker SR, Rosser R (Eds) Quality of Life: Assessment and Application. Lancaster: MTP/Kluwer.

Kaplan RM, Bush JW, Berry CC (1976) Health status: types of validity and the Index of Well-Being. Health Services Research 11: 478–507.

Katz S, Akpom CA (1976) Index of ADL. Medical Care 14: 116–18.

Katz S, Downs TD, Cash HR, Grotz RC (1970) Progress in development of the Index of ADL. Gerontologist 10: 20–30.

Katz S, Ford AB, Moskowitz RW, Thompson HM, Svec KH (1963) Studies of illness in the aged. The Index of ADL: a standardised measure of biological and psychosocial function. Journal of the American Medical Association 185: 914–19.

Kind P (1996) The EuroQol Instrument: an index of health related quality of life. In Spilker B (Ed) Quality of Life and Pharmacoeconomics in Clinical Trials. 2nd edn. Philadelphia: Lippincott-Raven.

Kind P, Carr-Hill R (1987) The Nottingham Health Profile: a useful tool for epidemiologists? Social Science and Medicine 25: 905–10.

Kind P, Gudex C (1991) The HMQ: Measuring Health Status in the Community. Centre for Health Economics Discussion Paper, number 93. York: University of York, Centre for Health Economics.

Klassen A, Fitzpatrick R, Jenkinson C, Goodacre T (1996) Should breast reduction be rationed? A comparison of the health status of patients before and after surgery. British Medical Journal 313: 454–6.

Kraus N (1991) The InterStudy Quality Edge, Volume 1, Number 1. Excelsior, Minneapolis: InterStudy.

Lansky D, Butler JBV, Frederick WT (1992) Using health status measures in the hospital setting: from acute care to 'outcomes management'. Medical Care 30 (Supplement): MS57–73.

Leigh P, Fries J (1991) Mortality predictors among 263 patients with rheumatoid arthritis. Journal of Rheumatology 18: 1298–306.

McGee HM, O'Boyle CA, Hickey A, O'Malley K, Joyce CRB (1991) Assessing the quality of life of the individual: the SEIQoL with a healthy and gastroenterology unit population. Psychological Medicine 21: 749–59.

McHorney CA, Ware JE, Lu JF (1994) The MOS 36-item short-form health survey (SF-36): III. Tests of data quality, scaling assumptions, and reliability across diverse patient groups. Medical Care 32: 40–66.

McKenna S, Hunt S, Tennant A (1993) The development of a patient-completed index of distress from the Nottingham health profile: a new measure for use in cost-utility studies. British Journal of Medical Economics 6: 13–24.

Meenan RF, Gertman PM, Mason JH (1980) Measuring health status in arthritis: the Arthritis Impact Measurement Scales. Arthritis and Rheumatism 23: 146–52.

Meenan RF, Mason JH, Anderson JJ, Guccione AA, Kazis LE (1992) AIMS2: the content and properties of a revised and expanded Arthritis Impact Measurement Scales health status questionnaire. Arthritis and Rheumatism 35: 1–10.

Meenan RF, Anderson JJ, Kazis LE, Egger MJ, Altz-Smith M, Samuelson CO, Willkens RF, Solsky MA, Hayes SP, Blocka KL, Weinstein A, Guttadauria M, Kaplan SB, Klippel J (1984) Outcome assessment in clinical trials: evidence for the sensitivity of a health status measure. Arthritis and Rheumatism 27: 1344–52.

Meenan RF, Gertman PM, Mason JH, Dunaif R (1982) The Arthritis Impact Measurement Scales: further investigations of a health status measure. Arthritis and Rheumatism 25: 1048–53.

Nelson EC, Landgraf JM, Hays RD, Wasson JH, Kirk JW (1990) The functional status of patients: how can it be measured in physicians' offices? Medical Care 1990: 28: 1111–26.

Nelson EC, Wasson JH, Johnson DJ, Hays RD (1996) Dartmouth COOP functional assessment charts: brief measures for clinical practice. In Spilker B (Ed) Quality of Life and Pharmacoeconomics in Clinical Trials. 2nd edn. Philadelphia: Lippincott-Raven.

O'Boyle C, McGee H, Hickey A, O'Malley K, Joyce CRB (1992) Individual quality of life in patients undergoing hip replacment. Lancet 339: 1088–91.

Oppenheim AN (1992) Questionnaire Design, Interviewing and Attitude Measurement. London: Pinter.

Oregon Health Services Commission (1991) Prioritization of Health Services. Salem: Oregon Health Commission.

Orley J, Kuyken W (Eds) (1994) Quality of Life Assessment: International Perspectives. Berlin: Springer-Verlag.

Patrick D, Peach H (1989) Disablement in the Community. Oxford: Oxford University Press.

Peto V, Jenkinson C, Fitzpatrick R, Greenhall R (1995) The development of a short measure of functioning and well-being for patients with Parkinson's disease. Quality of Life Research 4: 241–8.

Rosser RM (1988) A health index and output measure. In Stewart SR, Rosser RM (Eds) Quality of Life: Assessment and Application. Lancaster: MTP.

Rosser RM, Sintonen H (1993) The EuroQol quality of life project. In Stewart SR, Rosser RM (Eds) Quality of Life Assessment: Key Issues in the 1990s. London: Kluwer.

Ruta D, Garratt A (1994) Health status to quality of life measurement. In Jenkinson C (Ed) Measuring Health and Medical Outcomes. London: UCL Press.

Ruta D, Garratt A, Abdalla M, Buckingham K, Russell I (1993) The SF-36 health survey questionnaire: a valid measure of health status. British Medical Journal 307: 448–9.

Ruta D, Garratt A, Leng M, Russell I, Macdonald L (1994) A new approach to the measurement of quality of life: the Patient Generated Index (PGI). Medical Care 32: 1109–23.

Sheldon T (1993) Reliability of the SF-36 remains uncertain. British Medical Journal 307: 125–6.

Silver GA (1990) Paul Anthony Lembcke, MD, MPH: A pioneer in medical care evaluation. American Journal of Public Health 80: 342–48.

Spilker B (Ed) (1996) Introduction. In Spilker B (Ed) Quality of Life and Pharmacoeconomics in Clinical Trials. Philadelphia: Lippincott-Raven.

Szabo S, on behalf of the World Health Organisation Quality of Life (WHOQOL) Group (1996) The World Health Organisation Quality of Life (WHOQOL) assessment instrument. In Spilker B (Ed) Quality of Life and Pharmacoeconomics in Clinical Trials. 2nd edn. Philadelphia: Lippincott-Raven.

Thurstone L (1928) Attitudes can be measured. American Journal of Sociology 33: 529–54.

Torrance J (1986) Measurement of health state utilities for economic appraisal. Journal of Health Economics 12: 39–53.

Tugwell C, Bombardier C, Buchanan W, Goldsmith C, Grace E, Bennett K, Williams J, Egger M, Alarcon GS, Guttadauria M, Yarboro C, Polisson RP, Szydlo L, Luggen ME, Billingsley LM, Ward JR, Marks C (1990) Methotrexate in rheumatoid arthritis: impact on quality of life assessed by traditional standard item and individualised patient preference health status questionnaires. Archives of Internal Medicine 150: 59–62.

Van Agt, HME, Essink-Bot, M, Krabbe PFM, Bonsel GJ (1994) Test–retest reliability of health state valuations collecting using the EuroQol questionnaire. Social Science and Medicine 39: 1537–44.

Ware JE (1992) Measures for a new era of health assessment. In Stewart AL, Ware JE (Eds) Measuring Functioning and Well-Being. London: Duke University Press.

Ware J (1993) Measuring patients' views: the optimum outcome measure. SF-36: a valid, reliable assessment of health from the patient's point of view. British Medical Journal 306: 1429–30.

Ware JE, Brook RH, Stewart AL, Davies-Avery A (1980) Conceptualisation and Measurement of Health for Adults in the Health Insurance Study: Volume I, Model of Health and Methodology. Santa Monica, CA: The RAND Corporation.

Ware JE, Kosinski M, Keller SD (1994) SF-36 Physical and Mental Health Summary Scales: A User's Manual. Boston, MA: The Health Institute, New England Medical Center.

Ware JE, Kosinski M, Keller SD (1995a) SF-12: How to Score the SF-12 Physical and Mental Health Summary Scales. 2nd edn. Boston, MA: The Health Institute, New England Medical Center.

Ware JE, Kosinski M, Keller SD (1995b) A 12-item short-form health survey. Construction of scales and preliminary tests of reliability and validity. Medical Care 34: 220–33.

Ware JE, Kosinski M, Keller SD (1996) SF-12: an even shorter health survey. Medical Outcomes Trust Bulletin 4: 2.

Ware JE, Sherbourne CD (1992) The MOS 36-Item Short-Form Health Survey 1: conceptual framework and item selection. Medical Care 30: 473–83.

Ware JE, Snow KK, Kosinski M, Gandek B (1993) The SF-36 Health Survey Manual and Interpretation Guide. Boston, MA: The Health Institute, New England Medical Center.

Wasson J, Keller A, Rubenstein L, Hays R, Nelson E, Johnson D and the Dartmouth Primary Care COOP Project (1992) Benefits and obstacles of health status assessment in ambulatory settings: the clinician's point of view. Medical Care 30: (Supplement) MS42–9.

Wilkin D, Hallam L, Doggett M (1992) Measures of Need and Outcome for Primary Health Care. Oxford: Oxford University Press.

Wilkin D, Hallam L, Doggett M. (1993) Measures of Need and Outcome for Primary Health Care. Revised edition. Oxford: Oxford University Press.

Williams A (1985) Economics of coronary artery bypass grafting. British Medical Journal 291: 326–9.

Ziebland S, Fitzpatrick R, Jenkinson C (1993) Tacit models of disability in health assessment questionnaires. Social Science and Medicine 37: 69–75.

Chapter 10
Statistical considerations in design and analysis

Nicola J. Crichton

Introduction

There are several stages to any study. These are, broadly, planning, design, conduct, analysis and interpretation. There is a need for statistical input at all stages, not just at the analysis stage. Indeed many serious errors are made at the planning and design stage that introduce biases that cannot be rectified later.

The importance of study design has been discussed in several earlier chapters and cannot be overemphasised. Two aspects of design that require careful statistical consideration are the method of sampling and the appropriate size for the study. These issues will be considered in this chapter. A statistical perspective on some other aspects of study design are discussed in Crichton (1990).

A major challenge for many researchers is how to get the best out of the data they have collected. This involves deciding which of the multitude of statistical analyses is appropriate, valid and useful for addressing their objective, how to interpret the results of the analysis and how best to present their results. This chapter will present some techniques for displaying data as graphs and summary statistics and will demonstrate some of the commonly used statistical tests, as well as giving guidance on the selection and interpretation of statistical tests and explaining the benefits of using confidence intervals to present results. In general, few or no mathematical formulae will be given as these are available in a wide variety of statistical textbooks and in the computer age the most important skills are knowing what analysis to request and how to make use of the results of the analysis, rather than how to calculate the results.

Sampling methods

In all studies we collect information from a limited number of people. Often we intend to go on and make inferences about what is happening or what will happen in a much larger group of people. That is, we wish to generalise the findings of our study to a target population, assuming that the study participants are representative members of that target population. The way in which we select our study members will greatly affect how well our sample represents the target population. Since we cannot guarantee that a sample is representative without learning about the whole target population, it is helpful to use sample selection methods that minimise bias.

There are two broad classes of methods of sample selection: probability sampling and non-probability sampling. If researchers use a non-probability method of sample selection, for example volunteers or convenience or quota sampling, they are always vulnerable to criticisms of bias, or non-representativeness, however careful the research has been. Probability sampling involves some component of random selection. Using a probability sampling method should reduce the risk of selection bias.

The most commonly used method of probability sampling is simple random sampling. The essential idea is that each member of the target population has an equal chance of being included in the sample. First we need a list of the population (a sampling frame), then we must give each member of the population a unique number. Next we select numbers at random using, for example, a computer or random number tables, as described by Moore (1991: 11–16). The population members who have been allocated those numbers are the members of the sample. The major difficulty is that we need a list of the population and such lists do not always exist! For example, for many conditions it is impossible to obtain a list of sufferers even at the general practice level, let alone regionally or nationally, and so random selection becomes impossible.

As part of a study exploring patients' experiences in hospital, the researcher needed to select four patients from a 20-bed ward to talk with about their stories. The researcher numbered the beds on the ward, wrote the numbers on pieces of paper, mixed them up and drew out four pieces of paper. The patients in these bed numbers were interviewed. This was a simple practical way of selecting a random sample of the patients. A nurse was heard to say 'I'd never have chosen to interview that patient'. It is exactly because of this sort of personal preference, often unexpressed, that we need the reassurance of lack of bias that is offered by random selection.

Stratified random sampling is a sophistication of simple random sampling carried out to make sure that there is appropriate representation of subgroups of the target population. The target population is divided into homogeneous groups (strata) – for example three age groups: less than 30, 30 to 60, over 60. A random sample of subjects is taken from each stratum in turn. The number of subjects selected from each stratum should generally be such that the proportion in the sample from that stratum is the same as the proportion in the target population. A difficulty with stratified random sampling is that in order to carry this out we not only need a list of the population but we also need to know to which stratum each member of the population belongs. If such a list is available it is an excellent way of sampling.

Cluster sampling is sometimes used when the population is large, widely dispersed and occurs in discrete clusters. We may have a list of the clusters but not of every member of the cluster. We randomly select some clusters then collect information from each subject in the selected cluster. For example, we could randomly select a specific number of hospitals, each of which is a cluster of wards, then collect information from each ward of the selected hospitals. Cluster sampling can be extended to several stages; for example, we could take a random sample of hospitals, take a random selection of wards from the chosen hospitals, then collect information from every patient in the selected wards.

The major difficulty with any of the probability sampling methods is the need for a population list, or a method of compiling a list that gives every population member an equal chance of being selected. Such lists often do not exist and this leaves the researcher with little option but to use a non-probability selection – for example all patients in a three-month period, or all cases in a particular hospital, or all convenient cases.

Sample size and power calculations

Perhaps the question a statistician is asked most frequently is 'How large should my study be?' The approach to answering this question will depend on the way the study is being conducted and how the outcome is being measured, as well as statistical quantities such as the level of significance and power that we require. In addition the researcher will need to provide information about typical outcome and variability of outcome, and needs to define what would be a clinically useful size of effect to detect.

Consider, for the purpose of illustration, that we are to conduct a clinical trial that aims to compare two treatments to determine whether the new treatment is better than the old; where better means there is an improvement in response that is clinically important. Individual patients will vary in their response to the treatments so there is always a possibility that we will draw the wrong conclusion on the basis of our trial because of this variability in response. The more patients we include in the trial the more certain we might expect to be about the conclusions we draw. However, our time and resources are limited and we would not wish to deny patients a worthwhile treatment indefinitely. The size of our trial will be decided by balancing statistical and practical considerations.

There are two types of error that we might make in drawing conclusions from our trial. First we could conclude, on the basis of our trial, that the new treatment is significantly better than the old when in fact there is no difference in response on the two treatments: this is called a Type I error. Second, we could fail to detect in our trial a clinically important difference, when in fact such a difference exists: this is a Type II error. We do not know what the truth is – that is why we need to do a trial. So we need to keep the probability of both types of error as small as possible. We are only able to reduce both types of error simultaneously by increasing the size of the study.

The value we decide is an acceptable probability for the Type I error determines the level at which we conduct any hypothesis tests. Commonly this is called α and is often taken as 0.05 and may be written as 5%. This would mean that when we analysed our study we would reject the null hypothesis if the p-value were less than 0.05 (see below for an explanation of the p-value). In practical terms, the Type I error (α) is the probability that we detect a treatment difference, when in fact there is no difference. The choice of $\alpha = 0.05$, although used in many published papers, is arbitrary and you should not feel bound to use $\alpha = 0.05$. However, taking α larger than 0.05 will give too high a chance of a false positive to be widely acceptable, whereas taking α smaller than 0.05 will increase the sample size required.

The power is a measure of how likely we are to produce a statistically significant result for a treatment difference of a given magnitude. In practical terms it indicates the ability to detect a true difference of clinical importance. The power is equal to one minus the Type II error probability, often written 1–ß. We would like the power to be near one (or near 100%). When planning a study we need to have a good chance of detecting a clinically important treatment difference, should it exist. If the power is low, we may well be wasting our time and putting patients at risk for no good reason because if the study fails to detect a treatment difference we could not be sure whether that was because there was no treatment difference or because the study was too small to detect the difference. In their review of studies of effectiveness of nursing, Thomas and Bond (1995) point out that the majority of studies in this area are too small. They found only one that considered power in determining the sample size.

Precisely how the sample size is determined depends not only on the study design but also on the outcome measure. The two most common types of outcome variables are a continuous measure (for example, blood pressure, see below for more detail), in which case we generally wish to compare the mean (average) response for the treatments, or a binary measure (response/no response) in which case we generally compare the proportions responding. In either case we will need to specify the treatment difference we wish to detect. By stating a treatment difference that we consider to be of clinical importance we ensure that 'statistically significant' equates to 'clinically important'.

In order to calculate the sample size for a two-group comparison with a continuous outcome variable you will need to provide the following information: the variability of response on the standard treatment, how large a treatment difference will be considered clinically important, the Type I error, α, you find acceptable and the power to be used. Generally people take α to be equal to 0.05 and the power should be greater than 0.8. Examples of calculating sample sizes for continuous measures are provided by Altman (1991: 455–8), who also provides a simple nomogram (a graph) to allow calculation of sample size.

The most widely used formula for calculation of study size when the trial will be assessed by comparing mean outcome in group one with mean outcome in group two is the following:

$$n = 2 \left(Z_{\alpha/2} + Z_\beta \right)^{2\sigma/2} / \left(\mu_1 - \mu_2 \right)^2$$

where n is the number of subjects required in each group (so study size is $2n$). The research proposal needs to specify the difference in mean considered clinically worthwhile $(\mu_1 - \mu_2)$ and the size of standard deviation (SD or variability) of outcome (σ) expected for each group. If we take $\alpha = 0.05$ and we are using a standard two tailed test then $z_{\alpha/2} = 1.96$. If we take power of $1 - \beta = 0.90$ then $z_\beta = 1.28$. The values of $z_{\alpha/2}$ and z_β will change with changes in α and β so it is necessary to consult tables of the normal distribution to obtain the appropriate values of $z_{\alpha/2}$ and z_β. In carrying out these calculations it is assumed that the outcome variable has a normal distribution.

For example, in their study comparing a homeopathic treatment for hayfever with a placebo, Reilly et al. (1986) used a 100 mm visual analogue scale to measure symptoms. They determined that a mean difference between the groups of 10 mm would be important to detect. They estimated that the variability of response would give an SD of 20 mm. Thus for power of 85% and significance tests at the 5% level they require

$$n = 2(1.96 + 1.03)^2 20^2 / 10^2 = 72 \text{ patients per group,}$$

leading to a total study size of 144 patients. If the power is increased to 90% the number of patients required increases to 84 per group. It is usually sensible to increase the sample size a little beyond this to allow for dropouts.

To calculate sample size for a two-group comparison with a binary response variable you will need to provide the following information: the proportion expected to respond on the standard treatment, how large a difference in response will be considered clinically important, the Type I error and power. This is discussed further by Altman (1991: 458–60) and a comprehensive series of tables giving the sample size required for common values of Type I error and power are provided by Fleiss (1981).

It is necessary to include sufficient information in your study report to justify the sample size and to demonstrate that the study was designed to have adequate power. For example, Reilly et al. (1986) give all the necessary information to justify their sample size.

Statistical analysis

Types of data

Before we can discuss how to analyse data we need to give some consideration to the different types of data that we might have in our study. The nature of the observations has important implications for how we will summarise, display and analyse the data, because different statistical methods are appropriate for different types of data. Broadly, data can be considered as either categorical or numerical, and there are several different types of data within these classifications.

Categorical data occurs as two major types, nominal and ordinal. For nominal data the category labels are just names and there is no inherent order of the categories. For example, 'sex: male/female', 'religion: Christian/Jewish/Muslim/Hindu', and 'blood group: A/B/AB/O', are all examples of nominal variables. Categorical data in which there is a natural or logical order for the values of the scale are called ordinal data. For example, the severity of pain recorded as 'none/mild/moderate/severe provides ordinal data. Questions recording information such as: How confident do you feel about your ability to critically review a research article?

1.   Not confident at all
2.   A little confident
3.   Fairly confident
4.   Very confident
5.   I could teach someone else

provide ordinal data.

Numerical data are often described as being data on the interval/ratio scale of measurement. That is, there is an inherent order in the values on the scale and the differences between successive values on the scale are all the same. Types of numerical data include data derived by counting and data derived by measuring. Some examples of count data are number of children and number of people on a waiting list. Count data are additionally described as discrete because they can only take certain numerical values. Data derived by measuring, such as height, blood pressure, age and serum cholesterol, are often additionally described as continuous. Such observations are not restricted to certain values except by the accuracy of the measuring instrument. It is often reasonable to treat discrete numerical data as if they were continuous as far as statistical analysis is concerned.

Further discussion of types of data (or scales of measurement) and more examples are provided by Altman (1991: 10–17), Moore (1991: 151–4), Everitt (1994: 22–5) and Tierney et al. (1988).

Graphical presentation of data

The first step in analysing data is to try to organise the data and to identify patterns. It is unwise to rush into testing hypotheses without first looking at the data, organised in tables and graphs. Graphical displays are an excellent way of getting a feel for the data and for checking out assumptions that we may need to make later in more sophisticated analyses – for example, many statistical tests will assume that the data are normally distributed.

A well thought-out graph can be a very useful way of explaining important findings and often has more impact than simply reporting the results of statistical tests. Working at a time when statistics was in its infancy, Florence Nightingale was amongst the earliest users of graphical displays as a method of communicating research findings. Indeed she designed some novel displays, most notably her coxcomb, which is a kind of polar area chart and is described in Grier and Grier (1978). Florence Nightingale worked closely with Dr William Farr, an eminent statistician of the time, and in a letter to Sidney Herbert, cited by Diamond and Stone (1981: 69), she wrote: 'I have written to Dr Farr for the diagram which is to affect thro' the eyes what we may fail to convey to the brains of the public through their word-proof ears', which beautifully summarises the advantage of graphical display.

Amongst the most widely used graphical displays are pie charts, bar charts, histograms, boxplots and scatterplots. Each of these will be briefly discussed and illustrated. All these graphical displays can be produced easily in statistical packages such as Minitab and SPSS (Statistical Package for Social Scientists). All the figures in this chapter have been produced in Minitab.

Pie chart

The pie chart is a suitable graphic for displaying nominal or ordinal data. It involves drawing a circle and dividing the circle into wedges. Each wedge represents a category of the variable. The size of each wedge depends on the proportion of the population the category covers. Moore (1991: 180–1) or Daly et al. (1995: 8–10) provide more detail on how to draw pie charts. Figure 10.1 shows a pie chart for the number of nurses from the three health authorities involved in the study by Roe et al. (1994). The study is a descriptive survey of current reported practice of community nurses for their nursing treatment of leg ulcers. This picture gives no extra information beyond the simple summary that there were 34 nurses from health authority A, 78 nurses from health authority B and 40 nurses from health authority C included in the survey. Although this can be a striking graphic, it is often difficult to extract useful information from the chart, particularly if there are many categories.

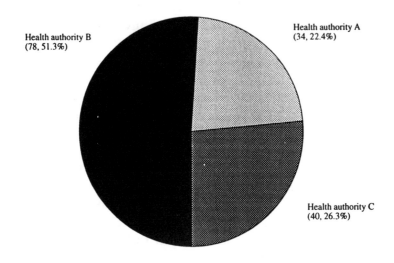

Health authority B
(78, 51.3%)

Health authority A
(34, 22.4%)

Health authority C
(40, 26.3%)

Figure 10.1: Pie chart showing the number of nurses from each health authority in a study of treatment of chronic leg ulcers (Roe et al., 1994).

Bar chart

The bar chart is a suitable graphic for displaying nominal or ordinal data. A bar represents each category. The size of the bar is equal to either the frequency of the category or the percentage in the category. There should generally be gaps between the bars reflecting the discrete categories. The bars may be drawn either vertically or horizontally. Examples are given in Daly et al. (1995: 10–12), Moore (1991: 184–6) and Altman (1991: 19–20). It is important that the frequency (or percentage) axis of the bar chart starts at zero, otherwise the visual impression can be misleading and will tend to exaggerate the differences between categories. In the study by Roe et al. (1994) considering community nurses' treatment of leg ulcers, nurses were asked which of a number of cleansers they used for leg ulcers. Figure 10.2 is a bar chart showing the percentage of community nurses selecting each solution.

Figure 10.3 is a bar chart of the cleansing solutions used, giving the three health authorities separately so we can look for any relationship between health authority and solution used. Since there are more nurses from some authorities than others it is necessary to do the comparison on a percentage (or proportion) scale. It is important

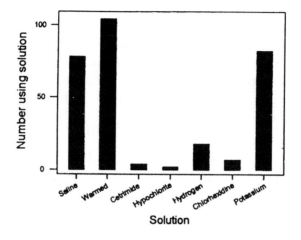

Figure 10.2: Bar chart showing the percentage of community nurses in three health authorities who use each of the solutions to cleanse leg ulcers (Roe et al., 1994).

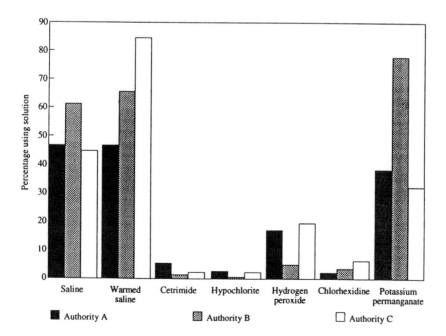

Figure 10.3: Solutions used by community nurses in three health authorities to cleanse leg ulcers (Roe et al. 1994, Table 3). (The number of nurses in the sample from each health authority is: A, $n = 34$; B, $n = 72$; C, $n = 40$.)

in graphs showing percentages that you state the group size so that readers can sensibly interpret the differences that they see. For example, a difference of 5% is quite large if the group size is 1000, but is far less impressive if the group size is 20.

In Roe et al. (1994) the data in Figure 10.3 are shown as part of a table. The most striking difference is that respondents from health authority B are more likely to use potassium permanganate. Although this information is available in the table in Roe et al. (1994), it is not as easy to spot as it is in Figure 10.3.

Histogram

The histogram is a suitable graphic for displaying numerical data but cannot be used for nominal or ordinal data. To produce a histogram, the range for the variable is divided into intervals of equal interval width, the number of observations in each interval is counted and then bars of height equal to the frequency or percentage (relative frequency) for the interval are drawn. There will not be gaps between the bars because we now have measurements on a proper numerical scale. Moore (1991: 191–4) and Altman (1991: 23–8) provide more detailed information about histograms, including a number of examples.

Figure 10.4 shows the histogram for the baseline pulse measurement for 92 students taking part in a pulse-rate study of response to exercise (Ryan and Joiner, 1994). The first histogram uses the intervals 48–52, 53–57, 58–62, and so on. The second histogram uses intervals 45–54, 55–64, 65–74, and so on. The choice of interval width is arbitrary and up to the researcher. The selection of different interval widths can make substantial changes to the look of the

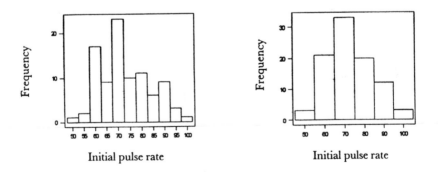

Figure 10.4: Histogram for initial pulse rate in the pulse-rate study for two different interval widths.

histogram, as Figure 10.4 illustrates.

Histograms are often used to make a judgement about whether data are roughly normally distributed. The normal distribution is symmetric, unimodal (has one peak) and has a characteristic 'bell-shape'. For more information about the normal distribution see Altman (1991: 51–7). We would generally be fairly safe in making an assumption of normality, provided the histogram looked roughly symmetric and we believed it to be unimodal.

Boxplot

The boxplot is a suitable graphic for displaying numerical data. A boxplot is a picture summarising the data by five values: the maximum value, the minimum value, the median, the lower quartile and the upper quartile. To calculate the median and the two quartiles we need to arrange the data in value order from smallest to largest (known as rank ordering the data). The value a quarter of the way through the size-ordered list, from the lowest value, is the lower quartile. The value halfway through the size-ordered list is the median, and the value three quarters of the way through is the upper quartile. In the boxplot, the lower and upper quartiles are indicated as a box, with the median shown within the box. Whiskers run from the box as far as the maximum and minimum observations. For more information see Moore (1991: 219–20) or Altman (1991: 33). Figure 10.5 shows a boxplot for the initial urinary knowledge score for nurses in a study investigating dissemination of research evidence

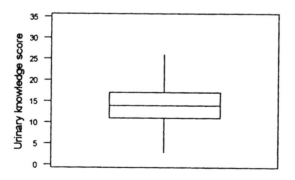

Figure 10.5: Boxplot of initial urinary knowledge score.

about continence care (Williams et al., 1997).

From the boxplot we observe that the median lies almost centrally in the box, telling us that the distribution of urinary knowledge scores is roughly symmetric. Figure 10.6 shows a boxplot for the urinary knowledge score displaying different grades of nurse separately. This is an easy way to compare the distribution of urinary knowledge score for different grades of nurse.

From Figure 10.6 we see that the median urinary knowledge score for grade D and below is lower than the lower quartile for all the other grades. The boxplots for grades E and F and above have very similar medians and lower quartiles. This suggests that those graded D and below have lower knowledge scores than the other grades. We also observe that the boxes (lower quartile to upper quartile) for all three grade groups are similar in size, indicating similar levels of spread (variability) in each of the grades.

What features are of interest in histograms or boxplots? Often what we need to know about a distribution is whether it is symmetric and unimodal in order to assess whether an assumption of normality is reasonable.

A distribution is symmetric if its two sides are approximately mirror images of each other about a centre line. For a boxplot this centre line is taken as the median and we are primarily interested in whether the median is roughly central in the box. For a histogram we have to imagine a centre line. Symmetry is often easier to determine from a boxplot than from a histogram because the shape of the

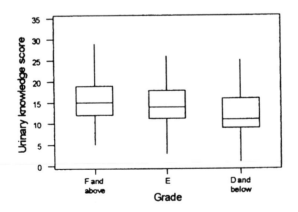

Figure 10.6: Boxplots of urinary knowledge score for different grades of nurse.

histogram can be very dependent on the interval width selected.

By unimodal we mean that the distribution has only one peak. A boxplot cannot tell us this. You also need to be careful with a histogram, particularly in small studies with relatively few subjects, since they may exhibit several peaks but these are often just an arte-fact of the small numbers. You should not reject the idea that a distri-bution is unimodal just because the histogram appears erratic, unless there are good theoretical reasons to expect a bimodal or trimodal distribution. Such distributions would be most likely to occur when we have two distinct subgroups, for example we consider blood glucose for a mixture of normal and diabetic individuals.

Scatterplots

If we are interested in ascertaining whether or not there is an associa-tion or a relationship between a pair of variables measured on an interval/ratio scale, we could use a scatterplot. We plot each subject's X variable value against his or her Y variable value. See Moore (1991: 255–6) and Altman (1991: 40) for examples. Figure 10.7 is a scatter-plot and shows the relationship between initial pulse rate and second pulse rate for the 92 students in the pulse rate study (Ryan and Joiner, 1994). The students randomly selected to exercise before the second measurement are indicated by circles, whilst those randomly selected to watch the others exercise are indicated by crosses. The line drawn on the figure indicates where initial pulse rate equals second pulse rate.

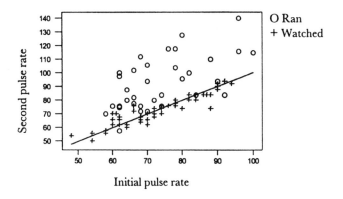

Figure 10.7: Scatterplot of initial pulse rate against second pulse-rate for the pulse-rate study. Circles are those who exercised; crosses are those who watched. The line shown is where initial pulse and second pulse are equal.

As expected, the value of second pulse rate is very close to the value of initial pulse rate for those who watched, that is the crosses all lie close to the line of equality. For those who ran we find second pulse rate is higher than initial pulse rate since all the circles are above the line of equality.

Describing data through summary statistics

The idea of descriptive or summary statistics is that we summarise data by a few carefully chosen numbers. Typically these consist of measures of centre or average and measures of variability or spread. The most commonly used type of average is the mean, which is calculated as the sum of all the observations divided by the number of observations. It should be noted that calculation of the mean is not sensible for categorical data.

The median, already mentioned in the discussion on boxplots, is another type of average. It is the value that comes halfway when the data values are in rank order, so it is the middle value. The mean is sensitive to the data at the extremes. However, the extreme values do not affect the median, so it is generally a better summary measure if there are outlying observations or if the distribution is skewed (non-symmetric, with a long tail on one side of the distribution).

A simple way of describing the spread of a set of data is to quote the lowest and highest values, or the range. However, this is not a satisfactory summary because it only takes account of the most extreme and perhaps most unusual values. Thus the range is not generally a good measure of spread. If we are summarising centre by the median, we generally indicate spread by the quartiles, or the numerical difference between them called the interquartile range. This indicates the spread of the middle 50% of the data. An alternative approach to quantifying variability is to consider the average distance of each observation from the mean, which is measured by the standard deviation (SD). Details of how to calculate the standard deviation are given in Altman (1991: 34–5).

The standard deviation has an important role in data analysis in both hypothesis testing and the calculation of confidence intervals. As a descriptive summary it is useful in two ways. First, if we are comparing two groups we can conclude that the group with the larger standard deviation is the more variable. Second, provided the distribution of the data is reasonably symmetric, about 95% of a set of observations will lie within two standard deviations of the mean.

Statistical hypothesis testing

In this section we will consider, in general, how we can attempt to obtain answers to specific questions or hypotheses. We are trying to predict, generalise, or infer information. For this we need to use one of the many inferential statistical techniques.

In order to be able to test ideas using a statistical test we will need to formalise our questions as hypotheses. This formalisation involves setting up a null hypothesis (H_0) and an alternative hypothesis (H_1). The null hypothesis is generally a statement of no change or no difference or no association. The alternative hypothesis is some other statement of interest, for example there is a difference or there is an increase or there is an association. The null hypothesis and the alternative hypothesis are the only statements under consideration.

The statistical test assesses how plausible the null hypothesis is in the light of the data we have gathered and the alternative that we have offered. If the null hypothesis does not seem plausible in the light of the data then we will wish to reject the null hypothesis in favour of the alternative. Thus a statistical test is simply a process of choosing between the null hypothesis and the alternative hypothesis.

To illustrate this process we can formalise some of the questions raised earlier when considering graphs. For example, when considering Figure 10.3 we questioned how nurses from different health authorities compared on the solutions they used to cleanse leg ulcers. This is a question of association: is use of a particular solution associated with health authority? We would formally state the hypotheses as, for example:

H_0: Use of potassium permanganate and health authority are not associated.

H_1: Use of potassium permanganate and health authority are associated.

When considering Figure 10.6 we asked whether urinary knowledge score was the same for all grades of nurse. This could be formalised as:

H_0: Mean urinary knowledge score for nurses graded D and lower is equal to mean urinary knowledge score for nurses graded E and above.

H_1: Mean urinary knowledge score for nurses graded D and lower is not equal to mean urinary knowledge score for nurses graded E and above.

There are many hundreds of different statistical tests. Which statistical test is appropriate depends on a number of important issues:

- The type of question (i.e. about difference or change or association).
- The type of data (i.e. the measurement scale).
- The assumptions that it is reasonable to make (e.g. that the distribution is normal).

If we can provide this information then we will be able to search through a statistical textbook and find an appropriate test. Table 10.1 summarises some of the most commonly encountered statistical tests and includes references for more detail.

A wide variety of statistical computer packages are available to carry tests – that is, to do the calculations. We are then left with having to interpret the output. Fortunately, most tests produce the same kind of final information. This is generally:

- The value of the test statistic.
- The p-value (probability value).
- A confidence interval (considered later).

When you are reading a paper these are the three pieces of information that the author is likely to report. Knowing the test statistic might help you identify the test the author used, which can be useful if the paper is unclear, but insufficient information is generally given in papers to allow you to check the calculation (even if you wanted to).

The p-value is central to the interpretation of the results. It is a measure of the plausibility of the null hypothesis. Strictly the p-value is *the probability of a result as extreme or more extreme than that observed, in the direction of H_1, when the null hypothesis is true.*

This precise definition might seem rather confusing. It will generally be adequate to simply regard the p-value as a measure of the plausibility of the null hypothesis. The p-value will, since it is a probability, always lie between zero and one. A probability of zero implies that the event is impossible. For example, if you do not buy a ticket for the national lottery, then the probability that you will win the jackpot is zero. (It is not much more than zero if you do buy a ticket!) A probability of one means that an event is certain. A low p-value (near zero) suggests that the null hypothesis is implausible; a high p-value (near one) suggests that the data we have observed are consistent with the null hypothesis.

Table 10.1: Examples of different statistical tests

Data type	Question	Test	Assumptions	Reference
Nominal	Association between two variables	Chi-square	Expected values all greater than five	Altman (1991: 241–53)
Nominal	Association between two variables	Fisher's exact	Both variables binary (only two categories)	Altman (1991: 253–8)
Nominal	Association between two variables	McNemar	Paired data, binary variables	Altman (1991: 258–9)
Ordinal or numerical	Equality of two medians	Mann-Whitney	Independent groups, same distribution shape	Altman (1991: 194–6)
Numerical	Equality of two means	t-test two sample	Independent groups, both normally distributed	Altman (1991: 194)
Ordinal or numerical	Equality of two medians	Wilcoxon signed rank	Paired data, distribution of differences is symmetric	Altman (1991: 191)
Numerical	Equality of two means	t-test paired	Paired data, difference normally distributed	Altman (1991: 191)
Numerical	Equality of several means	Analysis of variance (ANOVA)	Several independent groups, each normally distributed	Altman (1991: 205–9)
Numerical	Linear relationship	Pearson's correlation	Random sample of individuals. Both variables normally distributed	Altman (1991: 278–82)
Ordinal or numerical	Linear relationship in ranks	Spearman's rank correlation	Random sample of individuals	Altman (1991: 285–8)

What do we mean by a low p-value? Often people will take a p-value of less than 0.05 (that is $p < 0.05$) to be small and will reject the null hypothesis for such values. However, this is a totally arbitrary value to choose as the cut-off point. In some circumstances you might feel that you would want the p-value to be smaller than 0.01 before you would be prepared to reject the null hypothesis. Altman (1991: 167–9) and Gore and Altman (1987: 18 and 70–2) provide a more detailed discussion of the interpretation of p-values.

It is helpful if researchers report the exact p-value of their test (as given by their computer package) rather than simply reporting $p < 0.05$ because $p < 0.05$ covers a very wide range of possibilities. It could be that the p-value is 0.049 or that it is 0.00001. If the p-value is 0.049 then the evidence against the null hypothesis could be considered as very marginal, indeed we might not wish to reject the null hypothesis. However, if the p-value was 0.00001 then we would be convinced that there was evidence against the null hypothesis and would be happy to reject it. If researchers report the precise p-value they will give readers the opportunity to use their own judgement about the plausibility of the null hypothesis. However, if researchers simply report $p < 0.05$ they deny readers this opportunity.

It should be noted that if we reject the null hypothesis we are not saying that the alternative is correct – only that it is preferable to the null hypothesis in view of our data. If we fail to reject the null hypothesis this could be for any of three reasons:

1.   there is truly no difference/effect/change;
2.   the alternative offered is even less likely to be true in the light of our data;
3.   the study was too small to provide enough evidence to convince us that the null hypothesis was implausible.

In general it is unlikely that we will specify an alternative that is less tenable than the null hypothesis (reason 2). Unfortunately there is no easy way of establishing which of the other two explanations is correct. By carrying out pre-study sample size calculations, we can try to ensure that our study had a good chance of detecting a difference if it truly exists. If sample size calculations have been done, this would add support to an argument that reason 1 is the explanation of why we have not rejected the null hypothesis.

Parametric or non-parametric methods?

There are two main bodies of statistical testing techniques. These are known as parametric and non-parametric techniques. Parametric techniques are generally the most widely used. What is the difference between the two sets of techniques? Theoretical distributions are described by quantities called parameters, notably the mean and standard deviation, so methods that make distributional assumptions are called parametric methods. The t-test is an example of a parametric method. Methods that make no distributional assumptions are called non-parametric or distribution-free methods, and examples are the Mann-Whitney test, the Wilcoxon signed rank test and Spearman's rank correlation.

As they do not involve distributional assumptions, non-parametric methods are most often used to analyse data that do not meet the distributional requirements of parametric methods, usually that the data are normally distributed. Skewed data are commonly analysed by non-parametric techniques and data which are scores rather than measurements (so not on an interval/ratio scale) can often be handled by non-parametric techniques based on ranks.

Non-parametric techniques are considered more robust in the sense that they do not make many assumptions about the data. The cost is that they are less powerful, particularly in situations where the distributional assumptions of the equivalent parametric test would be fulfilled. The other disadvantage of non-parametric techniques is that estimation, for example, of the size of a treatment effect, can be difficult or impossible. As discussed by Altman (1991: 171–3), estimation, in particular confidence intervals, is generally much easier with parametric methods.

Frequently researchers select non-parametric tests because their sample size is small. This alone is a poor justification for the choice. If sample size is small it might be difficult to check out distributional assumptions, but it is unlikely that a small sample will convincingly violate distributional assumptions. With small samples the extra power of parametric tests is usually advantageous. In practice, unless distributional assumptions are clearly violated, it is unlikely that equivalent parametric and non-parametric tests will give vastly different results. In theory, we could perform both a non-parametric test and a parametric test and compare the results. In practice, we generally only perform one analysis, choosing between parametric or non-parametric methods. We usually use parametric methods unless there is some clear indication that the underlying assumptions are not met.

Examples of statistical tests

First let us consider again the study by Roe et al. (1994) and the question raised by Figure 10.3: do nurses from different health authorities make equal use of potassium permanganate to cleanse leg ulcers? The hypotheses under test are:

H_0:   Use of potassium permanganate and health authority are not associated.

H_1:   Use of potassium permanganate and health authority are associated.

As this is a situation in which we wish to consider association between two nominal variables, a chi-square test would be an appropriate test. The data under consideration are shown in Table 10.2.

Table 10.2: Nurses' use of potassium permanganate to cleanse leg ulcers

| | Health Authority | | | |
	A	B	C	Total
Use potassium permanganate	13	56	13	82
Do not use potassium permanganate	21	16	27	64
Total	34	72	40	146

We see that 78% of nurses in health authority B use potassium permanganate, but only 38% of nurses in A and 33% of nurses in C make use of this solution. Results of the chi-square test would be reported as $X^2 = 27.199$, degrees of freedom (DF) = 2, p = 0.000. X^2 is the test statistic and degrees of freedom relates to the number of rows and columns in the table. The number of degrees of freedom is used as part of the calculation that gets from the test statistic to the p-value. Neither X^2 nor DF is necessary for interpreting the test, provided we are informed of the p-value.

The interpretation of the test is that, since the p-value is small, certainly less than 0.05, we reject the null hypothesis and conclude that use of potassium permanganate is associated with health authority. There is significantly higher usage of potassium permanganate in health authority B than in A or C. The paper by Roe et al. (1994) contains several other illustrations of the chi-square test, which is one of the most widely used statistical tests.

Another widely used statistical test is the two-sample t-test. An example of a situation in which this would be an appropriate test is in determining whether urinary knowledge score is the same for different grades of nurse in the study by Williams et al. (1997). The hypotheses under test are:

H_0: Mean urinary knowledge score for nurses graded D and lower is equal to mean urinary knowledge score for nurses graded E and above.

H_1: Mean urinary knowledge score for nurses graded D and lower is equal not to mean urinary knowledge score for nurses graded E and above.

The mean knowledge score for the 67 nurses graded D and below was 12.39 (SD 4.77) whilst for the 166 nurses graded E or higher the mean score was 15.51 (SD 5.04). Carrying out the t-test, which assumes that the scores for each group of nurses follow a normal distribution, gives T = 4.34, DF = 231, p = 0.000. T is the test statistic and degrees of freedom (DF) relate to the number of nurses in the study. The number of degrees of freedom is used as part of the calculation that gets from the test statistic to the p-value and is of no direct help with interpreting the test.

The interpretation of the test is that, since the p-value is small, we reject the null hypothesis and conclude that the mean urinary knowledge score of nurses graded D and below is not equal to that of higher grade nurses. The paper by Williams, Crichton and Roe (1997) contains several other illustrations of the t-test, including some examples of the paired t-test. The paired t-test was used when nurses were repeatedly measured to look for change in knowledge following provision of a clinical handbook on continence care.

If we consider Figure 10.6 we could argue that it would be more appropriate to consider the three grade groups shown in the figure, in which case we would wish to test:

H_0: Mean urinary knowledge score for nurses graded D and lower is equal to mean urinary knowledge score for nurses graded E and is equal to mean urinary knowledge score for nurses graded F and above.

H_1: Mean urinary knowledge score is not equal for all three grade groups.

When we have more than two means to compare we use analysis of variance (ANOVA) rather than a t-test. For the 67 nurses graded D and below the mean knowledge score was 12.39 (SD 4.77), whilst for the 88 nurses graded E the mean score was 15.14 (SD 5.00) and for the 78 nurses graded F or higher the mean was 15.92 (SD 5.10). The results of the ANOVA would be reported as $F_{2,230} = 9.93$, p = 0.000.

The test statistic is $F_{2,230}$ and the values in the subscript are degrees of freedom for this test. Again, we reject the null hypothesis since the p-value is small, thus concluding that the mean urinary knowledge score is not equal for all grades. However, this test alone does not allow us to make claims about any particular grade being significantly different from any other.

Confidence intervals and estimation of size of effect

Nearly all statistical analysis is based on the principle that one obtains data on a sample of individuals and uses the information to make inferences about the wider population of all such individuals. For example, in the study by Williams et al. (1997) the nurses are assumed to be representative of hospital nurses. It was found that the mean urinary knowledge score for the nurses in the study was 14.61. The value 14.61 is a point estimate of the mean urinary knowledge score for the target population. Of course if the study were repeated and a different sample of nurses were selected to take part, then very likely we would get a different mean value. Thus based on a second sample we would make a different point estimate of the mean for the population.

We could also use the information in the study by Williams et al. (1997) to estimate the effect on knowledge of providing a research-based clinical handbook on continence. The mean change in knowledge score for those nurses provided with the handbook was an increase in score of 7.03. So we can infer that, for the nurses provided with the handbook, urinary knowledge score is increased by 7.03. Again, if this study were repeated with another sample, it is very unlikely that we would find that the mean change was precisely 7.03 in the second study. However, given that our only information comes from the one study we have done, our best estimate of the mean effect of the handbook on knowledge comes from the sample mean.

Rather than quoting a single value, which we believe from our study to be a reasonable estimate of the mean effect for the population, it would be preferable to quote a range of values within which we feel the mean effect for the population as a whole will lie. That is to quote:

Point estimate − margin of error; point estimate + margin of error

This is called a confidence interval. A single study usually gives an imprecise sample estimate of the overall population value of interest.

This imprecision is indicated by the margin of error – that is, by the width of the confidence interval. The larger the margin of error the lower the precision.

The width of the confidence interval (the margin of error) depends on three factors: the sample size, the variability of the characteristic being studied and the degree of confidence required. As far as sample size is concerned, the larger the sample size the more information we will have and therefore the more precise the result. Thus the margin of error should reduce as sample size increases. Wide confidence intervals thus emphasise the unreliability of conclusions based on small samples. With regard to variability, the less variable the characteristic the more precise our sample estimate and the narrower our confidence interval, so the margin of error should be reduced if the characteristic varies little from person to person. The higher we want the degree of confidence that our interval will include the true population value for the characteristic, then the wider we will need our confidence interval to be. For example, a 99% confidence interval will be wider than a 95% confidence interval because in order to be more confident that the true population value falls within the interval we will need to allow more potential values within the interval. The confidence level most commonly adopted is 95%, which will provide conclusions consistent with hypothesis tests carried out at the 5% level – that is, rejecting H_0 if $p < 0.05$.

We can calculate confidence intervals for a variety of estimators – for example, for the mean or mean change, or for a proportion or odds ratio. We will generally need to make some distributional assumptions in order to calculate a confidence interval. Gardner and Altman (1989) provide an excellent introduction to confidence intervals, and this also gives the mathematical details of how different confidence intervals are calculated.

When reading papers in the recent medical literature you will frequently encounter confidence intervals. Unfortunately they are currently rarely reported in the nursing literature, where the emphasis still tends to centre on whether 'results are significant' rather than on the size of the effect and its subsequent clinical relevance.

How are confidence intervals helpful? How are they interpreted?

Consider, again, the study by Williams et al. (1997) and the effect of the clinical handbook on knowledge score. A paired t-test carried out on the intervention group resulted in a p-value of 0.0000, so we rejected the null hypothesis and concluded that that mean urinary knowledge score was changed by having the handbook. The handbook produced a statistically significant improvement, but was it a clinically worthwhile improvement? We need to consider the actual size of effect that the handbook produced, i.e. a mean change in knowledge score of 7.03. The 95% confidence interval is from 5.68 to 8.34. That is we are 95% confident that the true mean change in urinary knowledge score is between these limits. This interval gives an idea of the size of effect, or the amount we might expect knowledge to change as a result of providing the handbook. From this interval we can conclude that it is extremely unlikely that urinary knowledge score is unchanged, since zero (no change) is not contained within the interval. By considering the range of values in the confidence interval we can assess whether there is significant clinical benefit resulting from the intervention under study.

Summary

In this short chapter it has only been possible to explore the general ideas behind statistical tests and confidence intervals. We considered some statistical aspects of designing research studies and introduced some ideas about how to analyse data. The advice of a statistician at the design stage of a study is likely to be beneficial not only with regard to sample size but also with planning for the analysis.

Statistical analysis has much more to offer, particularly with regard to exploring multivariate relationships and for developing statistical models to help explain or predict behaviour. However, the real benefit of modelling techniques such as linear or logistic regression or factor analysis can only be exploited if we carry out studies with a large enough number of subjects.

References

Altman DG (1991) Practical Statistics for Medical Research. London: Chapman & Hall.

Crichton NJ (1990) The importance of statistics in research design. Complementary Medical Research 4: 42–50.

Diamond M, Stone M (1981) Nightingale on Quetelet. Journal of the Royal Statistical Society Series A 144: 66–79.

Daly F, H, DJ, Jones MC, Lunn AD, McConway KJ (1995) Elements of Statistics. Wokingham: Addison-Wesley.

Everitt BS (1994) Statistical Methods for Medical Investigations. 2nd edn. London: Edward Arnold.

Fleiss JI. (1980) Statistical Methods for Rates and Proportions. 2nd edn. New York: Wiley.

Gardner MJ, Altman DG (1989) Statistics with Confidence. London: British Medical Journal Publishing.

Gore S, Altman D (1987) Statistics in Practice. London: British Medical Association.

Grier B, Grier M, (1978) Contributions of the passionate statistician. Research in Nursing and Health 1: 103–9.

Moore DS (1991) Statistics: Concepts and Controversies. 3rd edn. New York: WH Freeman & Co.

Reilly DT, Taylor MA, McSharry C, Aitchison T (1986) Is homoeopathy a placebo response? Controlled trial of homoeopathic potency, with pollen in hayfever as a model. Lancet ii: 881–6.

Roe BH, Griffith JM, Kenrick M, Cullum NA, Hutton JL (1994) Nursing treatment of patients with chronic leg ulcers in the community. Journal of Clinical Nursing 3: 159–68.

Ryan BF, Joiner BL (1994) Minitab Handbook. 3rd edn. Belmont, CA: PWS Publishing.

Tierney A, Closs J, Atkinson I, Anderson J, Murphy-Black T, Macmillan M (1988) On measurement and nursing research. Nursing Times 84(12): 55–8.

Thomas LH, Bond S (1995) The effectiveness of nursing: a review. Journal of Clinical Nursing 4: 143–51.

Williams KS, Crichton NJ, Roe BH (1997) Disseminating research evidence. A controlled trial in continence care. Journal of Advanced Nursing 25: 691–8.

PART THREE: DEVELOPMENT OF CLINICAL PRACTICE

Chapter 11
Developing practice through research

Ann McMahon

Introduction

This chapter is about the development of clinical nursing practice through research in the United Kingdom. It first examines why nurses develop their practice, the relationship between practice development and research, and the infrastructure that exists to support practice development in nursing. It then goes on to explore the process of practice development, along with some of the strategies that are deployed in nursing to develop practice through research.

Development of clinical nursing practice

The European Health Committee on Research states that research and development are inextricably linked in one continuous process. They are not, it is contended, 'distinct and separate types of activity' (European Health Committee, 1996: 10). This has not necessarily been seen to be the case in nursing in the United Kingdom (Kitson and Currie, 1996). There is a plethora of nursing literature about the development of clinical practice but the relationship between this activity and research is not always clear and, indeed, the evidence that development is a systematic activity is often lacking. In a review of clinical practice development and research activities across four district health authorities, Kitson and Currie (1996: 45) found that nurses were involved in a great deal of development activity but this was rarely based on research evidence, nor conducted as:

> a planned systematic activity, with clear objectives, an appropriate method-ology for evaluation and a clear understanding of the outcomes to be achieved.

To understand the relationship between research and development (R and D) in nursing it is necessary first to unpick the rationale for development and then examine nursing, research and development with the wider context of health care delivery.

Why do nurses develop their practice?

The most fundamental question that needs to be asked is why do nurses develop their practice? What motivates nurses to undertake activities associated with practice development? The Code of Professional Conduct for nurses in the UK states that nurses should

> act always in such a way as to promote and safeguard the well-being of patients and clients (UKCC, 1992).

Draper (1996) argues that, as a consequence of this, nurses are professionally bound to demonstrate development of their practice. If this is the case, nurses must also be professionally bound to substantiate practice developments with evidence that demonstrates that quality of patient care has improved as a consequence. Thus if the major driver for development in nursing is professional accountability, it should by definition be inextricably linked to research activity.

The influence of central policy on developments in nursing

The focus of nursing practice development initiatives has been greatly influenced by central policy developments (Graham, 1996). When systematically examining four nursing development units (NDUs) in the Yorkshire region, Graham (1996) uncovered examples where nurses were using recent health care policy to define their work and clarify the nature of their interventions. In addition, during the first phase of an external review of the Department of Health NDUs Redfern et al. (1994) identified eight policy documents that were considered to have had an impact on NDUs, their staff and their managers. These were:

- Working for Patients (Secretaries of State for Health, 1989).
- Caring for People (Secretaries of State for Social Services, 1989).
- Promoting Better Health (Secretaries of State for Social Security, 1987).
- Health of the Nation (Department of Health, 1992a).
- Tomlinson Review (Department of Health, 1992b).
- A Strategy for Nursing (Department of Health, 1989).

- A Vision for the Future (Department of Health, 1993a).
- The Patients' Charter (Department of Health, 1991a).

Central policy initiatives that endeavour to give a strategic direction for the development of the NHS clearly steered and will continue to steer nurses to develop their practice in a specific direction. Despite the claims of authors such as Meerabeau (1996) that the concept of evidence-based practice includes a notion of evidenced-based policy making, a review of the policy documents cited above would lead one to conclude that:

> particular economic, political or ideological factors may either stifle, or give rise to, new policy initiatives without any evidence from research informing the process. (Mullhall, 1995: 580).

With reference to the NHS reforms (Secretaries of State for Health, 1989), Closs and Cheater (1994) concur with this assessment of the policy formulation process. They argue that the NHS reforms were based entirely upon ideology with no regard whatsoever for research evidence, that nurses work in a culture which does not value research, and so it should come as no surprise that nurses themselves do not appear to value research evidence.

There has equally been a major force from within the profession shaping the focus of developments in nursing through influencing the content of central policy initiatives for the profession (Department of Health, 1989, 1993a). For example, Luker (1996) examined some of the developments associated with 'new nursing', such as primary nursing, and concluded that much of the change that has taken place has not been underpinned by research evidence, but has in fact been driven forward by evangelical zeal.

Thus it can be concluded that, to date, the drivers for development in nursing have lacked an evidence base (Luker, 1996) and research and development (R and D) skills have rarely been applied in the process of development (Kitson and Currie, 1996). Perhaps this is because research has traditionally been seen to lie within the domain of academic life and development has been safely guarded as the property of nurses in practice. As an explanation for the gap between research activity and development activity in nursing, the cultural differences between academic activity and practice are but one dimension of this complex issue. What is most striking is that, when examining the literature that identifies policy that has influenced the direction and nature of development activities in nursing, no reference is found to the National Health Services Research and Development Strategy (Department of Health, 1991b).

The National Health Service Research and Development Strategy

The National Health Service Research and Development Strategy was developed in response to a House of Lords select committee on science and technology which was critical of the absence of a coherent strategy within the NHS for the articulation of its research needs. In addition, the committee noted that there were no mechanisms in place to facilitate the uptake of research evidence into the service (House of Lords Select Committee on Science and Technology, 1988).

Research for Health – a research and development strategy for the NHS – was launched in April, 1991 (Department of Health 1991b). The primary objective of this strategy was 'to ensure that the content and delivery of health care in the National Health Service is based on high quality research relevant to improving the health of the nation.' (Department of Health, 1991b: 2). With reference to development, the strategy states that:

> emphasis will . . . be given to the systematic development within the NHS of the results of research . . . and that three stages in this process will be supported. (Department of Health, 1991b: 5)

These are:

- the development of new methods of care;
- the experimental introduction of these methods into services and evaluation in trials;
- the establishment of their use throughout the NHS.

Development is thus viewed as a logical progression from research. This approach to development is limited by the paucity of rigorously validated evidence to support interventions in use and the complexity of the implementation process (Kitson et al., 1996a). As an alternative to this 'implementation model', Kitson et al. (1996a) outline the 'practice development model'. This is an inductive approach to practice development through which theory may be generated. It is, however, frequently dismissed as subjective, due to its lack of rigour.

The development of nursing practice within the NHS is recognised as 'service development', not as an R and D activity. As a service or managerial responsibility it has to be funded from patient care budgets and has not benefited from the supportive R and D infrastructure created within the NHS through the R and D strategy. Yet it has been claimed that policy initiatives such as the Strategy for

Nursing (Department of Health, 1989) and the Vision for the Future (Department of Health, 1993a) require R and D skills to deliver them effectively (Luker, 1996).

There appears to be little acknowledgement in practice of the complexity of skills required to ensure that practice development is done well and that it is effective. This should have come as no surprise, when Kitson and Currie (1996: 45) revealed that

> nurses are still being encouraged to be individual champions of change without the supportive infrastructure around them to ensure that their efforts are beneficial.

If policy and practice objectives are to be delivered, nurses require access to supportive infrastructures.

National initiatives to support practice development in nursing

The Practice and Service Development Initiative

The NHS R and D strategy acknowledges the importance of a robust information strategy to avoid unnecessary duplication of effort. There is an important facet of this information strategy that endeavours to forge a link between research and developments in nursing and in the therapy professions. The 'Practice and Service Development Initiative' (PSDI) has been established within the NHS Centre for Reviews and Dissemination at the University of York. The aim of the PSDI is to co-ordinate the development of regional databases of practice and service development initiatives in order to facilitate networking, celebrate good practice and prevent nurses and their therapy colleagues from 're-inventing the wheel'. This is the only part of the R and D strategy that specifically focuses on development in nursing and therapy practice. It does not discriminate between research-based developments and other innovations in practice. What it does endeavour to do is identify areas of practice where nurses and therapists are in need of evidence to underpin practice developments. The PSDI feeds this information into research commissioning agendas but it can offer no guarantees that research will be commissioned in those fields identified. This initiative focuses on identifying research evidence required by nurses and therapists to support a deductive approach to practice development. In this way it is working towards cementing the relationship between research and practice development in nursing. Contact details for the PSDI are listed at the end of this chapter.

Outside of the NHS and the R and D strategy there have been a number of national initiatives that have specifically supported the development of nursing practice. These include the Kings Fund Nursing Development Units programme, the work of the Foundation of Nursing Studies and the Royal College of Nursing (RCN) Dynamic Quality Improvement (DQI) Network and the Network for Psychiatric Nursing Research (NPNR). Contact details for each of these initiatives are also listed at the end of this chapter.

King's Fund Nursing Development Units Programme

The nursing development unit (NDU) is the most commonly cited formal environment or laboratory for the initiation or application of practice development initiatives. They have been described as 'a fulcrum for change' (Graham, 1996: 266). NDUs were first established in the early 1980s (Neal, 1994). They are units recognised by the King's Fund nursing developments team as 'any defined clinical area where a group of nurses are striving to develop the service they offer to patients/clients, with the added responsibility of researching and evaluating practice, then disseminating their findings' (King's Fund Centre, 1992).

Although this is clearly a national initiative co-ordinated and supported by the nursing team at the King's Fund Centre, the focus for the development of nursing is within a clinical team. Neal (1994: 31) states that NDUs exist

> almost anywhere where the independent contribution of nurses can be explicitly defined.

NDUs and the activity that takes place in them can be thought of as existing on a continuum of stages of development (see Figure 11.1). Neal (1994) argues that the stage of development of the unit influences the type of activity that takes place within it and the degree of impact it is likely to have on the profession. She describes those at the beginning of their development as 'nurture' units and highly developed units are considered 'mature'. The more mature the NDU, the greater likelihood of there being evidence of development through research.

The Nursing Developments Network at the King's Fund has recently been renamed the Practice Development and Research Network. Membership of the network, it is claimed, helps nurses to keep up to date with innovations and the latest practice. Network members receive a newsletter and are afforded opportunities to attend networking days.

Type of unit	*Nurture*	*Mature*
Focus of activity	practice development and evaluation	research
Area of impact	resource to parent organisation – unlikely to have impact on the profession	national resource with an appreciable contribution to the nursing profession and health care

Figure 11.1: The continuum of nursing development units (after Neal, 1994).

The Foundation of Nursing Studies (FONS)

The *raison d'être* of the Foundation of Nursing Studies is 'to help the nursing profession to disseminate, use and implement proven research findings to improve patient care' (Foundation of Nursing Studies, 1994).

To this end their strategy focuses on supporting both research dissemination and implementation. To support research dissemination, the FONS runs conferences, supports a network of nurses engaged in practice development and offers advice and support to those wishing to run local conferences and study days. In recognition of the complex nature of research utilisation and the need to evaluate the effectiveness of strategies to promote the use of research in practice, FONS have developed an ongoing strategy to investigate these issues and disseminate their findings (Foundation of Nursing Studies, 1994). In addition FONS have commissioned expert researchers to run a series of workshops focused on the effective utilisation of research and its funds and supports projects which are committed to putting research into practice.

Royal College of Nursing Institute Dynamic Quality Improvement (DQI) Progamme

A whole range of activity takes place under the auspices of the network programme, which supports practice development through research.

DQI Programme

The expressed aims of the DQI Programme are:

- to facilitate networking and communication on issues relating to the quality of health care;

- to provide a framework of support, information and education to nurses and other health care professionals striving to improve the quality of health provision;
- to act at the interface between clinical practice and policy development at a local, national and international level.

The network operates on both a national and a regional level and links into the European Nursing Quality Network (Euroquan). Activities of the network include workshops, seminars, conferences, networking events and the production and dissemination of newsletters. Membership of the network is open to nurses and other health care professionals.

Nursing and Midwifery Audit Information Service

The Nursing and Midwifery Audit Information Service is a joint initiative with the Royal College of Midwives and is funded by the Department of Health. The service is staffed by information specialists who facilitate project networking opportunities and provide help and support to nurses and midwives endeavouring to develop evidenced-based practice through the application of clinical audit.

Education programmes

The DQI Programme team provide a range of educational packages from one-day awareness raising workshops through to week-long residential courses.

Research and development activity

The team undertakes a large amount of activity 'behind the scenes' that supports the development of practice through research. It is involved in leading the development and testing of national multidisciplinary guidelines, the conduct of systematic literature reviews, evaluating the effectiveness of its products (Morrell et al., 1995) and updating them accordingly.

Network for Psychiatric Nursing Research (NPNR)

The Network for Psychiatric Nursing Research is a project funded by the Department of Health to support practising nurses trying to make sense of mental health research. The NPNR holds both a membership database and a projects database and organises conferences to facilitate networking amongst members with shared interests.

Other initiatives to support practice development in nursing

Other initiatives reported in the literature to support the development of practice include, for example, the comprehensive approach taken by the former Yorkshire NHS Region. In the first instance, an audit of research activity amongst nurses and those in the professions allied to medicine (PAMS) was conducted in 1991 (Yorkshire Regional Health Authority, 1991). Using information gleaned from this, a strategy was formulated to develop the research resource in nursing and PAMS across the region (Hamer, 1992).

This region-led approach gave rise to a number of initiatives including

- the establishment of networks for trust based personnel with a lead responsibility for R and D;
- the establishment of networks for those engaged in practice development initiatives;
- a regional learning network for clinical leaders (Malby, 1996).

Thus, the Yorkshire region effectively developed a supportive infrastructure to nurture the research and development activities of nurses (and PAMS) across the region.

The notion of a nursing development unit was further developed within the Yorkshire region to encompass the full involvement of the multidisciplinary health care team in what were known as practice development units (PDUs) (Malby, 1992). Part of the Yorkshire Regional strategy included encouragement and support of the development of an organisational approach to R and D. This strategy recognised that unit-based approaches and organisational approaches were by no means mutually exclusive (Draper, 1996).

There are scant references to organisational approaches in the literature, perhaps because such approaches have not had the same high profile associated with being part of a national network that, for example, the NDUs have enjoyed through the King's Fund. Nor have organisational approaches been 'pump-primed' with funding, conditional upon dissemination strategies beyond the organisations they have been set up to support. However, what little information there is concerning organisational approaches offers some useful insights.

Reflecting on his own experience, Knight (1994: 35) argues that the development of nursing practice on an organisation-wide scale requires:

- clear distinction between the management of nurses and the leadership of nursing;
- a structure that cultivates the development of nurses and their practice;
- active encouragement for practising nurses to participate in the formulation of clinical policies and standards;
- development of audit awareness amongst nurses;
- promotion of research partnerships between the trust and institutions of higher education;
- strategies for the sharing of ideas innovations and outcomes.

Malby (1996) states that an organisational approach to R and D could lead to the integration of R and D, clinical audit and nursing strategy. This was my personal experience as Assistant Director of Nursing Services and Head of Research and Development in Mid-Staffordshire from 1989 to 1995 (McMahon and Darby, 1993). In addition, a number of nurses with lead responsibility for R and D within their respective trusts have begun to share their experiences within the Royal College of Nursing Research Society's twice-yearly newsletter. Without exception, the nurses who hold trust-based R and D roles are in support positions to the trust Executive Director of Nursing. Some nurses are a 'one (wo)man band' and others manage teams of R and D nurses. The sorts of activities that they are engaged in are listed under four headings in Figure 11.2. These are planning activities, activities to raise the profile of R and D in nursing, practical steps and strategic intent.

Knight (1994) and others (for example Thomas and Ingham, 1995) acknowledge that the focus of their work is on the 'D' end of the R and D continuum. With the notable exception of a service evaluation for a respite care provision (Darby et al., 1991), initiatives undertaken in Mid-Staffordshire by the nursing R and D team between 1989 and 1995 also focused on development and dovetailed with the quality assurance initiatives within the trust. One example of the work undertaken was the development and implementation of a clinical risk-management programme (McMahon and Jackson, 1992), which included a trust-wide research-based approach to the prevention, management and evaluation of pressure sores (McMahon and Smith, 1993; Jackson et al., 1993). Other areas examined included use and management of urethral catheters, monitoring and prevention of falls in the elderly and monitoring and prevention of cross infection. The appropriate clinical nurse specialists and I made up the core team for the clinical risk-management programme. The development activity and subsequent publications were drawn from initiatives conceived and developed by practitioners in clinical practice on wards within the trust. When policy-driven developments such as the Patients' Charter (Department of Health, 1991) were high on the agenda, the R and D team was called upon to support the development and evaluation of practice. Consultancy was provided on a ward-by-ward basis and unit networking meetings were facilitated to encourage the sharing of difficulties encountered and solutions discovered. In order to provide a hospital-wide picture of the implementation of the 'named nurse' concept, an instrument developed by Bowman et al., (1991) was applied across the trust. A full report of this initiative is available elsewhere (McMahon, 1995).

PLANNING ACTIVITIES
- developing an R and D strategy for nursing or ensuring nursing features in the Trust R and D strategy
- identifying priorities for research
- conducting R and D needs analysis

ACTIVITIES TO RAISE THE PROFILE OF RESEARCH AND DEVELOPMENT IN NURSING
- building and maintaining a research culture for nursing
- promoting research-based practice
- promoting nursing research projects
- developing local networks
- facilitating research fora and interest groups

PRACTICAL STEPS
- managing a research support unit
- running research awareness and critical appraisal courses
- running skills workshops
- providing opportunities to shadow nurse researchers
- developing and maintaining databases of Trust R and D activity
- producing a local newsletter
- supporting nurses conducting research

STRATEGIC INTENT
- formalising links with Higher Education
- working towards clearly defined research career ladders for nurses
- working towards multidisciplinary integration
- ensuring that nursing R and D activity features in the new funding arrangements for NHS R and D (McMahon, 1997)

Figure 11.2: Organisational approach.

To further develop the research activity within trust-based R and D teams, Knight (1994) argues for stronger links with academic institutions. There is already emerging evidence of the development of research partnerships between both acute and community trusts and institutions of higher education in the form of joint appointments at professorial level (McMahon, 1997). With the final implementation of the recommendations of the new funding arrangements for NHS research and development (Culyer, 1994), this is a trend that is likely to continue.

The evidence used to underpin practice development

By definition, a deductive approach to practice development requires evidence to underpin it. Research evidence or findings are most often disseminated through publications. This evidence is traditionally assessed by conducting literature searches and reviewing the evidence. These require searching and appraisal skills. Searching has become an increasingly complex activity as there has been a notable increase in the numbers of research-based publications in the field of nursing over the last 40 years (Brown et al., 1983; Van Cott et al., 1991). A comprehensive search of the literature therefore now requires sophisticated library and information management skills. In turn, critical appraisal of the literature has become an increasingly more complex activity. Roe (1993: 31) states that: 'Systematic . . . reviewing of the literature . . . has now developed as a method in its own right.'

Access to quality systematic reviews therefore clearly offers a good short cut for nurses wishing to develop their practice through research. Through its information strategy, the NHS R and D Directorate has identified two centres of excellence in the conduct of systematic reviews. These are the NHS Centre for Reviews and Dissemination at the University of York and the UK Cochrane Centre in Oxford. A systematic review is defined as:

> the process of systematically locating, appraising and synthesising evidence from scientific studies in order to obtain a reliable overview' (NHS Centre for Reviews and Dissemination, 1996: 90).

It is effectively a highly controlled and rigorous review of the evidence. A systematic review may include a meta-analysis, which is the application of a range of statistical techniques to combine data from a range of studies incorporating randomised controlled trials (RCTs) (see Chapter 6).

All good nursing libraries will have abstracts of the work of this centre, known as the Cochrane Library and DARE (Database of Abstracts of Reviews of Effectiveness), on CD-ROM. For those with access to the Internet, DARE can be accessed online on URL http://www.york.ac.uk/inst/crd/info.htm: username and password crduser. For those who prefer hard copy, the centre have produced abstracts of their reviews under the titles 'Effectiveness Matters' and 'Effective Health Care Bulletins'. A number of reviews which have been completed to date are of particular relevance to nursing. These include the following titles, which have been published as a compilation (Nursing Standard, 1997):

- Non-Pharmacological Interventions for Acute Pain.
- Use of Compression Stockings.
- The Prevention and Treatment of Pressure Sores.
- Preventing Falls and Further Injury in Older People.
- Pre-Operative Patient Instruction: Is It Effective?
- Use of Naso-Gastric Tubes for Effective Laparotomy.
- Managing Primary Breast Cancer: a Review of Care.
- Psycho-Educational Care for Adults with Cancer.
- Psychosocial Interventions for Coronary Artery Disease.

More reviews of relevance to nursing are in the pipeline. For further information the centre can be contacted at the address given at the end of the chapter.

For the majority of topics there is not an up-to-date, definitive systematic review of the evidence ready to be translated into practice. In order to assist practitioners, those involved in the evidence-based nursing movement have developed the concept of 'levels of evidence' as applied to nursing. Morgan and Fennessey (1996) have developed a model that examines the role of information, guidelines, standard setting and audit in the dissemination and implementation of research into practice (see Figure 11.3).

Their model represents a matrix that identifies sources of evidence, namely the availability of national guidelines or local guidelines, the availability of sources of critically appraised or collated research, or indeed any research on the topic under consideration. Clinical guidelines are a means of making research evidence more accessible to practitioners by packaging it in a sympathetic manner. Guidelines represent a step-by-step description of how research findings should be used in practice (Closs and Cheater, 1994). They also act as a framework for evaluating the appropriateness of care that

SOURCES OF EVIDENCE

1. ARE NATIONAL GUIDELINES AVAILABLE ?

- Royal colleges and professional organisations
- Primary information sources (journals etc.) accessed through electronic sources or libraries
- NHSE
- Agency for health care policy and research (USA)
- St. George's Hospital, London
- Conferences and exhibitions
- Scottish Intercollegiate guidelines network
- Nursing and midwifery audit information service
- Networking and word of mouth
- Potentially a new service will be developed in the future

YES →

NO

2. ARE LOCAL GUIDELINES AVAILABLE ?

- Local audit and quality departments
- Local and regional databases
- Health and nursing information sources
- Regional audit co-ordinators local CHC's etc.
- Professional bodies and royal colleges
- Conferences and exhibitions
- St. George's Hospital, London
- Nursing and midwifery audit information service

YES →

NO

3. ARE THERE SOURCES OF APPRAISED OR COLLATED RESEARCH ?

- Systematic reviews published in primary information sources (journals etc.) accessed through libraries, electronic searches
- Professional organisations and royal colleges
- Journals which collate research results such as Bandolier, Evidence based medicine, ACP Journal Club, organisations which collect 'good' appraised research such as Cochrane Centre and York Centre for reviews and dissemination
- Various projects such as promoting action on clinical effectiveness (Pace; Kings Fund)
- Nursing and midwifery audit information service

YES →

NO

4. IS THERE ANY RESEARCH AVAILABLE ?

- Primary literature (journals etc.), accessed through electronic literature search, library service or other information providers
- Department of Health
- Academic institutions and independent research organisations
- Local databases
- Professional bodies and royal colleges
- International nursing organisations
- Conferences and exhibitions
- Internet and computer networks
- Networking and word of mouth, practice development departments

YES →

NO →

Figure 11.3: Levels of evidence (Morgan and Fennessey, 1996). (Reproduced with permission of the authors, Nursing and Midwifery Audit Information service Royal College of Nursing, 1996).

CONSIDERATIONS   ACTION

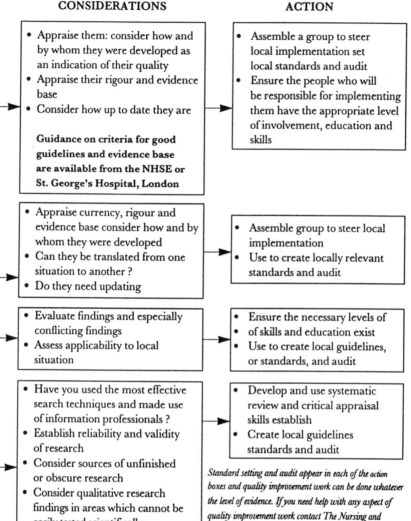

- Appraise them: consider how and by whom they were developed as an indication of their quality
- Appraise their rigour and evidence base
- Consider how up to date they are

Guidance on criteria for good guidelines and evidence base are available from the NHSE or St. George's Hospital, London

- Assemble a group to steer local implementation set local standards and audit
- Ensure the people who will be responsible for implementing them have the appropriate level of involvement, education and skills

- Appraise currency, rigour and evidence base consider how and by whom they were developed
- Can they be translated from one situation to another ?
- Do they need updating

- Assemble group to steer local implementation
- Use to create locally relevant standards and audit

- Evaluate findings and especially conflicting findings
- Assess applicability to local situation

- Ensure the necessary levels of
- of skills and education exist
- Use to create local guidelines, or standards, and audit

- Have you used the most effective search techniques and made use of information professionals ?
- Establish reliability and validity of research
- Consider sources of unfinished or obscure research
- Consider qualitative research findings in areas which cannot be easily tested scientifically
- Establish group to steer local implementation of good research

- Develop and use systematic review and critical appraisal skills establish
- Create local guidelines standards and audit

Standard setting and audit appear in each of the action boxes and quality improvement work can be done whatever the level of evidence. If you need help with any aspect of quality improvement work contact The Nursing and Midwifery Information Service, Room 521, 20 Cavendish Square, London, W1M 0AB. We can also provide contact names and addresses for any of the organisations mentioned in the diagram.

SOURCES OF EVIDENCE

5. WHAT TO DO WHEN NO RESEARCH EXISTS

- Consensus and expert opinion professional bodies, academic and nurse specialists
- Textbooks, journals and non-research literature (check author, currency etc.)
- Use patient feedback or complaints or other local information as part of quality improvements based on agreement at local level
- Conduct your own research
- Feed into policies affecting research prioritisation
- Choose another area for audit
- Contact nursing and midwifery audit information service

DON'T DO NOTHING

health professionals deliver and patients receive (Dickson, 1996). Other sources of research can be accessed through literature searching, searching databases of research in progress such as the NHS research register, and through consulting colleagues. This may be face-to-face consultation through professional networks, conferences and educational events or it may be through exploring Internet Web pages and subscribing to Internet discussion groups. Based on the sources of evidence available, Morgan and Fennessey (1996) have identified what needs to be considered and what action needs to be taken in order to develop research-based practice.

The Nursing and Midwifery Audit Information Service have produced a number of factsheets in response to their most commonly asked questions. The levels of evidence matrix (Figure 11.3) has been reproduced in Information Factsheet number 3 and is available upon request. Contact details for the Nursing and Midwifery Audit Information Service are available at the end of this chapter.

The strategies adopted to enable practice development through research

Strategies that enable practice development through research are about both knowledge and skill. When pursuing a deductive approach to practice development the first stage is to gain knowledge of the evidence required to underpin the practice development. This activity is simplified considerably when effective research dissemination strategies are in place. Knowledge, once gained, then has to be translated into practice. This is aided by deploying a tried-and-tested research utilisation strategy. On the other hand, if an inductive approach to practice development is pursued, a tried-and-tested approach to practice development, from which theory may be generated, should be deployed. At the Royal College of Nursing Institute, Kitson et al. (1996) have successfully amalgamated the deductive and inductive models within their practice development programmes. They argue that: 'practice development should not be separate from systematic evaluations of those changes, nor should only one approach be advocated: more important is the clarity and rigour with which the projects are set up' (Kitson et al., 1996b: 436)

Research dissemination in nursing is a complex activity that requires collaborative action between nurses in practice, researchers and those who are responsible for ensuring that nurses have access to research information (Dickson, 1996). To be effective this must include research appreciation programmes incorporating workshops in critical appraisal skills.

Journal clubs have been reported as an effective means of supporting research dissemination (Shelton, 1988; Lindquist et al., 1990; Tibbles and Sandford, 1994; Kirchhoff and Beck, 1995; Hammick, 1991). They are a tool that can be utilised in any branch of nursing. Just like any group activity, establishing the purpose of the journal club at the outset is fundamental. Once this is clear, a framework can be established outlining group membership and leadership. Terms of reference incorporating ground rules can then be drawn up. Important practical decisions must be made at the outset regarding the venue for meetings, the scheduling of meetings, the process of article selection and their distribution and how the activity will be resourced. It may be appropriate to develop guidelines for participation.

Research dissemination is subsumed within research utilisation strategies, but the importance of robust approaches to dissemination and appreciation must not be overshadowed by a utilisation strategy. A dissemination strategy can be viewed as a crucial part of the planning stage of any utilisation strategy but it can also stand alone as an independent educational activity. This is why, as with the journal club example illustrated above, clarity of purpose is essential if the desired outcome is to be attained. Kirchhoff and Beck (1994) have developed a useful matrix of types of activity undertaken in journal clubs, their advantages and disadvantages and their potential for research utilisation. They discuss the merits of reviewing a single journal article: it requires minimal preparation time and has a high potential for group participation with short, frequent sessions. Reviewing a single journal article serves as a useful introduction to the journal club environment. Such a narrow coverage, however, has no potential for research utilisation. At the other extreme, reviewing a single topic with an exhaustive preparatory search clearly requires more time to prepare and conduct the session but has high potential for research utilisation as the scientific merit of the evidence can be appraised and conflicting findings identified. The opportunity is also afforded to compare current practice with the evidence uncovered.

Whether working in the inductive domain, the deductive domain or deploying an integrated approach, there are a range of research methods and management strategies that can be deployed to support the development of practice through research. Supportive and enabling strategies include collaboration (Tierney and Taylor, 1991; Kelly et al., 1996), secondments and joint appointments (Closs and Cheater, 1994). Process management methods include clinical audit and other quality improvement initiatives. Research methods include action research.

Research utilisation was not the primary focus of the experiment in researcher-practitioner collaboration in a breast-care unit in Edinburgh (Tierney and Taylor, 1991). However upon completion of a study examining the benefits of scalp cooling as a means of preventing alopecia in patients receiving chemotherapy, the ward sister, who was the lead practitioner in the collaboration, encouraged her staff to read the final report. She led discussion and drew up a plan to implement a number of the research recommendations and Tierney and Taylor (1991) were able to report that change had taken place. In another study examining the work of Macmillan paediatric nurses, collaboration between the Macmillan nurses within a regional paediatric oncology unit and academic colleagues led to the development of a new method of recording care for children with cancer (Kelly et al., 1996). When identifying strategies to enhance the utilisation of research, Closs and Cheater (1994) advocated secondment into research teams on a full-time or indeed a part-time basis as a means of exposing practitioners and/or their managers to research. Joint appointments were also cited as a means of facilitating implementation of research into the practice arena (Closs and Cheater, 1994).

Clinical audit is defined by the Department of Health as:

> The systematic and critical analysis of the quality of care, including the procedures used for the diagnosis, treatment and care, the associated use of resources and the resulting outcomes and quality of life for the patient. (Department of Health, 1993b: 3)

It is a dynamic process where quality is defined, performance is measured and, when indicated, action is taken to improve performance. Evidence is sought when defining quality and the levels of evidence matrix developed by Morgan and Fennessey (1996) and reproduced in Figure 11.3 serve as a useful guide to identifying sources of evidence and what to do when research evidence is not available. Research and development skills are also required for the measurement phase of the cycle. Unbiased and precise sampling methods must be determined and valid and reliable data on performance must be collected (Russell and Wilson, 1992). Management skills are then required to bring about change, when indicated.

Action research, research and development

Greenwood (1984) was amongst the first to argue the case for action research in nursing. It is a method based on the work of Kurt Lewin (1946), which has become increasingly popular in nursing (Webb, 1993). Its distinguishing features are that action research is situational, collaborative and participatory and self evaluative (Greenwood, 1984). Holter and Schwartz-Barcott (1993) state that the major goals of action research are to create change in practice and to develop or refine existing theory. However not all authors are convinced that these two goals should be given equal footing. Elliott (1991) is emphatic in his claims that the primary purpose of action research is to improve practice and that knowledge generation is of secondary importance. On the other hand, Cunningham (1992: 166) is anxious that an action researcher may become obsessed with action to the point that he or she 'ceases to do research'. This scenario, he argues, may give rise to 'an interesting impressionistic case study, but not a contribution to wisdom' (Maxwell, 1984). Luker (1992) argues that action research studies polarise towards either a research or a development focus. She likens the research focus to evaluation research and the development focus to action learning.

Three main approaches to action research found in the literature are the technical collaborative approach, the mutual collaborative approach and the enhancement approach (Holter and Schwartz-Barcott, 1993). With the technical collaborative approach, the problem and the solution are identified prior to the engagement of the researcher. A deductive approach is therefore adopted and the researcher's role is that of technical expert and facilitator. With the mutual collaborative approach, the researcher(s) and the practitioner(s) work inductively towards a mutual understanding through the process of collaboratively identifying possible problems, their underlying causes and potential solutions. The enhancement approach takes this a step further, the aim being to raise the collective consciousness of the practitioners. The researcher facilitates a process of critical reflection to enable the practitioners to challenge some of the underlying assumptions and values they hold about their practice. It is argued that change in practice is more likely to be sustained with the enhancement approach because of the fundamental challenge of underlying assumptions and values.

Examples of the application of action research include research utilisation strategies (Hunt, 1987), the implementation of innovations in practice (Bellman, 1996) and the development of 'new' roles in nursing (Jones, 1996). Hunt's (1987) frequently cited study sits somewhere between the technical collaborative and the mutual collaborative approaches in that the overall aim of equipping nurse teachers with the skills to find and utilise research data in practice was explicit from the outset. However the selection of specific topics was determined by the nurse teachers themselves, namely mouth care and pre-operative fasting. When it came to the implementation of the pre-operative fasting research findings, once again Hunt adopted an approach in between the technical collaborative and the mutual collaborative approach. Based on the research evidence traced by the nurse teachers, hospital anaesthetists formulated a policy on pre-operative fasting. However, ward sisters experienced difficulty translating the policy into practice. Hunt therefore acted as a facilitator, working with the ward sisters to identify why they were experiencing difficulty and what could be done about it. Analysis of this approach led Hunt to believe that 'nurses tend(ed) to be very pessimistic about the co-operation expected in collaborative change activities . . . nurses appeared to view themselves as victims rather than initiators of change' (Hunt, 1987: 108). However, Hunt also advised that 'changing inappropriate organisational contexts and resources and negotiating with a range of other disciplines are generally beyond the capacity of any one individual' (Hunt, 1987: 109).

Bellman (1996) used the enhancement approach to action research on a surgical ward. Following a period of group reflection on the nursing model identified in the ward philosophy, Bellman, as a co-researcher with the ward team, facilitated the introduction of three innovations in practice, namely patient self-medication, patient-controlled analgesia and patient information leaflets. Having initiated and participated in the enhancement approach to action research, Bellman (1996) concluded that this approach gave practitioners confidence, demonstrated co-researchers' contribution to professional practice and knowledge development, raised awareness of – and demystified – the research process and strengthened relationships within the multidisciplinary team. In addition Bellman (1996: 137) identified six criteria that, once met, enhanced the likelihood of a successful action research study:

- continuous management support;
- a known and credible facilitator;
- endorsement of the change by patients and the multidisciplinary team;
- a knowledge of the change process;

- a commitment to group shared reflection and learning;
- the implementation of the enhancement approach to action research.

Jones (1996) adopted a technical collaborative approach to action research in order to introduce a service development, namely implementation of the role of the emergency nurse practitioner (ENP) in a paediatric accident and emergency department. The drivers for this change in practice are outlined in Figure 11.4. This study illustrates the incongruence between policy initiatives in the NHS. There is a host of policy initiatives embedded within the drivers for this initiative, but the reality of market forces and the impact they have had on the skill mix within the department seriously curtailed the progress of this feasibility study. As a consequence, this study illustrates the crucial requirement of securing full managerial support for the development of practice through research.

needs assessment	commentators had reported that a significant proportion of patients attending A & E do not need to be seen by a doctor
professionalisation strategy	nurses desire to extend their skills
policy development	reduction in junior doctors' hours
managerial concerns	long waiting times for patients with minor injuries
tested solution with proven outcomes	other A & E departments had reported successful outcomes when introducing this service development

Figure 11.4: Drivers for service development (after Jones, 1996).

Summary

This has argued that nurses are professionally accountable for the development of their practice and for justifying the development of practice with evidence of improvements in the quality of patient care. On this basis the relationship between research and development must be inextricably linked, not 'in one continuous process' as suggested by the European Health Committee (1996), but in two, perhaps interlinking circles, acknowledging the place of inductive knowledge generation as well as the traditional deductive approaches (Kitson et al., 1996). The focus of developments in nursing has largely been influenced by two major facets: 'professional evangelism' and government policy. Neither of these appears to take research evidence as its primary reference. Developments associated with 'professional evangelism' appear to be driven by beliefs that new is better than old (Luker, 1996) and, indeed, those that have greatest impact are underwritten by policy (Butterworth et al., 1996). However the argument here is not that policy should be informed entirely by research evidence, but that R and D skills, coupled with management skills and management support, are required to deliver many of the policy agendas (Luker, 1996). The picture, currently identified in the literature is one of polarised activity. On the one hand we have the development as espoused within the NHS R and D strategy (Department of Health, 1992b), with a narrow definition of development (Kitson et al., 1996). On the other hand, within nursing there is clearly a great deal of development activity that has been criticised for lacking clarity of purpose and rigour (Lorentzen, 1994; Draper, 1996).

The major implication for the profession is that it should recognise the importance of this division or polarisation of thinking and activity and first acknowledge and then realise the benefits of finding and claiming the middle ground (See Figure 11.5). It is interesting to note that, in policy terms, this synthesis is beginning to emerge. There appears to be evidence of a shift from disparate policy developments towards integration, particularly and most importantly in this case, with reference to the NHS R and D strategy.

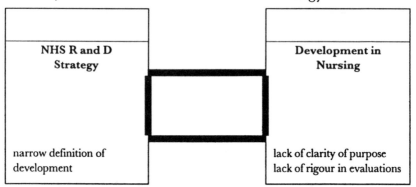

Figure 11.5: Polarisation between NHS R and D strategy and development in nursing.

In the most recent White Paper, *The National Health Service – A Service with Ambitions* (Secretary of State for Health, 1996), Stephen Dorrell, the then Secretary of State advised that:

> It is important that the service which is delivered to patients reflects the latest advances in clinical understanding ... The NHS Research and Development Programme, reinforced by clinical audit and continuing

professional education, will play an increasingly important role in this process. (Secretary of State for Health, 1996: 6).

This could be of great significance to the development of practice through research within the profession, particularly because of the interest in evidence-based practice. Policy statements such as this legitimise the synthesis of R and D with practice development, and indicate a realisation of the fact that the success of NHS R and D programmes does depend on an understanding, at all levels within the National Health Service, of the power of R and D to promote improvements in health care (Department of Health, 1991b).

It is argued here that the significance of this depends upon how the profession manages the challenges such an opportunity creates. Figure 11.5 suggest that a two-pronged strategy is required. Graham (1996) endeavoured to make explicit the nature and purpose of nursing through the systematic review of four nursing development units. He claimed that:

> In investigating the art and science of nursing practice within NDUs we are aware of the validity and evaluation issues in such an investigation. Often we utilise research methods born out of new research paradigms which often don't carry the stamp of official approval or recommendation. Yet we have found traditional research methods lacking when trying to understand the nature of nursing practice, as the methods are often divorced and distant from certain realities which are important in understanding nursing intervention and interactions. (Graham, 1996: 262)

The nursing profession is not alone in its frustration with the definitions of R and D within the NHS R and D Strategy (Pope and Mays, 1993). The profession must develop and implement strategies to influence thinking at all levels about the importance and relevance of both inductive and deductive research and development strategies. Such strategies should include the formation of strategic alliances with like-minded individuals and ensure that the quality of nursing research and development activity is of a high standard. Ensuring that the quality of research and practice development activity in nursing is of a high standard depends upon each of these activities being regarded of equal importance and in turn being adequately supported. This requires the provision of an infrastructure that offers supervision, resources and technical advise (Kitson and Currie, 1996).

The new funding arrangements for NHS R and D (Culyer, 1994) claim to offer access to NHS R and D funds for all parts of the NHS. If this proves to be the case, it clearly creates an opportunity for the profession (Robinson, 1996) in affording it the opportunity to develop an infrastructure to support and develop the necessary R and D skills required throughout the profession to effectively develop practice through research (McMahon, 1997). Only trusts can bid for funds, and universities are not eligible. However, one of the criteria against which bids will be assessed will be evidence of collaboration with the university sector. Consequently we are likely to see more evidence of the bringing together of these two cultures in nursing which, in itself, will require evaluation (Graham, 1996).

Sharing and networking of experiences of linking research and practice development must continue through publication and networking. Kitson et al. (1996) argue for the establishment of practice development and research centres which should include the following features:

- A range of methodologies to implement research into practice and to develop practice.
- Formation of multi-disciplinary and multi-methods teams working in partnership with clinical practice.
- Acceptance of the value of deductive and inductive approaches to knowledge generation and testing.
- Practice development based on theoretical frameworks conducted systematically and committed to generation of new knowledge.
- Implementing research into practice based on sound knowledge, undertaken within clearly defined organisational contexts and carefully evaluated.
- A commitment to developing highly skilled teams of research and development staff to work in partnership with clinical staff.
- A commitment to education and training to disseminate methods of evaluating practice.
- Provision of practical, realistic, desirable improvements in clinical practice that are theoretically sound. (Kitson et al., 1996: 438).

Only when the necessary structures and resources are in place will the profession have the confidence to state that practice developments that are promulgated throughout the service are based on sound evidence both in terms of their content and their methods of introduction.

Appendix 11.1: useful addresses

Dynamic Quality Improvement Programme
Royal College of Nursing Institute
Radcliffe Infirmary
Oxford
OX2 6HE
tel. 01865 224667

King's Fund Nursing Developments Programme
King's Fund Development Centre
11–13 Cavendish Square,
London W1M OAM
tel. 0171 307 2400

Network for Psychiatric Nursing Research
Royal College of Nursing Institute
Radcliffe Infirmary
Oxford
OX2 6HE
tel. 01865 228489

Nursing and Midwifery Audit Information Service
Room 521
20 Cavendish Square
London
W1M 0AB
tel. 0171 629 7464

Practice and Service Development Initiative
NHS Centre for Reviews and Dissemination
University of York
York YO1 5DD
tel. 01904 433636

The Foundation of Nursing Studies
154 Buckingham Palace Road
London
SW1W 9TR
tel. 0171 824 8182

References

Bellman LM (1996) Changing nursing practice through reflection on the Roper, Logan and Tierney model: the enhancement approach to action research. Journal of Advanced Nursing 24: 129–38.

Bowman GS, Webster RA, Thompson DR (1991) The development of a classification system for nurses' work methods. Internatinal Journal of Nursing Studies 28(2): 175–87.

Brown JS, Tanner CA, Padrick KP (1983) Nursing search for scientific knowledge. Nurse Researcher 33: 26–32.

Butterworth T, Bishop V, Carson J (1996) First steps towards evaluating clinical supervision in nursing and health visiting. I. Theory, policy and practice development. A review. Journal of Clinical Nursing 5:127–32.

Closs SL, Cheater FM (1994) Utilization of nursing research: culture, interest and support. Journal of Advanced Nursing 19: 762–73.

Culyer A (1994) Supporting Research and Development in the NHS. London: HMSO.

Cunningham I (1992) Interactive holistic research: researching self managed learning. In Reason P (Ed) Human Inquiry in Action. London: Sage Publications.

Darby M, Lam B, McMahon A (1991) An evaluation of the respite care services at a hospital for the elderly. Research Advisory Group, Royal College of Nursing, London.

Department of Health (1989) A Strategy for Nursing. London: Department of Health.

Department of Health (1991a) The Patients' Charter. London: HMSO.

Department of Health (1991b) Research for Health: A Research and Development Strategy for the NHS. London: HMSO.

Department of Health (1992a) Health of the Nation. London: HMSO.

Department of Health (1992b) Tomlinson Review. London: HMSO.

Department of Health (1993a) A Vision for the Future. Report of the Chief Nursing Officer. London: HMSO.

Department of Health (1993b) Clinical Audit. London: HMSO.

Dickson R (1996) Dissemination and implementation: the wider picture. Nurse Researcher 4(1): 5–14.

Draper J (1996) Nursing development units; an opportunity for evaluation. Journal of Advanced Nursing 23: 267–71.

Elliott J (1991) Action Research for Educational Change. Buckingham: Open University Press.

European Health Committee (CDSP 95) (1996) Nursing Research Report and Recommendations. Strasbourg: Council of Europe.

Foundation of Nursing Studies (1994) Annual Report: Where does nursing fit into your life? London: The Foundation of Nursing Studies.

Graham I (1996) A presentation of a conceptual framework and its use in the definition of nursing development within a number of nursing developments units. Journal of Advanced Nursing 23: 260–6.

Greenwood J (1984) Nursing research: a position paper. Journal of Advanced Nursing 9: 77–82.

Hamer S (1992) Developing the Research Resource in the Nursing and Therapy Professions. Harrogate: Yorkshire Regional Health Authority.

Hammick M (1995) A research and journal club: a medium for teaching, professional development and networking. European Journal of Cancer Care 4: 33–7.

Holter IM, Schwartz-Barcott D (1993) Action research: what is it? How has it been used and how can it be used in nursing? Journal of Advanced Nursing 18: 189–304.

House of Lords Select Committee on Science and Technology (1988) Priorities in Medical Research. London: HMSO.

Hunt M (1987) Translating research findings into nursing practice. Journal of Advanced Nursing 12: 101–10.

Jackson S, McMahon A, Cage R (1993) Prevention and management of pressure sores. British Journal of Nursing 2(13): 672–7.

Jones S (1996) An action research investigation into the feasibility of experienced registered nurse sick children's nurses (RSCNs) becoming children's emergency nurse practitioners (ENPs). Journal of Clinical Nursing 5: 13–21.

Kelly P, Evans M, Jordan A, Orem V (1996) Developing a new method to record care at home for children with cancer: an example of research and practice collaboration in a regional paediatric oncology unit. European Journal of Cancer Care 5: 26–31.

King's Fund Centre Nursing Developments Programme (1992) Nursing, Midwifery or Health Visiting Development Units. Guidelines for preparation of proposals. London: King's Fund Centre.

Kirchhoff KT, Beck SL (1994) Using the journal club a component of the research utilisation process. Heart and Lung 23(3): 246–50.

Kitson A, Currie L (1996) Clinical practice development and research activities in four district health authorities. Journal of Clinical Nursing 5: 41–51.

Kitson A, Ahmed LB, Harvey G, Seers K, Thompson DR (1996) From research to practice: one organisational model for promoting research based practice. Journal of Advanced Nursing 23: 430–40.

Knight S (1994) An organisational approach. Nursing Times 90(41): 33–5.

Lewin K (1946) Action research and minority problems. Journal of Social Issues 2: 34–46.

Lindquist R, Robert RC, Treat D (1990) A clinical practice journal club: bridging the gap between research and practice. Focus on Critical Care 17(5): 402–6.

Lorentzen M (1994) Nursing Development Units: professionalization strategy for nurses, cheap service option or genuine improvement in patient care? Journmal of Advanced Nursing 19:835–6.

Luker K (1992) Research and development in nursing. Journal of Advanced Nursing 17: 1151–2.

Luker K (1996) Research and the configuration of nursing services. Journal of Clinical Nursing. 6(4): 259–68.

McMahon A (1997) Implications for nursing for the NHS R&D funding policy. Nursing Standard 28(11): 44–8.

McMahon A, Darby M-A (1993) Research and Development – Nurse Led, Unit Wide. Madrid: International Congress of Nurses.

McMahon A, Jackson S (1992) A Clinical Risk Management Programme. Harrogate: Quality Assurance Network Annual Conference.

McMahon A, Smith, K (1993) Evaluation in practice. British Journal of Nursing 2(12): 625–30.

Malby R (1992) A credit where it's due. Nursing Times 88(43): 48–50.

Malby R (1996) In Baker M, Kirk S (Eds) Research and Development for the NHS. Evidence, Evaluation and Effectiveness. Oxford: Radcliffe Medical Press.

Maxwell N (1984) From Knowledge to Wisdom: a revolution in the aims and methods of science.Oxford: Blackwell.

Meerabeau L (1996) Managing policy research in nursing. Journal of Advanced Nursing 24: 633–39.

Morgan L, Fennessey G (1996) Levels of Evidence. DQI Network News 4: 3.

Morrell C, Harvey G, Kitson K (1995) The Reality of Practitioner-Based Quality Improvement. National Institute for Nursing Report no. 14.

Mulhall A (1995) Nursing research: what difference does it make? Journal of Advanced Nursing 21: 576–83.

Neal K (1994) The function and aims of nursing development units. Nursing Times 90(41): 31–3.

NHS Centre for Reviews and Dissemination (1996) Undertaking systematic reviews of research on effectiveness. CDR guidelines for those carrying out or commissioning reviews. York: NHS Centre for Reviews and Dissemination.

Neal K (1994) The function and aims of nursing development units. Nursing Times 90(41): 31–3.

Nursing Standard and NHS Centre for Reviews and Dissemination (1997) Systematic Reviews: Examples for Nursing. London: RCN Publishing Company.

Pope C, Mays N (1993) Opening the blackbox: an encounter in the corridors of health services research. British Medical Journal 306(6873): 315–8.

Redfern S, Norman I, Murrells T, Christian S, Gilmore A, Normand C, Langham S (1994) External review of the Department of Health Funded Nursing Development Units: Consultation Seminar – Project Paper 1. London: Department of Health.

Robinson K (1996) Funding sources for nurse researchers. Nurse Researcher 4(2): 57–64.

Roe B (1993) Undertaking a critical review of the literature. Nurse Researcher 1(1): 31–42.

Russell IT, Wilson BJ (1992) Audit: the third clinical science? Quality in Health Care 1: 51–5.

Secretaries of State for Health (1989) Working for Patients. Cm 555. London: HMSO.

Secretaries of State for Health and Social Services (1989) Caring for People: Community Care in the Next Decade and Beyond. London: HMSO.

Secretaries of State for Social Security (1987) Promoting Better Health. London: HMSO.

Secretary of State for Health (1996) The National Health Service: a service with ambitions. London: HMSO.

Shelton SE (1988) Keeping pace with nursing literature through a professional gerontological nursing journal club. Journal of Geronological Nursing 14(11): 16–28.

Thomas S, Ingham A (1995) The unit based clinical practice development: a practitioner's and a manager's perspective. In Kendrick K, Weir P, Rosser E (Eds) Innovations in Nursing Practice. London: Edward Arnold.

Tibbles L, Sanford R (1994) The Research Journal Club: a mechanism for research utilization. Clinical Nurse Specialist 223–6.

Tierney AJ, Taylor J (1991) Research in practice: an 'experiment' in researcher–practitioner collaboration. Journal of Advanced Nursing 16: 506–10.

UKCC (1992) Code of Professional Conduct for the Nurse, Midwife and Health Visitor. 3rd edn. London: UKCC.

Van Cott ML, Tittle MB, Moody LE, Wilson ME (1991) Analysis of a decade of critical care nursing practice research: 1979–1988. Heart and Lung 20: 394–7.

Webb C (1993) Action research: philosophy, methods and personal experience. In Kitson A (Ed) Nursing, Art and Science. London: Chapman & Hall.

Yorkshire Regional Health Authority (1991) A report of an audit of research activity of nurses and professions allied to medicine. Harrogate: Yorkshire Regional Health Authority.

Chapter 12
The dissemination and utilisation of research

Sheila Rodgers

Introduction

The dissemination and utilisation of research findings has become an area of great interest to practitioners, managers and policy makers in all areas of the health services. Previously, the efforts of individuals were needed for dissemination and utilisation but this was haphazard and ineffective and more active implementation of research was required (Department of Health, 1995). The number of practices based on research is thought to be quite low in all aspects of health care delivery. It has been estimated that only 15 per cent of medical interventions carried out in the NHS in the UK have been proven to be effective in improving the health of patients (Smith, 1991). Yet, in nursing, little evidence exists on the extent of research utilisation although there has been extensive speculation about ritualistic practice (Walsh and Ford, 1989).

Nursing has been plagued by the assumption that if researchers identify an area of interest, conduct and publish research, practising nurses will read it and use it. This assumption must be challenged if nursing is to move forward to becoming a research-based profession.

The impact of NHS policies

Hunter and Polit (1992) argue that the use of research and its influence in health policy has been minimal at even the highest level in the Government: 'the direct deliberate and systematic use of research findings is so rare as to be negligible' (Hunter and Polit, 1992: 164).

The lack of research implementation in practice and policy making was recognised with the first strategy for research and development (R and D) in the NHS in 1991, which aimed to change health care so that it would become based on relevant high quality research (Department of Health, 1991):

> The prime objective is to see that R&D becomes an integral part of health care so that clinicians, managers and other staff find it natural to rely on the results of research in their day to day decision making and longer term strategic planning. (Department of Health, 1991: 1)

Research was proposed to look at how to promote the uptake of good projects once developed and evaluated in clinical trials, along with an information strategy and a projects register to centralise information about ongoing and completed research.

Sir Michael Peckham (Director of R and D) had firm views that health service practice should become research based, with new approaches being carefully trialled and evaluated against existing practices. He advocated extended trials to take into account economic feasibility and commercial viability (Peckham, 1991). This policy was to a great extent driven by the need for cost containment. This continues to be a strong motivating factor as escalating costs outstrip resources. Rapid technological developments in health care, a need to introduce objectivity into health care services planning and seeing the patient as an informed consumer have also raised the profile of quality issues. All of these factors drive the need for a research-based health service (Luker and Kenrick, 1995).

In 1991, the Scottish Strategy for Nursing Research was also published (SOHHD, 1991). Whereas the move toward research utilisation was supported, there was little comment on how this was to be achieved. There was no specification of who was to take responsibility for the process, nor of the resources that would be available. In contrast, the English Strategy for Nursing Research (Department of Health, 1993) placed more emphasis on the development of a research culture by health service managers (Closs and Cheater, 1994).

In 1995, 20 priority areas covering many aspects of implementation were identified for study by the Department of Health (1995). Throughout this report the orientation is stated as health services research yet the detail refers to clinicians and relies heavily on publications relating to the implementation of medical research. Whereas many of the priority areas could be of equal concern to nursing and midwifery practice, the tone of the report is clearly medically focused and the relevance for nursing, midwifery and professions allied to medicine (PAMs) is only established in a few of the priority areas. These priorities have now been used to set the research agenda in the study of dissemination and implementation of research in the health services.

Effectiveness and efficiency

In the drive for cost containment and value for money, effectiveness and efficiency have become key goals of the health service. Clinical effectiveness would seem to be based upon the application of sound research to practice. However, several definitions exist and other similar terms co-exist.

Effectiveness may be defined as the likelihood of desired outcomes resulting from some type of intervention, whereas clinical effectiveness is the likelihood of desired relevant clinical outcomes. Efficiency concerns the value and extent of the outcome compared to the costs of carrying out the intervention. The costs should include not only financial costs and the time of health care staff involved but also the costs to the patient in terms of any undesired effects. Efficiency is not just about whether something is value for money – although this is important, especially in policy and resource allocation decisions. Deykin and Haines (1996) caution against an assessment of effectiveness alone and argue that effective practices can be used inappropriately or with the wrong client group. Appropriateness is a more subjective factor but it is essential to take it into consideration.

The term 'evidence-based practice' is also used to describe practice based on information or knowledge. French (1996) sees evidence-based practice as synonymous with research-based practice. However, many different types of evidence can and have to be used as a basis for practice. Mulhall (1996) argues that knowledge is not only derived from empirical research but also from nursing theory and clinical knowledge encompassing both life events and nursing experience.

Yet personal experience and anecdote can lead to strong personal beliefs that can significantly influence practice. Closs and Cheater (1994) argue that too much health service practice is based upon personal belief rather than research-based evidence. However, when experience includes a process of reflection, analysis and evaluation, this can lead to the development of great expertise on which much of health care has been based. There are some difficulties with this in that extraneous variables may lead to invalid conclusions, or an insufficiently critical analysis of the experience may occur. There is a need for thorough reflection and analysis as well as much caution when relying on personal evidence.

Randomised controlled trials (RCTs) are often seem as the gold standard of evidence, especially in medical research (Woolf et al., 1990). Yet RCTs may not always be the most appropriate method to study a problem in health care. Nursing, in particular, embraces a more eclectic approach and other forms of research are viewed as being relevant and rigorous.

When there is no research, expert opinion may have to be used, along with patient opinion. Neither should be discounted in the face of research evidence as expert and patient opinion will be contextually based and this may be more important in some instances. When research is generalised, assumptions can be made about what might happen in similar prescribed circumstances. However, only the expert knowledgeable practitioner can assess the particular circumstances. Individual cases are not only complex and multi-factorial but are also subject to the patient's informed choice and moral and ethical decision making. Levels of probability of outcome or calculations of numbers of patients needed to be treated before any significant effect is seen can be applied to populations but when a practitioner is caring for an individual, this information has to be considered alongside the expert assessment of the patient by the practitioner and the patient's wishes. Policy makers and purchasers may find the 'evidence' more compelling when considering a generic issue or a population, where it must have economic, professional and social benefit (Cavanagh and Tross, 1996).

The discussion so far has assumed that research evidence is used directly in some type of new intervention or practice. Directly applicable research may lead to the development of protocols but this may not be the case for all research outcomes. Not all research is directly or 'instrumentally' applicable but some may be more indirect or conceptually influential on practice:

> they may extend the way that nurses think about what they do, how they relate to the people they care for, and generally stimulate more reflective and questioning practice (Closs and Cheater, 1994: 762).

Richardson et al. (1990) recognised the existence of research that might be of indirect use or illuminating, but subsequent policy papers have neglected this important application of research.

A study by Rodgers (1994) led to the definition of research utilisation given in Table 12.1.

Table 12.1: A definition of research utilisation

Research utilisation:

A process directed toward the transfer of research-based knowledge into nursing practice.

Research-based knowledge results from corroborated studies and may be of:

- Direct use – explanatory and predictive findings immediately applicable to practice.
- Indirect use – enlightening, extending understanding of practice.
- Methodological use – measurement scales, outcome measures or tools that may be used in practice.

Evidence-based practice, then, is required politically in order to make the best use of available resources, including technology, and to link clinical effectiveness and cost efficiency. Professionally, it is required for accountability, to promote research-based practice and to involve and inform patients.

Nurses and nursing research

The definition of accountability has moved on as practice knowledge was previously sufficient to justify practice whereas now there is a drive for knowledge derived from research:

> Practitioners are under an implicit and sometimes explicit obligation to demonstrate that they are acting according to the most up to date and available knowledge, and there is now an expectation that health care should be informed by research as well as practice based knowledge. (Luker and Kenrick, 1995: 60)

There is now also an expectation with PREP that registered nurses will be well informed (UKCC, 1990). Pre-registration education of nurses is almost exclusively at diploma level since the introduction of the 1992 Project 2000 programmes. However, one might ask whether this equips them sufficiently to be able to read, critically analyse and synthesise findings from research papers. It could be argued that nurses require these skills if they are to be meaningful consumers of research. The majority of existing nurses were trained prior to 1992 and are unlikely to have had much formal education in research. Unless this situation is addressed the likelihood is that most nurses will continue to be mystified by research, see it as someone else's business and continue to base their practice on social norms and personal beliefs.

Nursing research, then, is essential for accountable professional practice and practice that is clinically effective and efficient. However doubts exist as to whether there is a sufficient body of research knowledge in nursing on which to base practice. The Briggs report is generally acknowledged as the first call in the UK for nursing to become a research-based profession (Briggs, 1972), yet progress has been slow.

There is some concern that nursing research is under-resourced, both in terms of funding for projects and in lacking sufficient post-doctoral expertise. Large-scale, fully funded, multi-centre, post-doctoral research appears to be the exception rather than the rule in nursing. There has been a proliferation of small-scale one-off studies that, although of value, should not be considered as a basis for changes in practice without at least some attempt at replication. In the English Strategy for Nursing Research (Department of Health, 1993) it was recognised that there were a large number of small, poorly supported studies in nursing.

The dissemination of research

Traditionally, research has been disseminated through journal publications but the literature is now so vast that information overload has resulted for many health care professionals (Deykin and Haines, 1996). Nursing is no exception to this. There has been a real increase in the volume of nursing literature:

> which threatens to swamp competent researchers in specialised fields let alone practitioners who may hold more general interests (Mulhall, 1996: 191).

As well as coping with the volume of literature, the language and complexity of reports causes further difficulties. Much research is written in a manner that makes it difficult to understand or it may be of poor quality (Peters, 1992; Rodgers, 1994). Research tends to be reported in the research journals for academic scrutiny, whereas practitioners tend to read other types of nursing journals. In particular, practitioners may find it difficult to comprehend what the implications for practice may be unless these are made clear by researchers. The wider use of short reports in professional journals might therefore be a particularly useful strategy.

Much of the literature is of very varied quality and many practitioners may feel that they lack the skills to appraise the reports. It is possible to use reviews on a topic where an author has drawn together and interpreted some of the literature in an area. French (1996) cites indwelling urinary catheter care as a case in point.

Accessing the original research may be difficult and in some cases unlikely if there are no systematic reviews in the area. Unsystematic reviews have limited value but again the problem is not exclusive to nursing. Deykin and Haines (1996) report that many traditional review articles in medical journals are also of poor quality:

> The use of unsystematic reviewing procedures results in the possibility that practice becomes based on unquestioned popular consensus rather than rigorous reliable evidence (French, 1996: 114).

Sources of information

In contrast, a systematic review critically reviews all the research in one particular subject area. Another form of synthesising research knowledge in an area is meta-analysis, where all the results from a number of studies are combined (see Chapter 6). Such rigorous synthesis can provide important and useful knowledge but the statistical procedures and methods used are very complex and are difficult for many nurses to understand and appraise and it is not easy for them to work out what the practice implications are, unless these are made clear by the researcher.

The NHS Centre for Reviews and Dissemination (CRD) was set up in 1994 as part of the information strategy of the NHS R and D strategy. The Centre aims to promote research-based practice in the NHS by providing systematic reviews on selected topics. These reviews are maintained on databases and an information service is provided. Bulletins such as the *Effective Health Care Bulletin,* newsletters and patient information leaflets are produced to disseminate the findings of the reviews. The Database of Abstracts of Reviews of Effectiveness (DARE), produced by CRD, is a bibliography of published research that has been subject to systematic review. Within CRD, the Practice and Service Development Initiative focuses on disseminating relevant research to nurses, midwives and health visitors and other PAMs.

The Cochrane Collaboration was also part of the NHS R and D information strategy and has similar aims to CRD but focuses solely on the review of randomised controlled trials (RCTs) and has strong international links. The Cochrane database of systematic reviews is available on-line or on CD-ROM. Separate databases exist on pregnancy and childbirth and on effective professional practice. However the vast majority of topics reviewed are based on clinical treatments for different pathologies, which is perhaps not surprising given that it deals exclusively with RCTs. Some reviews in the

Cochrane Collaboration on Effective Professional Practice (CCEPP) do have a much broader remit and also specifically address nursing practice.

The aim of these centres is to produce information for evidence-based health care but there is a concern that practitioners must be able to retain clinical freedom to pursue care for the individual as they see best and to follow what the individual wants. It may be difficult to go counter to government-sponsored research and any guidelines produced from it (Deykin and Haines, 1996). Chapter 13 provides a full discussion on the use of guidelines and protocols. A National Projects Register at the Department of Health has also been developed and should prove a useful resource to search out ongoing or unpublished research. (Contact details for CRD and the Cochrane centres are given at the end of the chapter.)

French (1996) argues that nurses are not using these new databases as they are not generally available to all clinical staff in the Trusts. All the midwives in a study by Meah et al. (1996) knew about the Cochrane database but they had difficulty gaining access to it. Part of the problem may be the difficulty in accessing libraries as nursing moves into higher education.

Few studies in nursing have examined the effect of different forms of dissemination but one such study has been conducted by Luker and Kenrick (1995). One hundred and thirty district nurses completed pre- and post-test questionnaires to test their knowledge on leg ulcer care; 109 of the nurses received a research-based information pack on leg ulcer care, with the remainder acting as controls. A significant knowledge gain was demonstrated six weeks after receipt of the pack in the experimental group, but this was not evident in the control group. Unfortunately the authors did not enquire to what extent the nurses were basing their practice on the research-based knowledge.

Pearcey (1995) surveyed 398 nurses and found that 69 per cent had current research information distributed to their place of work, but 59 per cent felt it was inadequate in some way. They said it was not distributed sufficiently widely, there was a lack of time to read and no discussion took place.

Mugford et al. (1991) reviewed studies on feedback designed to change practice. Feedback was more effective when clinicians already had an interest in the area or were conducting a review, whereas unsolicited feedback was found to have little effect. Both Pearcey and Draper (1996) and Armitage (1990) found that, even when great efforts were made to provide nurses with what seemed to be relevant research, the information was either rejected or ignored.

It is perhaps a little disappointing, but not surprising, that printed material such as journal publications and information sent by mail have been ineffective in changing practice (Freemantle and Watt, 1994). Many other methods of distributing information about research findings have been proposed such as audit and feedback, conferences, education and educational material, use and development of practice guidelines, marketing, opinion leaders, academic detailing and reminder systems (Department of Health, 1995). Unfortunately they all tend to be focused on one particular approach and on one particular topic, rather than using a 'whole system' approach to shift to a research culture. Most have only just begun to be evaluated and this is mainly in relation to medical practice.

Critical appraisal skills

Although providing information alone seems to have little effect on practice, the ability to critically appraise research papers seems to be a prerequisite for implementation. In the report of the task force on R and D, it was clearly stated that research literacy is needed before a move to research-based practice can be made (Department of Health, 1992).

The provision of research courses for nurses would seem to be essential. Not only does education in research create a more positive attitude to research (Harrison et al., 1991) but it can make research more accessible and easier to read. Closs and Cheater (1994) do not support the separate teaching of a methods course in research but prefer the teaching of topics throughout the curriculum from a research base. Such a form of teaching from a research base was found to be significantly associated with a higher level of research-based practice in a recent survey of 680 nurses (Rodgers, 1997).

The expertise of nurses in critically evaluating reported research has to be questioned. Both Hunt (1987) and Armitage (1990) found that nurses were hampered by their lack of critical reading skills when trying to implement research, whereas French (1996) suggests that nurses seem to have a positive attitude to research but lack confidence and the ability to evaluate and use it. Pearcey (1995) surveyed 398 nurses to ask them what they perceived their needs were for research skills training. She found that 97 per cent were not satisfied with their research skills, and felt they needed the basic skills of searching the literature, reading and evaluating reports and the application of research.

One project that has attempted to address this issue with health service staff is the Critical Appraisal Skills Programme (CASP). This is part of the Getting Research into Practice Project (GRiPP), which began in Oxfordshire in 1993 and looked at how selected topics could become more research-based in practice. CASP uses multidisciplinary workshops where clinical problems are discussed and research literature is reviewed in order to appraise the evidence on potential solutions to a problem. These workshops are described in detail by Milne (1995). Contact details are also given at the end of the chapter.

Nursing research utilisation

The fact that the findings of research or any innovation appear to have significant advantages for practice does not mean to say that they will sell themselves to the target audience. Peters (1992) suggests that we would only have to implement what we know from current research to give significant improvements in health, without conducting any further research. It seems that the problem of lack of utilisation is the one that needs to be addressed:

> There are more difficulties in implementing the results of health services research into practice then there are with the results of clinical research (Chief Scientist Reports, 1992: 66).

In the knowledge-driven model or rational deductive approach, new knowledge is created, made known and then its use is assumed. Williamson (1992) suggests that failure results if practitioners do not perceive that there is a problem that requires change, and so may dismiss the research as of no consequence. Kitson et al. (1996) argue that the knowledge-driven model neglects the complexity of organisational issues, contextual and organisational factors. Rogers (1983) described a model of adoption of innovations to explain how new findings come to influence behaviour. The first stage in the model is one of knowledge or awareness, where the individual learns about the new practice or innovation. Following an assessment of the potential advantages and disadvantages of the practice and other characteristics such as its complexity, a decision is reached about whether this would be a good practice to adopt. This is called the stage of persuasion or belief in a practice. A decision is then made about whether or not to try out the practice – the stage of *implementation*. Following this, there will be an evaluation of the innovation in use and a decision taken concerning whether or not to continue with the innovation – the stage of *confirmation*. This model has been used quite widely in the study of nursing research utilisation (Brett, 1987; Coyle and Sokop, 1990; Pearcey and Draper, 1996; Rodgers, 1994; Michel and Sneed, 1995).

Most studies to date on nursing research utilisation have been carried out in North America. There is limited information about the extent of research utilisation in the UK, much of which has been small scale and ungeneralisable (Cullum, 1996). This has now become a rapidly expanding area of research. Some of the findings from key North American studies are presented here, followed by a review of important studies conducted in the UK.

North American studies

Ketefian (1975) was one of the first to look at research in practice. The use of the research finding that nine minutes were required for an accurate recording of oral temperature using a mercury thermometer was assessed. Only one out of 87 nurses used the practice. Kirchhoff (1982) looked at the extent to which coronary precautions had been discontinued following research that showed they were no longer necessary. Twenty-four per cent had discontinued iced water restrictions whilst 35 per cent no longer recorded rectal temperature.

Brett (1987) surveyed 279 nurses on their level of adopting 14 research-based nursing practices. The practices were thought to be important findings, to be useful in the context of acute hospital nursing, to have scientific merit, to be suitable to apply to practice, and to be usable independently by nurses. The nurses were asked to report whether they were aware of each practice, whether they were persuaded that they should use it, and whether they used it sometimes or used it always, according to Rogers' (1983) model of adoption of innovation. Levels of adoption were scored from 0 to 4 points. Level of adoption varied according to the nursing practice concerned. On average, only four of the nursing practices were used 'sometimes' and only one was 'always' used. Nine of the practices were therefore infrequently used by the nurses. The total mean adoption score across all practices was 2.17, which suggests that the nurses were somewhere around being persuaded and just beginning to use the practices sometimes. Coyle and Sokop (1990) replicated the study with 112 nurses. Their findings were consistent with Brett's, the total mean adoption score being 1.96 indicating that the nurses were only in the stage of persuasion.

Champion and Leach (1989) achieved a response from 59 (39 per cent) out of 150 nurses to their questionnaire, assessing variables thought to be linked with utilisation. Ten questions related to self report of use of research were included. A moderate level of research utilisation was reported, with a slight tendency to agree that they used research in practice. However the validity of self reporting on use of research has to be questioned.

Michel and Sneed (1995) studied 200 graduate nurses from one hospital. An 84 per cent response rate was achieved. They assessed the adoption of five nursing practices based on Rogers (1983) adoption of innovation model. The mean adoption score was 2.21, indicating that the nurses were mostly only persuaded about using the practices and in the very early stages of beginning to use them. However, this study included a significant number of non-clinical staff (43 per cent). The relevance of use of the research findings by managers and educators may be limited and the results are not comparable with other studies where the focus is on the practice of clinical nurses.

None of these studies attempted to look at research findings that may be more conceptual or indirect in their application. Practices that may require the co-operation of other staff were also purpose excluded, further limiting the generalisability of any of these results.

UK studies

Hunt (1987) attempted to use an action research project to look at the translation of research findings into practice beginning with a group of nurse teachers undertaking literature searches. They then produced summaries and guidelines, held study days and went through hospital committees to affect a policy change on mouth care. A triad of ward sister, manager and teacher was created to address changes at ward level. However, there was only very limited success, with scant uptake of new mouth-care practices and no change in pre-operative fasting regimes.

Armitage (1990) reports a study in which a small working group aimed to seek out examples of research-based practice. However, they found that very little research was being used and even this was without any real understanding:

> it was established that research was not being used with any depth of understanding except in a very few isolated instances (Armitage, 1990: 12).

Lacey (1994) conducted a small study to look at research utilisation. A survey of 20 nurses was conducted using the questionnaire developed by Champion and Leach (1989). Interviews were also conducted as part of the study aimed at establishing whether this would be a useful instrument for a UK context. A positive attitude to research was generally found. When the nurses were asked about what sort of research-based practice they used, wound care, pressure sore prevention, pre-operative care and control of cross infection were mentioned most often. Seven out of 20 knew about research in pre-operative fasting but only two out of 20 were able to use these findings.

All the studies described here are based on self report of research utilisation. In their study of community nurses, Luker and Kenrick (1995) found that nurses could not easily distinguish between research-based and practice-based knowledge, seeing this as an artificial distinction.

In a recently completed study, 680 clinical nurses working in general medical and surgical wards in Scotland responded to a questionnaire designed to assess their research utilisation (Rodgers, 1997). A methodology based on Rogers' (1983) model of adoption of innovations was developed for a UK context through an exploratory study (Rodgers, 1994). The issue of the validity of self-reported use of research was resolved through interviews in a pilot study. Scores on individual practices ranged from 60 per cent of nurses never having heard of a practice to 84 per cent always using a practice. The mean score for all nurses across all 14 nursing practices was 2.65 suggesting that, on average, nurses in this survey had heard of, believed in and were making progress using the practices. The study included research findings of indirect or conceptual use as well as those of direct or instrumental use. The nurses tended to score quite highly on the practices that were of more indirect use.

Influences on the utilisation of research

Much of the early literature on influences on research utilisation focused on the characteristics of individual nurses, rather than of the organisation in which they were working, based on the assumption that utilisation of research was an individual responsibility (Champion and Leach, 1989). All studies conducted to date have collected elements of demographic and personal details but few correlations with levels of research utilisation have been found. Most studies have highlighted the importance of education and reading and the need to have sufficient ownership and authority over the introduction of new practices.

Michel and Sneed (1995), in their study of graduate nurses, found that nurses who had a higher level of education and perceived a policy to exist were more likely to base their practice on research. What is not clear is whether education leads to research-based practice or whether higher education attracts particular types of nurses who have research-based practice. Ehrenfield and Eckerlings (1991) found that higher education degrees were related to use of research findings in that the nurses were more able to cope with research activities and had more positive attitudes towards research. The association between a higher educational level and research utilisation was also found in a survey in Scotland, and was followed up in interviews with the nurses (Rodgers, 1997). Here the nurses explained how completing degree studies not only gave them the knowledge and skills to appraise research and demonstrate their use in justifying practice but also that they felt more confident and assertive and would be more likely to question practice.

Studying research has been identified in several studies as being associated with more positive attitudes to utilisation (Champion and Leach, 1989; Pearcey, 1995). Comparing different types of education, Lacey (1994) found nurses felt that courses led to an increase in knowledge of research and improved morale, whereas degree courses often involved engagement in some type of research. In another study, nurses said that on courses, as opposed to study days, they were expected to engage in study and read and complete course work whereas attendance at study days and conferences could be an entirely passive experience and was often more of a morale booster (Rodgers, 1997).

Brett (1987) found significant relationships between research utilisation and the time a nurse spent reading and attending research conferences. These findings were confirmed in the replication study by Coyle and Sokop (1990) who also found that greater job satisfaction was correlated with higher research utilisation, although they offer no explanation for this. Rodgers (1997) also found that nurses who read at least one journal regularly, had attended more study days and conferences, or had greater job satisfaction, had a higher level of research utilisation. These relationships were explored further in interviews with a sub-sample. Greater job satisfaction seemed to be related to feelings of autonomy and carrying out individualised patient care. A lack of autonomy has been cited by nurses in several studies as being a barrier to research utilisation:

> Nurses who have ideas about how they wish to alter practice at times feel powerless to act as the final decision is not theirs to make when other disciplines are involved, for example with drug administration and pre-operative fasting. (Armitage, 1990: 13)

There is a lack of role models in nursing for those who use research, question practice and challenge the status quo (Phillips, 1986) although the charge nurse can be a powerful role model for nurses in a ward setting (Rodgers, 1997). Lacey (1994) found one of the biggest barriers to implementation to be lack of autonomy and not feeling able to challenge medical colleagues. The nurses perceived a lack of co-operation from medical and theatre staff in the same way as nurses in the study by Hunt (1987). However, when doctors and theatre staff were approached by nurses in Hunt's study, they were actually found to be co-operative. These findings were confirmed in a later study, where perceived lack of co-operation of medical and other staff was not associated with a lower level of research utilisation (Rodgers, 1997). More important was the lack of self confidence, skills to appraise research, assertiveness and the ability to question practice, including that which required medical staff involvement. A higher level of self confidence was associated with higher perceived autonomy. This suggests that if a nurse has the knowledge, education and experience then questioning others, including medical staff, will be more likely.

Hunt (1987) suggested that charge nurses had a high degree of autonomy as many chose to ignore new guidelines on mouth care. Another interpretation might be that the charge nurses did not perceive a problem with mouth care and so saw no need to change. One of the reasons for the rejection of information on research-based practices is thought to be a lack of ownership by nurses (Armitage, 1990). It would seem more important that a climate for nurses to question and solve their own problems needs to be created to effect research-based practice. Important features of the type of climate where research-based practice was promoted were thought to include being given the authority for practice and the ward being organised to deliver individualised patient care (Rodgers, 1994, 1997). Nurses felt that when care was patient centred, they were able to practise at a higher level, making decisions about individual patients' care rather than following routine or ritual. Where the charge nurse used a participative management style, teamwork, peer accountability, reflective practice and research utilisation were facilitated (Rodgers, 1997). The creation of this type of ward culture or climate seems to be very much the responsibility of the charge nurse although support from senior managers and a similar approach to the management of the organisation is also required.

Pearcey and Draper (1996) support the notion of staff involvement and used action research to study utilisation in one ward. The nursing staff identified the area of practice for development as preoperative information-giving, as practice was very varied and had no clear rationale. The nurses agreed to change practice and introduce protocols and, at this stage, were left to do this themselves. However, three months later they had failed to produce any protocols. Exactly why they failed to develop protocols is unclear, but there is mention that the ward was just beginning to use team nursing. Presumably task nursing was in place previously, which may not have led to any perceived individual responsibility for patient care but rather to rote, unthinking performance. This type of climate may be unlikely to succeed in changing to research-based practice. Efforts to move toward individualised patient care, greater autonomy and responsibility of nurses, and the creation of an open questioning climate by the charge nurse may have led to more research-based practice in general.

The effect of the ward climate was profound in one study (Rodgers, 1997). In a stepwise multiple regression of factors influencing research utilisation, the one factor that accounted for more variance than any other was if the nurse worked in a surgical ward as opposed to a medical ward. Based on nurses' interviews, reasons for this were thought to be that the nature of surgical care was more precise and predictable, and there was also often fast changing technology which urged the nurses to be receptive to change and aware of research. It was also suggested that there was a lack of research in medical nursing and that medical wards could have a very heavy workload, as opposed to the high turnover of the surgical wards. Several nurses also suggested that surgical nurses may be more assertive and more likely to question practice.

Haines and Jones (1994) support the view that the use of research in practice is less of an individual effort and more an organisational issue and that changes in practice can therefore be brought about through changes in the organisation and its culture. Such a view now seems to be the consensus in nursing (Closs and Cheater, 1994; Cavanagh and Tross, 1996; Kitson et al., 1996). The education of nurses without attention to the organisational climate is foolhardy:

> Individuals who have attended post basic and continuing education courses are often fired with enthusiasm for change. It is well recognised by many senior nurses that on their return to the work place it is often quenched by

the same system and circumstances from which they came. (Armitage, 1990:14)

One accepted method of introducing a new practice in an organisation is to introduce a new policy or procedure. However, such a strategy appears to be of little value. Brett (1987) and Rodgers (1997) found that there was no relationship between utilisation of research and the existence of a hospital policy.

Coyle and Sokop (1990) and Michel and Sneed (1995) both concluded that hospital policy may be an effective means to influence practice as they found a correlation between the adoption of a practice and nurses' perception that a hospital policy exists. However Brett (1987) and Rodgers (1997) found that there was no significant correlation between existence of a hospital policy and nurses' perception that a policy existed. It seems that nurses had little knowledge of the policies and procedures. In interviews, they were quite open that the policy and procedure manuals were either too large to read, out of date or just not part of everyday practice (Rodgers, 1997). Much greater use of policy and procedure manuals was reported when nurses had been involved in drawing them up using research to inform the policies. They were then highly motivated to put them into practice.

The mix of different types of nurses employed in the hospital setting has been found to have an influence on research utilisation. Brett (1987) found that when there was a higher percentage of nurses with a first degree in nursing, the level of research utilisation was higher. In the study by Rodgers (1997) research utilisation was higher where a greater proportion of the total nursing workforce was first-level registered nurses (RNs). During interviews, directors of nursing from the high-scoring hospitals in this study were strongly committed to employing a high percentage of first-level nurses. However, these directors were also notable in their commitment and strategic planning to achieving research-based practice and an autonomous professional nursing workforce. The clinical nurses argued that a higher proportion of first-level RNs enabled peer discussion and individualised patient care, which has also been associated with research utilisation. It seems that when a high proportion of high quality nurses are employed, not only does this reflect the commitment of the senior nurse executive to promoting the value of high quality professional nursing but that real opportunities for research-based care are facilitated in the clinical areas through peer discussion and the potential for systems of delivering individualised nursing care.

The size of an organisation may affect the ability of staff to make changes in practice. In the hospital setting, one might expect that large, acute specialist teaching hospitals might have a higher level of research-based practice. However Brett (1989) found that nurses in large hospitals, where there were many mechanisms to support research utilisation, had the lowest scores for research utilisation. Nurses in small hospitals with similar levels of support had the highest level of research utilisation. However, there is no evidence that any of the support mechanisms were actually used by and were affecting nurses at ward level in any of the hospitals. It would seem that, while mechanisms designed to create a climate for research utilisation, such as nurse research posts, attendance at conferences and access to journals may be introduced, size and complexity of an organisation may override any positive effects of these influences.

This finding is supported by a later study in the UK (Rodgers, 1997). A direct correlation was found between hospital size and utilisation of research, although two atypical hospitals were excluded from this analysis. The tendency was that the smaller the hospital, the higher the level of research utilisation. One of the atypical hospitals was one of the very largest ones, which also had the highest research utilisation score of all 25 hospitals in the study. Although this opposes the general trend, it was clear from the interviews conducted with nurses in this hospital that it was possible to overcome the negative effects of size through the use of other facilitative factors. A small size appeared to facilitate research utilisation because communication was thought to be easier, there was less bureaucracy and managers had to be more supportive of staff to ensure recruitment and retention.

The support of managers has been identified as one of the most important factors in facilitating research utilisation (Hunt, 1987; Armitage, 1990; Funk et al., 1991; Lacey, 1994; Rodgers, 1997). The main constituent of such support seems to be facilitation – providing access to ongoing education, encouraging staff to take ideas forward, representing staff within the bureaucracy, promoting a participative management style, ensuring a high proportion of first level RNs, disseminating research information and devolving authority for action to nurse/ward level.

In a study of variables thought to be linked with utilisation, Champion and Leach (1989) found that attitude was most highly correlated with utilisation, followed closely by availability of research. Support was not significantly correlated but when they broke down the scale into individual items, they found that the support of key managers including the director of nursing and head nurse was significantly correlated with use of research. Their support was needed to provide time for studying and reading, for access to courses and to show that they valued research utilisation by including it in appraisals and rewarding its use.

Funk et al. (1991) studied 924 clinical nurses, and found the two greatest barriers to utilisation were the feeling of not having enough authority to change patient care procedures and insufficient time to implement new ideas. Both barriers were of the work setting. All eight items relating to work setting were in the top 10 barriers including lack of support from doctors, managers and other staff, and lack of facilities and time. Presentation and accessibility of research were the next largest barriers. Funk et al. (1991) argue that those who use research in practice have enhanced perceptions of themselves as professionals and are more satisfied. This may be the case but it may be more related to the autonomy associated with, and proposed as a prerequisite for research-based practice. Nurses with a high level of autonomy may also be using their skills to their full extent in terms of discretion over decision making rather than being bored and unchallenged in a setting where the work is task orientated and there is no individual responsibility for patient care. Thus there has to be a complete climate shift to participative management, individualised care with individual nurse responsibility, ownership of change and management support:

> Decentralised administration and shared governance offer ways to give greater authority over practice to clinicians (Funk et al., 1991: 93).

Research utilisation has to be seen, then, as an organisational responsibility. As research utilisation is so complex and interdisciplinary, it requires a whole culture shift in the organisation and the NHS, including government bodies, to a climate where research is valued in informing practice. This valuing needs to be expressed in terms of taking a firm responsibility for utilisation, including the provision of resources.

Summary

The impact that the post 1992 diploma-level education will have on the ability of nurses to utilise research has yet to be assessed. What is clear is that utilisation is more likely when nurses have attended research courses and higher and further education. It seems that more education and higher levels of education enable nurses to gain not only knowledge and skills of appraisal but also the confidence and ability to be more questioning and reflective, leading to a higher level of research-based practice. A commitment to the higher and further education of nurses is essential.

Close involvement of staff in implementation is essential for sustained change and for staff to be truly committed to the change. There must be a shift in the overall organisational climate in relation to team building, the organisation of care, education and priority setting before any attempts at utilisation of research are conducted (Kitson et al., 1996).

Accountability in nursing may be redefined so that rather than practice being based on knowledge, it will be based on research. Along with this, systems of nursing that promote individual responsibility for patient care further a sense of accountability of the nurse to the patient. Autonomy for research-based practice is essential if nurses are to change their practice to becoming research based. The ability to justify practice not only to patients but also to peers seems important. A sufficiently high proportion of first level RNs must exist within the workforce and have opportunity for discussion for research utilisation, as one element of professional practice, to develop.

Managers must accept the responsibility for research utilisation in their organisations whilst devolving the necessary authority and providing sufficient resources to enable clinical nurses to utilise research. Strategies and action plans to co-ordinate a shift to research-based practice as the day-to-day norm must originate from senior nurse managers or the executive nurse and have the commitment and enthusiasm of the executive nurse in order to ensure that plans are taken forward. Research utilisation in nursing must be identified by the director of nursing as an issue and facilitated through a bottom-up process of change (Rodgers, 1997). Top-down centralised control of diffusion and utilisation is unlikely to lead to practice change. Discussion and ownership by practitioners are essential (French, 1996).

The influence and interaction of organisational factors on research utilisation need to be further explored in the UK. Action research has been advocated (Michel and Sneed, 1995) as the way forward for studying research utilisation. Attempts to use this approach in the UK have so far proven unsuccessful, however (Hunt, 1987; Pearcey and Draper, 1996). However this may be because the studies were both concerned with introducing 'one-off' practice changes rather than addressing the organisational climate. Focusing on only one area of practice at a time does not create the climate for research-based practice, and is slow and very time-consuming. A whole culture shift is required to inculcate new ways of thinking and working so that change is sustained and research-based practice becomes a way of life in all aspects of care.

Appendix 12.1: contact details

Getting Research into Practice Project (GRiPP) and Critical Appraisal Skills Programme
(CASP) Project Manager
GRiPP
Anglia and Oxford Regional Office
Old Road
Headington
Oxford
OX3 7LF

Centre for Reviews and Dissemination (CRD)
Information Officer
NHS Centre for Reviews and Dissemination
University of York
Heslington
York
YO1 5DD

Cochrane Collaboration
UK Cochrane Centre
NHS R&D Programme
Summertown Pavilion
Middle Way
Oxford
OX2 7LG

References

Armitage S (1990) Research utilisation in practice. Nurse Education Today 10(1): 10–15.

Brett JL (1987) Use of nursing practice and research findings. Nursing Research 36(6): 344–9.

Briggs A (1972) Report of the Committee on Nursing, Cmnd 5115. London: HMSO.

Cavanagh SJ, Tross G (1996) Utilising research findings in nursing: policy and practice considerations. Journal of Advanced Nursing 24: 1083–8.

Champion VL, Leach A (1989) Variables related to research utilisation in nursing. An empirical investigation. Journal of Advanced Nursing 14: 705–10.

Chief Scientist Reports (1992) Dissemination and Implementation of Research. Health Bulletin 50(1): 66–67.

Closs SJ, Cheater FM (1994) Utilisation of nursing research; culture interest and support. Journal of Advanced Nursing 19: 762–73.

Conduct and Utilisation of Research in Nursing Project (1983) Using Research to Improve Practice. MI, New York: Grune & Stratton.

Coyle LA, Sokop AG (1990) Innovation behaviour among nurses. Nursing Research 39(3): 176–80.

Cullum N (1996) Review: networking for research dissemination. NT Research 1(2): 119.

Department of Health (1991) Research for Health: A research and development strategy for the NHS. London: HMSO.

Department of Health (1992) Report of the task force on Research and Development. London: Department of Health.

Department of Health (1993) Report of the task force on the Strategy for Nursing Midwifery and Health Visiting 04/93. London: Department of Health.

Department of Health (1995) Methods to promote the implementation of research findings in the NHS: priorities for evaluation. Leeds: NHS Executive.

Deykin D, Haines A (1996) Promoting the use of research findings. In Peckham M, Smith R (Eds)The Scientific Basis of the Health Services. London: BMJ Publishing.

Ehrenfield M, Eckerlings S (1991) Perceptions and attitudes of registered nurses to research: a comparison with a previous study. Journal of Advanced Nursing 169(2): 224–320.

Freemantle N, Watt I (1994) Dissemination: Implementing the findings of research. Health Libraries Review 11: 133–7.

French B (1996) Networking for research dissemination; collaboration between research education and practice. NT Research 1(2): 113–18.

Funk SG, Champagne MT, Wiese RA, Tornquist EM (1991) Barriers to using research findings in practice. Applied Nursing Research 4(2): 90–5.

Haines A, Jones R (1994) Implementing research findings. British Medical Journal 308: 1488–92.

Harrison LL, Lowery B, Bailey T (1991) Changes in nursing students' knowledge about and attitudes towards research following an undergraduate research course. Journal of Advanced Nursing 16: 807–12.

Hunt M (1987) The process of translating research findings into nursing practice. Journal of Advanced Nursing 12: 101–10.

Hunter DJ, Polit C (1992) Developments in health services research: perspectives from Britain and the United States. Journal of Public Health Medicine 14(2): 164–8.

Ketefian S (1975) Application of selected nursing research findings into nursing practice. Nursing Research 24: 89–92.

Kirchhoff KT (1982) A diffusion survey of coronary precautions. Nursing Research 31: 196–201.

Kitson A, Ahmed LB, Harvey G, Seers K, Thompson D (1996) From research to practice: one organisational model for promoting research based practice. Journal of Advanced Nursing 23: 430–40.

Lacey E (1994) Research utilisation in nursing practice – a pilot study. Journal of Advanced Nursing 19: 987–95.

Luker KA, Kenrick M (1995) Towards knowledge based practice; an evaluation of a method of dissemination. International Journal of Nursing Studies 32(1): 59–67.

Meah S, Luker KA, Cullum NA (1996) An exploration of midwives' attitudes to research and perceived barriers to research utilisation. Midwifery 12: 73–84.

Michel Y, Sneed NV (1995) Dissemination and use of research findings in nursing practice. Journal of Professional Nursing 11(5): 306–11.

Milne R (1995) Piloting short workshops on the critical appraisal of reviews. Health Trends 27(4): 120–3.

Mugford M, Banfield P, O'Hanlon M (1991) Effects of feedback of information on clinical practice. British Medical Journal 303: 398–402.

Mulhall A (1996) Epidemiology Nursing and Health Care. Basingstoke: Macmillan.

Pearcey P (1995) Achieving research-based nursing practice. Journal of Advanced Nursing 22: 33–9.

Pearcey P, Draper P (1996) Using the diffusion of innovation model to influence practice; a case study. Journal of Advanced Nursing 23: 714–21.

Peckham M (1991) Research and development for the National Health Service. Lancet 338: 367–71.

Peters DA (1992) Implementation of research findings. Health Bulletin 50(1): 68–77.

Phillips LRF (1986) A Clinicians Guide to the Critique and Utilisation of Nursing Research. Norwalk, CT: Appleton Century Crofts.

Richardson A, Jackson C, Sykes W (1990) Taking Research Seriously. London: HMSO.

Rodgers SE (1994) An exploratory study of research utilisation by nurses in general medical and surgical wards. Journal of Advanced Nursing 20: 904–11.

Rodgers SE (1997) A study into the extent of, and factors influencing research utilisation by nurses in general medical and surgical wards in the Scottish health service. Unpublished Final Report Summary, Department of Nursing Studies, University of Edinburgh.

Rogers E (1983) Diffusion of Innovation. New York: Free Press.

Smith R (1991) Where is the wisdom? Editorial. British Medical Journal 303: 798–9.

SOHHD (1991) A Strategy for Nursing Research in Scotland. Edinburgh: SOHHD.

UKCC (1990) The report of the Post Registration Education and Practice Project.

London: United Kingdom Central Council for Nursing, Midwifery and Health Visting.

Walsh M, Ford P (1989) Nursing Rituals Research and Rational Action. Oxford: Butterworth-Heinemann.

Williamson P (1992) From dissemination to use: management and organisational barriers to the application of health services research finding. Health Bulletin 50(1): 76–8.

Woolf S, Battista R, Anderson G, Logan A, Wang E (1990) Assessing the clinical effectiveness of preventative manoeuvres: analytic principles and systematic methods in reviewing evidence and developing clinical practice recommendations. Journal of Clinical Epidemiology 43(9): 891–905.

Chapter 13
Use of clinical guidelines in the development of practice

Kate Seers

Introduction

It seems obvious that health care professionals all want to give patients the best possible care. However, the rationale for many of the things undertaken in day-to-day practice is not always clear nor is it based on sound evidence, but there is an increasing emphasis on providing efficient and effective care (Department of Health, 1991, 1993). Movement towards basing care on sound evidence is likely to be a very gradual process, and at the moment this evidence may not exist in many areas. However, it seems important to make sure there is an awareness of good evidence that does exist and, where there is no evidence, to know that care is based on current opinion so that one is thus more cautious in its application.

In the current drive towards making care evidence based, a plethora of terms have evolved, such as evidence-based medicine, nursing or health care (for example Sackett et al., 1997) and clinical effectiveness (NHSE,1996a). It is sometimes difficult to know how all these terms relate to each other and which to use. Sackett et al. (1997: 2) define evidence-based medicine as 'integrating individual clinical expertise with the best available external clinical evidence from systematic research'. This definition thus emphasises the integration of research evidence and professional judgement. Hicks (1997: 8) goes further and says that

> evidence based health care takes place when decisions that affect the care of patients are taken with due weight accorded to all valid, relevant information.

271

A more global interpretation can be found in the definition of clinical effectiveness as

> The extent to which specific clinical interventions, when deployed in the field for a particular patient or population, do what they are intended to do – i.e. maintain and improve health and secure the greatest possible health gain from the available resources (NHSE, 1996a: 45).

One could thus try to achieve clinical effectiveness by using evidence-based health care.

An indication of increasing activity in this area is the recent publication of journals such as *Clinical Effectiveness in Nursing*, launched in March 1997 and *Evidence Based Medicine* launched in November 1995 with *Evidence Based Nursing* due for publication in November 1997. Newell (1997: 1) described clinical effectiveness as providing nursing with 'its greatest challenge and its most powerful opportunity'. The whole area of using evidence and having it put into practice is an exciting opportunity, and this chapter will focus on one way of starting to use evidence in practice: clinical guidelines.

Development and use of guidelines

When practitioners identify a clinical problem, they increasingly want, or are urged, to try to solve that problem by finding the best available evidence. For most problems in practice that can be the beginning of a long process of trying to focus the clinical problem so it can become an answerable question, then finding the evidence, appraising that evidence, then trying to see whether it applies to those for whom you care. There may already be a methodologically sound systematic review of the area. To date these have been mainly, although not exclusively, based on evidence from randomised controlled trials (see Cochrane Library, 1997 version 2). Although this evidence can be extremely useful for answering questions about effectiveness (see Cullum (1997) for a review of randomised controlled trials in nursing), some questions in nursing and health care more generally will only be answerable using evidence from qualitative research. The science of developing a systematic review from qualitative research is in its infancy, although some guidance does exist, for example Noblit and Hare (1988).

Finding and using research evidence can be quite time consuming and requires a person (or team) skilled in asking focused clinical questions, searching for evidence, appraising that evidence and then deciding whether or not it applies to those for whom they care. Even then the process of having such evidence put into practice is not straightforward. There are often many barriers and delays, described, for example, by Funk et al. (1991) as including the individual and setting as well as the actual research being used. Haines and Jones (1994) argue that clinical guidelines are one possible way to speed up implementation of research findings. There have been a variety of suggestions for best practice over the years. For example, ward procedure manuals, mainly based on expert opinion, were once common, then standards of care emerged that were sometimes but not always based on research and, more recently, clinical guidelines are being developed and used (see Duff et al. (1996a) for a discussion of the difference between guidelines, protocols and standards). It may be that methodologically sound clinical guidelines already exist for a particular work based problem.

Definition

Clinical guidelines are

> systematically developed statements to assist practitioner decisions about appropriate health care for specific clinical circumstances (Field and Lohr, 1990: 50).

They should

> convert science-based knowledge into clinical action in a form accessible to practitioners . . . (AHCPR, 1990: 1).

They aim to reduce unjustified variations in practice, helping practitioners to base their decisions on the best available evidence, and thus improving patient outcomes. Grimshaw and Russell (1993b) outline how guidelines can have mandatory elements, for example when elements are scientifically robust and have important implications for patient outcome. When there are alternative management strategies with no scientific evidence as to their relative effectiveness, they argue the element should be considered optional. A key element of a guideline is that it is based on the best available evidence. This would be research evidence when such evidence exists, but may be expert opinion if this is the only evidence available. The important point here is that the guideline user should know what is based on research evidence and what on expert opinion. A guideline based on expert opinion should be used more tentatively than one based on sound research evidence: experts have been wrong in the past. Reasons for the popularity of guidelines are listed by Hopkins (1995) and include

- results of clinical research have not béen taken up and used in practice;
- there is enormous variation in practice in the management of common conditions;
- attempts are being made to control the costs of health care; and
- there is a link with audit, which needs to take place against some sort of standard.

The Royal College of General Practitioners (1995) highlight the point that many clinical guidelines have been produced but often have not followed any clear development protocols, and thus it is unclear on what evidence they are based. They set out the methodological scientific issues involved in guideline development. They caution that guidelines call for 'careful reflection on their function and critical appraisal of their quality'.

How are guidelines developed?

Guidelines can be developed locally or nationally. National guidelines are likely to be broad statements that will need to be adapted locally. The NHS Executive (1996b) outlines the NHS approach to development, appraisal and application of guidelines. They put the development, publication and maintenance of guidelines very firmly at the door of the professions. Since the production of guidelines is likely to be time consuming and expensive, the selection of a topic involves concentrating on areas where the greatest improvements in patient care are likely. The five key reasons outlined by the NHSE (1996b) for choosing a topic are:

- there is excessive morbidity, disability or mortality;
- treatment is likely to reduce morbidity, disability or mortality;
- there is wide variation in clinical practice around the country;
- the services involved are high volume and low cost or low volume and high cost; and
- there are, for example, primary/secondary care or professional boundaries involved.

They outline key characteristics in the development of good guidelines. These include the following:

- the guidelines must be based on a systematic, critical review of the literature. There are some useful sources of guidance in this area, including NHS Centre for Reviews and Dissemination (1996), Chalmers and Altman (1995) and the Cochrane Handbook in the Cochrane Library (1997);
- they should specify the patient population, how any recommendations affect patient care, clearly state whether they are based on research or expert opinion, make clear both costs and benefits of implementation, and state the implications for all those involved;
- the guidelines should be endorsed before publication by the relevant professional bodies. Simple language is important.

The NHSE then use the *Effective Health Care Bulletin* (1994) on implementing clinical guidelines to suggest guidelines should be:

- valid (when they are followed, they lead to improvements in patient outcomes);
- reproducible (given the same evidence, another group would produce similar recommendations);
- reliable (in the same clinical circumstances, health professionals apply them similarly);
- cost effective (they lead to improvements in health at acceptable costs);
- based on representative development (all key disciplines and interests contributed to guideline development, including patients);
- clinically applicable (the target population is defined in accordance with scientific evidence);
- flexible (they identify exceptions and how patient preferences can be incorporated);
- clear (they use precise definitions, unambiguous terms and are in user friendly formats);
- reviewable (when and how they will be reviewed is explicit);
- amenable to clinical audit (they suggest ways adherence could be monitored);
- based on meticulous documentation (of patients, assumptions and methods. The recommendations are linked to available evidence).

The *Effective Health Care Bulletin* had in turn adapted these suggestions from Field and Lohr (1992).

Levels of evidence

The extent to which one can feel confident in the recommendations of guidelines depends, amongst other things, on the research designs used in the studies supporting the guideline statements. The NHSE uses three levels of evidence for guidelines:

- randomised controlled trials;
- other robust experimental or observational studies;
- more limited evidence, expert opinion endorsed by respected authorities.

It is helpful to have evidence graded in this way but one of the problems with these levels of evidence is that they focus on, for example, the effectiveness of an intervention. Many areas of nursing research will use qualitative methodologies to answer questions such as 'what is it like to . . .'. Exactly where this sort of study fits into such levels is unclear, and more work is needed in this area to facilitate the inclusion of rigorous, systematic qualitative research findings. However, the NHSE (1996b) states that only those recommendations based on randomised controlled evidence should be used in contract specification.

The NHS has a firm view that guidelines are the responsibility of those who develop them, and acceptance and use will be at the discretion of clinicians, purchasers and providers.

Using guidelines in practice

The NHSE (1996b) suggests that experts be available to advise on implementing guidelines and adapting guidelines for local needs. This implies that implementing guidelines in practice is not as straightforward as it may seem. Although the development of guidelines is still in its infancy, implementing them, using national guidelines locally and knowing which strategy to use, is even less well developed. There are many reasons why research is not used in practice, and just providing clinicians with the evidence does not necessarily mean that they will use that research in practice. There is a difference between the distribution or dissemination of guidelines and the implementation or use of guidelines. It seems logical that if people are provided with what seems to be a rational argument, they should adopt that evidence. However, it seems to be more complex than this: Grimshaw et al. (1995) showed that just distributing guidelines was of limited value in affecting the quality of care. Potential users will not make use of guidelines simply because they are given to them. There are many reasons why they are not used, including concerns over workload, lack of clarity about their evidence base and the legal implications of their use, as well as all the factors that affect the introduction of any change into clinical practice. Mansfield (1995) asked 268 hospital doctors (of all grades) about their attitudes to guidelines. Reasons for not using guidelines included being unaware of the guidelines (80%), and that guidelines were poorly developed (67%) or were impractical (49%). Ways of promoting guideline use were described as encouragement from senior doctors (72%) and from peers (59%) and by monitoring behaviour and feedback (68%). So a range of factors seems to be important. This is supported by The Royal College of General Practitioners (1995), who divide reasons for the failure of guidelines to influence health care and health outcome into

- internal factors related to the actual guidelines; or
- external factors related to the context in which they are introduced.

The internal barriers they identify are based on the reverse of the characteristics of good guidelines listed above. Guidelines lack validity, reproducibility, reliability, representativeness and so on. The external barriers are grouped into two sections: problems of distribution, dissemination or implementation and problems of resistance to their use. Not only do guidelines need to be disseminated to appropriate groups, but the ground must be carefully prepared first so the potential user has thus a more active role (in, for example, educational or professional initiatives) rather than being just a passive recipient of guidelines. The importance of clear, easily utilised presentation of guidelines is stressed.

User resistance to guidelines is divided into failure from passivity and failure from active resistance. Passive failure includes lack of ownership, the guideline being seen as irrelevant, unhelpful or impractical, a lack of incentives or the guideline may simply be ignored. Active resistance is described as including rival guidelines in use, hostility to an outsider, guidelines being seen as extra work with no reward or an unusual way of working or as eroding clinical autonomy or interfering with the doctor–patient relationship. Fears that use would encourage external audit or may result in litigation are also listed.

Ownership of guidelines seems important. Humphris and Littlejohns (1995) discuss how national guidelines are likely to be valid (if correctly applied they lead to expected improvements in health status) but not used, whereas local guidelines are likely to be used but may not be valid. They argue that 'the human factor' needs to be taken into account and 'the final result is as much one of professional politics as it is of science' (1995: 221). Grimshaw and Russell (1994) suggest that if guidelines are developed by the clinicians who will use them, then few resources are needed to disseminate and implement them. However, guidelines developed externally need a greater emphasis on dissemination and implementation. It seems that the context into which guidelines are introduced, comprising the setting and the individuals, is important. The representativeness of guideline development may be important in how a guideline is perceived. Lomas (1993) argues that interpretations of stakeholders are needed to supplement information available, and that legitimate conflicts over values need to be resolved. He feels that, to introduce a guideline successfully, all key professionals need to contribute to its development to ensure ownership and support. Of course, the key professional would need to be seen as acceptable and credible by others in the group for this to work.

Appraisal of guidelines

It is important to assess the validity of guidelines before embarking on any implementation. Grimshaw and Russell (1993a) outlined three factors that affect validity. First the scientific evidence should be systematically derived, using explicit search strategies and inclusion criteria and rigorous methods of data synthesis. Second, the panel developing the guideline should include most, if not all, of the relevant disciplines but few end users of the guideline, and, third, the recommendations should be explicitly linked to the evidence from which they are derived. They conclude there is little evidence on dissemination and subsequent implementation of guidelines. The NHSE (1996b) clearly states that the acceptance and use of guidelines will be at the discretion of individual clinicians, health authorities and trusts. Thus some sort of appraisal of a guideline will be crucial.

One way guidelines may be assessed is using a tool described by the Royal College of General Practitioners (1995). This report includes as an appendix a draft appraisal instrument for clinical guidelines developed by the Health Care Evaluation Unit at St George's Hospital, London. It addresses the validity of guidelines, with sections on who was responsible for development, objectives, the guideline development group, background evidence used, interpretation and assessment of the evidence, group consensus processes used, likely costs and benefits, peer view used, updating mechanisms, other guidelines in existence, a summary and a global assessment of the development process, their applicability and their clarity. Each of the total 37 items is scored 'Yes', 'No', 'Not sure' or 'Not applicable'. There is also a second section on the application of guidelines, which covers local protocol development, dissemination and implementation, and the monitoring of guidelines or clinical audit.

In addition, the *Journal of the American Medical Association* has published two users' guides for the critical appraisal of guidelines. These look at whether the guideline recommendations are valid (Hayward et al., 1995), what the recommendations are and whether they will help caring for a patient (Wilson et al., 1995). These guides include a series of questions. To address whether the recommendations are valid, the questions to ask include:

- Were all important options and outcomes clearly specified?
- Was an explicit and sensible process used to identify, select and combine evidence?
- Was an explicit and sensible process used to consider the relative value of different outcomes?
- Is the guideline likely to account for important recent developments?
- Has the guideline been subject to peer review and testing?

When looking at what the recommendations are, the questions include:

- Are practical, clinically important recommendations made?
- How strong are the recommendations?
- What is the impact of uncertainty associated with the evidence and values used in the guidelines?

Finally, when considering whether the guidelines will help in caring for patients, questions include:

- Is the primary objective of the guideline consistent with your objective?
- Are the recommendations applicable to the patients?

Can guidelines affect practice?

A systematic review of 59 evaluations of clinical guidelines suggested that they can change medical practice if they are appropriately developed, disseminated and implemented, although the size of improvements varied considerably (Grimshaw and Russell, 1993a). This review was updated by Grimshaw et al. (1995) (based on the *Effective Health Care Bulletin* No. 8) and included another 32 studies, making a total of 91 studies. They concluded that 43 out of 44 studies classified as providing grade I evidence (rigorous evaluations) reported significant changes in process and 8 out of 11 showed significant changes in outcome. This suggests that properly developed guidelines can change clinical practice and may lead to changes in patient outcome.

Cheater and Closs (1997) undertook a selective review of the effectiveness of methods of dissemination and implementation of clinical guidelines for nursing practice. They concluded that there was a large amount of anecdotal or descriptive material, but very little research evidence. Thomas et al. (1997) are currently undertaking a systematic review to try to identify rigorous evaluations of clinical practice guidelines in professions allied to medicine, including nursing.

Strategies for implementing guidelines

It is a considerable challenge to change practice through the use of guidelines (Grimshaw and Russell, 1994). Implementing guidelines means that those affected need not only knowledge about the guidelines, but also the recognition that change needs to happen. Managerial and professional support is also needed to facilitate this process. Education, not only about the content of the guidelines but also about the ways in which people change, may well be very important. Mittman et al. (1992) outline possible guideline implementation strategies. Humphris and Littlejohns (1996: 7) conclude that

> apparently simple and straightforward changes are set within a complex chain of interdependent units and may block progress.

For example, Kalunzy et al. (1995) outline how there must be a recognition that expectations are not being fully met at present if people are to start using guidelines. In addition, organisational characteristics, such as structure, formalisation of decision making, existing communication, co-ordination and resources all affect how a guideline might be implemented. Kalunzy et al. (1995) suggest a core of factors that may help in implementing guidelines, which include:

- be clear who is targeted (for example, individuals or organisations);
- stage the implementation and invest time to develop a perception of a performance gap;
- manage supporters and detractors – for example, identify key stakeholders, assess their attitudes towards the change, assess their power to affect the change;
- set achievable small goals so that progress can be seen fairly quickly;
- build on existing structures, such as audit;
- be proactive – develop a plan and timetable for formulation and implementation.

They conclude that 'without managerial commitment and organisational strategy, guidelines will remain an irritant and perceived threat . . .' (1995: 351).

How the introduction of guidelines is managed seems crucial to the success of implementation. For example, Oxman et al. (1995) undertook a systematic review of 102 trials of interventions to improve professional practice. These included educational materials, conferences, opinion leaders, reminders, audit and feedback. All the interventions showed some effect some of the time. They concluded there were no magic bullets but interventions, used appropriately, could improve use of research and effectiveness of health care.

The Cochrane Collaboration for Effective Professional Practice has a useful systematic review in this area (Freemantle et al., 1997). This looks at printed educational materials and their effect on behaviour of health care professionals and on patient outcomes. They conclude that it is difficult to assess effectiveness because of methodological problems with the primary studies. However, their tentative conclusions include that the effects of printed educational materials are small, and the additional impact of active interventions such as audit and feedback or workshops and conferences is also small. Educational outreach and opinion leaders have greater effects, which are likely to be of practical importance. Future work on opinion leaders is currently under way (Thomson et al., 1997).

Limitations of guidelines

Guidelines do not provide the answer to clinical problems. They are there to help with decisions about care. Clinical judgement and patient preferences also form an important part of the decision making process.

Hopkins (1995) outlined some reservations about clinical guidelines. These include that guidelines tend to be written for a clinical diagnosis, rather than a clinical problem. Hopkins points out that patients present with problems, not a diagnosis. A problem-focused guideline is thus more appropriate and certainly more helpful for those in training. He also argues that the target health professional audience and the target patient population are often not adequately identified in many guidelines. He highlights how the central tenet of guidelines is that they are based on good scientific evidence yet, in many areas of care, support and reassurance, rather than any technical intervention, are a large part of day-to-day work. Although Hopkins seems to see this as detracting from the usefulness of guidelines, presumably the most effective ways of giving support and reassurance could be the focus of research that would inform future guidelines. Following on from this, he stresses the importance of an outcome from the patient's perspective, with guidelines needing to reflect the values of those who use the NHS. Work is being developed in this area – for example Duff et al. (1996b). He also points out that co-morbidity, especially in an older population, is likely to be important and is often not taken into account. Other reservations include the fact that updating of guidelines is essential but rare.

Other concerns about guidelines include the legal implications of their use. Hurwitz (1995) argues that they will increasingly be used in court. However, this does not mean an unquestioning approach: guideline adherence does not automatically equate with reasonable practice. There are sometimes legal concerns over, for example, the position of a practitioner who has not followed a guideline. The NHS Executive (1996b: 10) argues that the Bolam principle (where there can be two or more acceptable ways of viewing any aspect of care) could be used, where a professional would show that others in the field supported the course of action. The *Effective Health Care Bulletin* (1994: 4) argues that compliance with clinical guidelines is unlikely to prove decisive in medical negligence 'unless the intervention concerned is so well established that no responsible doctor acting with reasonable skill would fail to comply with it'.

Another possible limitation of a guideline may be that it can be much more difficult to implement a guideline in practice than one might imagine. For example, Ellrodt et al. (1992) assessed the impact of a guideline that required the categorisation of patients admitted for chest pain into high or low risk groups. The person categorising had to accurately interpret seven explicitly defined guideline criteria.

Nurses applying the guideline were knowledgeable and trained and chosen for their past expertise in guideline implementation. Nevertheless 7 per cent of patients were misclassified as a low risk when they were at high risk, and 4 per cent were misclassified as high risk when they were at low risk. This highlights the legal and ethical risks for patients, health professionals and the institution of these misclassifications. These misclassifications occurred despite an explicit guideline, many hours of training and expert consultation being continuously available. Hospitals without these resources may fare much worse. Moreover, this guideline was quite simple, with seven explicitly defined criteria and a dichotomous outcome (high or low risk) at one point in time. A complex guideline with multiple branches applied at multiple times with less explicit criteria would be a concern.

National initiatives

There are several national initiatives to help with development and implementation of guidelines.

The Royal College of Nursing (RCN) has a clinical effectiveness initiative and, within this programme, the development, use and evaluation of clinical guidelines is a focus. The programme is also developing and piloting multiprofessional education modules for implementing clinical guidelines (in collaboration with other royal colleges and professional organisations) and is developing and evaluating a framework to promote patient involvement in clinical guidelines (in collaboration with patient and professional organisations). The RCN has established a steering group for its clinical guidelines work. In May 1994 its aims were to

- provide an information service on clinical guidelines for RCN members and people involved in the development and use of guidelines;
- provide education and facilitation to enable nurses to implement clinical guidelines and audit clinical practice;
- participate in clinical appraisal and approval of guidelines;
- collaborate in the development of multiprofessional guidelines;
- monitor and evaluate the development, implementation and effectiveness of the clinical guidelines developed by the RCN in collaboration with other professions and patients' representatives.

This group's remit was broadened in May 1995 to include issues related to clinical effectiveness (Royal College of Nursing, 1996). The NHS Executive has a clinical outcomes group that oversees the selection, development and appraisal of guidelines that the NHSE can commend to the NHS and it identifies gaps in care covered by clinical guidelines. It also has an interest in the implementation of guidelines (NHSE, 1996a).

The Cochrane Collaboration is involved in the production of systematic reviews (Cochrane Database of Systematic Reviews – CDSR) available in the Cochrane Library (1997). They have 196 completed reviews and 208 protocols for reviews currently being undertaken. As part of this process, the Cochrane Collaboration on Effective Professional Practice is working on systematic reviews that include the effectiveness of various approaches to implementation.

The NHS Centre for Reviews and Dissemination at York is involved in compiling a Database of Abstracts of Reviews of Effectiveness (DARE). There are currently 1686 entries on this database, which are also available in the Cochrane Library (1997), and the Centre has been involved in the production of effective health care bulletins, including Bulletin Number 8, Implementing Clinical Practice Guidelines (*Effective Health Care Bulletin*, 1994).

The Clinical Resource and Audit Group (1993) in Scotland have developed an integrated approach to guidelines in both primary and secondary care.

One other initiative of interest, which predates activity in the UK, is the establishment in 1989 of the Agency for Health Care Policy and Research in the United States. This agency was set up to improve the effectiveness of health care, and as part of this initiative it has been involved in facilitating the development of clinical practice guidelines (see AHCPR, 1990). Its web site address is

http://www.ahcpr.gov/guide

and 19 guidelines are currently available, covering such areas as acute and cancer pain management, cardiac rehabilitation and urinary incontinence.

There is also ongoing research in this area. For example, in April 1997 there was a call for proposals on the evaluation of methods to promote the implementation of research findings from the NHSE North Thames Research and Development Directorate.

Key documents

Two documents from the NHSE (1996a, 1996b) on Promoting Clinical Effectiveness and Clinical Guidelines respectively have provided a useful overview of the issues involved. The Royal College of General Practitioners (1995) report on the development and implementation of clinical guidelines and the Royal College of Nursing Clinical Effectiveness Initiative (1996) are also useful resources. For an example of a guideline developed in the UK, see North of England Asthma Guideline Development Group (1996).

Transferability of guidelines between clinical settings and health professionals

Much of the work undertaken to look at both the development and implementation of clinical guidelines has had a medical focus – for example Grimshaw and Russell (1994) and Mansfield (1995). However, there is a move towards including all key stakeholders in guideline development and use. It might be that factors affecting behaviour vary between different health professionals. However, there are also likely to be many similarities. Although one may want to be cautious in applying research and/or guidelines from other clinical areas and settings or which focus on other professions, at the same time it would seem prudent not to throw the baby out with the bathwater. Both Cheater and Closs (1997) and Thomas et al. (1997) have been looking at this area with a non-medical focus, as discussed earlier. Closer interdisciplinary working on guideline development and implementation, as well as more generally, should help all professions and settings learn from well-conducted research and well-constructed guidelines. Mutual respect for the contribution of all those involved in care will facilitate this process, but the success of such an approach would seem depend on the individuals involved and is likely to be variable.

Summary

There is a need to monitor the introduction of guidelines so that there is an evaluation of their effect on health of patients. A clearly documented methodology of development is crucial so that their robustness can be judged (see Eccles et al., 1996, for example). Developing skills in guidelines appraisal, as suggested by Hayward et al. (1995) and Wilson et al. (1995), will be important. There is currently little evidence about how best to implement the recommendations of guidelines and more research is needed to increase our understanding and effectiveness. Grimshaw and Russell (1994) conclude that guidelines can only succeed if they are rigorously developed and if appropriate development, dissemination and implementation strategies are adopted. They highlight the need to introduce the principles of change management and the need for leadership, energy, avoiding unnecessary uncertainty, good communication and time.

Well-developed guidelines have the potential to improve patient care by helping practitioners to base their care on the best available evidence. They are not there to constrain practice. Indeed, the Royal College of General Practitioners (1995: 5) describe guidelines as having the

> dual function of recommending evidence based good practice, as well as legitimising acceptable variations in practice where the evidence is weak and its interpretation controversial.'

Guidelines are a tool to support the good practice of individual practitioners, in consultation with those for whom they care.

References

Agency for Health Care Policy and Research (1990) Nursing Advisory Panel for Guideline Development: Summary. Rockville: US Department of Health and Human Services.

Chalmers I, Altman D (Eds) (1995) Systematic Reviews. London: BMJ Publishing.

Cheater FM, Closs SJ (1997) The effectiveness of methods of dissemination and implementation of clinical guidelines for nursing practice. Clinical Effectiveness in Nursing 1(1): 4–15.

Cochrane Library (1997) Issue 2. Update Software.

Clinical Resource and Audit Group (1993) Clinical Guidelines: A report by a Working Party set up by the Clinical Resource and Audit Group. Edinburgh: Scottish Office.

Cullum N (1997) Identification and analysis of randomised controlled trials in nursing: a preliminary study. Quality in Health Care 6: 2–6.

Department of Health (1991) Research for Health. A Research and Development Strategy for the NHS. London: HMSO.

Department of Health (1993) Research for Health. London: Department of Health.

Duff LA, Kitson AL, Seers K, Humphris D (1996a) Clinical guidelines: an introduction to their development and implementation. Journal of Advanced Nursing 23: 887–95.

Duff LA, Kelson M, Marriott S, McIntosh A, Brown S, Cape J, Marcus N, Traynor M (1996b) Clinical guidelines: involving patients and users of services. Journal of Clinical Effectiveness 1(3): 104–12.

Eccles M, Clapp Z, Grimshaw J, Adams PC, Higgins B, Purves I, Russell I

(1996) North of England evidence based guidelines development project: methods of guideline development. BMJ 312: 760–2.

Effective Health Care (1994) Implementing Clinical Practice Guidelines. Bulletin Number 8. Leeds: University of Leeds.

Ellrodt AG, Conner L, Riedinger MS, Weingarten S (1992) Implementing practice guidelines through a utilisation management strategy: the potentials and the challenges. Quality Review Bulletin 18(2): 456–60.

Field MJ, Lohr KN (1990) Clinical Practice guidelines: A Direction of a New Agency. Washington, DC: Institute of Medicine.

Field MJ, Lohr KN (Eds) (1992) Guidelines for Clinical Practice. From Development to Use. New York: National Academy Press.

Freemantle N, Harvey EL, Wolf F, Grimshaw JM, Grilli R, Bero LA (1997) Printed educational materials to improve the behaviour of health care professionals and patient outcomes. In Bero L, Grilli R, Grimshaw J, Oxman A. Collaboration on Effective Professional Practice Module of the Cochrane Database of Systematic Reviews, updated 3 March 1997. Available in The Cochrane Library (database on disk and CD-ROM) The Cochrane Collaboration, Issue 2, Oxford. Update Software. Updated quarterly.

Funk SG, Champagne MT, Wiese RA, Tornquist EM (1991) Barriers to using research findings in practice: the clinician's perspective. Applied Nursing Research 4(2): 90–5.

Grimshaw JM, Russell IT (1993a) Achieving health gain through clinical guidelines. I: Developing scientifically valid guidelines. Quality in Health Care 2: 243–8.

Grimshaw JM, Russell IT (1993b) Effects of clinical guidelines on medical practice: a systematic review of rigorous evaluations. Lancet 342: 1317–22.

Grimshaw JM, Russell IT (1994) Achieving health gain through clinical guidelines II: Ensuring guidelines change medical practice. Quality in Health Care 3: 45–52.

Grimshaw J, Freemantle N, Wallace S, Russell I, Hurwitz B, Watt I, Long A, Sheldon T (1995) Developing and implementing clinical practice guidelines. Quality in Health Care 4(1): 55–64.

Haines A, Jones R (1994) Implementing the findings of research. BMJ 308: 1488–92.

Hayward RSA, Wilson MC, Tunis SR, Bass EB, Guyatt G (1995) Users' guide to the Medical Literature: VIII How to use clinical practice guidelines. A. Are the recommendations valid? JAMA 274(7): 570–74.

Hicks N (1997) Evidence based health care. Bandolier 39 4(5): 8.

Hopkins A (1995) Some reservations about clinical guidelines. Archives of Disease in Childhood 72: 70–5.

Humphris D, Littlejohns P (1995) The development of multiprofessional audit and clinical guidelines: their contribution to quality assurance and effectiveness in the NHS. Journal of Interprofessional Care 9(3): 207–25.

Humphris D, Littlejohns P (1996) Implementing clinical guidelines: preparation and opportunism. Journal of Clinical Effectiveness 1(1): 5–7.

Hurwitz B (1995) Clinical guidelines and the law: advice, guidance or regulation? Journal of Evaluation in Clinical Practice 1(1): 49–60.

Kalunzy AD, Konrad TR, McLaughlin CP (1995) Organisational strategies for implementing clinical guidelines. Journal of Quality Improvement 21(7): 347–51.

Lomas J (1993) Making clinical policy explicit: legislative policy making and lessons for developing practice guidelines. International Journal of Technology Assessment in Health Care 9: 11–25.

Mansfield CD (1995) Attitudes and behaviours towards clinical guidelines: the clinicians' perspective. Quality in Health Care 4: 250–5.

Mittman BS, Tonesk X, Jacobson PD (1992) Implementing clinical practice guidelines: social influence strategies and practitioner behavior change. Quality Review Bulletin 18(2): 413–22.

Newell R (1997) Towards clinical effectiveness in nursing. Editorial. Clinical Effectiveness in Nursing 1(1): 1–2.

NHS Centre for Reviews and Dissemination (1996) Undertaking systematic reviews of research on effectiveness. CRD guidelines for those carrying out or commissioning reviews. CRD report 4. York: CRD.

NHS Executive (1996a) Promoting clinical effectiveness: a framework for action in and through the NHS. Leeds: NHSE.

NHS Executive (1996b) Clinical guidelines. Using clinical guidelines to improve patient care within the NHS. Leeds: NHSE.

Noblit GW, Hare RD (1988) Meta-ethnography: Synthesising Qualitative Studies. Newbury Park: Sage Publications.

North of England Asthma Guideline Development Group (1996) North of England evidence based guidelines development project: summary version of evidence based guidelines for the primary care management of asthma in adults. BMJ 312: 762–6.

Oxman AD, Thomson MA, Davis DA, Haynes RB (1995) No magic bullets: a systematic review of 102 trials of interventions to improve professional practice. Canadian Medical Association Journal 153(10): 1423–31.

Royal College of General Practitioners (1995) The development and implementation of clinical guidelines. Report of the Clinical Guidelines Working Group. Report from General Practice 26. London: RCGP.

Royal College of Nursing (1996) Clinical Effectiveness Initiative. A Strategic Framework. London: RCN.

Sackett DL, Richardson WS, Rosenberg W, Haynes RB (1997) Evidence Based Medicine. How to Practice and Teach EBM. Edinburgh: Churchill Livingstone .

Thomas L, Cullum N, McColl E, Rousseau N (1997) Guidelines in professions allied to medicine (protocol). In Bero L, Grilli R, Grimshaw J, Oxman A. Collaboration on Effective Professional Practice Module of the Cochrane Database of Systematic reviews, updated 3 March 1997. Available in The Cochrane Library (database on disk and CD-ROM) The Cochrane Collaboration, Issue 2, Oxford. Update Software. Updated quarterly.

Thomson MA, Oxman AD, Haynes RB, Davis DA, Freemantle N, Harvey EL (1997) Local opinion leaders to improve health care professional practice and health care outcomes (protocol). In Bero L, Grilli R, Grimshaw J, Oxman A.Collaboration on Effective Professional Practice Module of the Cochrane Database of Systematic reviews, updated 3 March 1997. Available in The Cochrane Library (database on disk and CD-ROM) The Cochrane Collaboration, Issue 2, Oxford. Update Software. Updated quarterly.

Wilson MC, Hayward RSA, Tunis SR, Bass EB, Guyatt G (1995) Users' guide to the Medical Literature: VIII How to use Clinical Practice Guidelines. B. What are the recommendations and will they help you in caring for your patient? JAMA 274(20): 1630–2.

Chapter 14
Action research: the debate moves on

Christine Webb, Pat Turton, David Pontin

Introduction

Action research is an approach that has been attracting more and more interest in nursing in recent years, as can be seen from the numbers of articles published and PhD theses completed. This chapter will look at what action research is, why this rise in its take-up has occurred in nursing, some issues and debates that are taking place about its use, and two examples from different fields of nursing that illustrate the approach, its strengths and some criticisms.

Action research: definitions and categories

Various writers have discussed different types of action research and debated which types can be justified as 'real' action research. A brief look at these debates will help in coming to a definition on which to base the chapter.

Kurt Lewin (1946) is generally credited with being the main founder of action research in the USA, with researchers at the Tavistock Institute of Human Relations in London as the initiators in the UK (Susman and Evered, 1978). Lewin defined action research as a spiral of steps, each involving planning, acting, observing and evaluating the process. These cycles involve the overlapping of action and reflection so that changes in plans can be made as people learn from experience. Group decision-making and commitment to improvement are crucial in Lewin's approach (McTaggart, 1994) and what distinguishes action research from traditional forms is involvement of both the researcher and 'researched'. 'Subjects' become active participants in the project and the research is done by, with and for them instead of on them.

Subsequently action research has been much used in education in the UK and Australia (Carr and Kemmis, 1986; McTaggart, 1994) and in a variety of industrial or organisational settings in the USA and elsewhere (Whyte, 1989). As a result of these differing experiences, a number of classifications of action research have been drawn up. Carr and Kemmis (1986) identify three different types, which are technical, practical and emancipatory, while Holter and Schwartz-Barcott (1993) have a similar scheme involving technical collaborative, mutual collaborative and enhancement approaches. In the first, or technical form, the researcher persuades practitioners to apply findings from other research in their own work. This is more like a traditional experiment. Practical or mutual collaborative action research involves outside researchers assisting participants to analyse, change and evaluate their own practice. Emancipatory or enhancement action research is based on joint collaboration and responsibility for practice development. In Hart and Bond's four-category scheme, the experimental and organisational types seem to parallel the technical type, professionalising action research is similar to mutual collaboration or practical action research, while their empowering form is the emancipatory or enhancement type (Hart and Bond, 1995). This is illustrated in figure 14.1.

Carr and Kemmis 1986	Holter and Schwartz-Barcott 1993	Hart and Bond 1995
Technical	Technical collaborative	Experimental
		Organisational
Practical	Mutual collaborative	Professionalising
Emancipatory	Enhancement	Enhancement

Figure 14.1: Types of action research.

These classifications have in turn been criticised and different examples of action research projects have been given different labels. For example, Meyer (1995a) questions the categorisations and believes that 'action research should be viewed more as an approach to research which can incorporate a variety of methodologies'. McNiff (1988) also finds the classifications unsatisfactory and prefers the term 'generative action research' to emphasise the creative elements for participants, while Whyte (1989) and others increasingly use the term 'participatory action research'. Rather than becoming diverted by semantic arguments (Meyer, 1995b), it is probably better to agree with Meyer and call projects 'action research' if they are democratic, collaborative, and use both quantitative and qualitative evaluation methods.

This fits with the six characteristics of action research put forward by Susman and Evered (1978), which must be present if a project is to qualify for the description 'action research'. It must:

- be future oriented
- be collaborative
- involve system development
- generate theory grounded in action
- be agnostic
- be situational.

Thus, researcher and participants collaborate to change the ways things work in the future by developing the system within which they work. Their project produces theories based on their actions, but these theories are themselves subject to further change and development because they apply to the particular situation and need to be re-tested and possibly modified to fit in other situations.

Action research in nursing

The theory–practice gap and why nurses do not use research findings in their practice has been the subject of many articles (Webb and Mackenzie, 1993). It is commonly reported that nurses do not read research-based articles in journals because they find them difficult to understand and do not see their relevance to their own work. Webb and Mackenzie (1993) used action research to pursue these very issues. They ran a research methods course for trained staff during which questionnaires using open and closed questions and care plan analysis were designed by students and then carried out as a joint project. The findings confirmed that levels of reading, understanding and application of research in clinical practice were low in the areas studied. Evaluation of students' experiences of the course, using open-ended questions, elicited an extremely positive outcome, with nurses who undertook the course changing towards having very positive attitudes and understandings of the research process, one stating:

> This has given me a clearer insight into the mechanisms of research. It made me realise that much thought and planning goes into the research process and that nothing can be taken for granted. This small piece of

research took a lot of time and planning and made us all think long and
hard about what we were trying to achieve.

This example fulfils the criteria identified earlier for action research
in that it was undertaken by, with and for the nurses involved, was
conducted democratically and collaboratively and used a variety of
research methods.

Other action researchers have also used the method to involve
practising nurses in understanding and implementing research findings. These include introducing the nursing process (Lauri, 1982),
primary nursing (Titchen and Binnie, 1993a), improving stroke care
(Gibbon and Little, 1995), developing ophthalmic nursing
(Waterman, 1994; Waterman er al.. 1995) and providing respite care
(Nolan and Grant, 1993).

From this growing body of experience in using action research in
nursing, a number of issues and questions have emerged. It is important that these are debated and that action researchers reflect on
their successes and difficulties so that what is learned is passed on for
the benefit and learning of future researchers. Indeed such reflection
is part of the actual action research approach (Kemmis and
McTaggart, 1988). Some of these issues will be discussed in the
following section.

Ethical issues: informed consent, anonymity and confidentiality

Action research differs from traditional approaches in that there is
not a tightly drawn-up and agreed research proposal at the start of
the project. By the very nature of collaborative research, it is impossible to be certain at the start what will actually happen, what the
direction of the research will be, and what changes in practice may
be negotiated along the way. This means that not only do those in at
the start not have a completely clear picture, but that others joining
the setting after the process has begun do not have a real choice
about whether to participate because the work is already ongoing.
Meyer (1993a) had this problem, with 85 new staff joining and 89
leaving over the one-year period of her multi-disciplinary attempt to
introduce lay participation in a hospital ward. Similarly, Pontin had
31 joiners and 29 leavers over a two-year period of implementing
primary nursing (Pontin, 1996).

Attempting to maintain informed consent through the progress
of a study involves frequent briefings of new people to bring them up

to date and to try to ensure that the changes achieved do not get whittled away. This process can be very time-consuming.

Most action research projects are like case studies in that they involve intensive study of one particular setting. This raises problems of anonymity and confidentiality when the findings are reported in articles, books and theses because it can be difficult to disguise data enough to prevent the setting and participants being identified (Meyer, 1993a).

A related issue is confidentiality when there is more than one researcher involved (Titchen and Binnie, 1992) or when an action researcher needs to discuss the project with a supervisor or other adviser. Apart from the need for academic supervision, it is widely agreed that undertaking action research can be stressful and that support is needed for researchers who are dealing with the tensions of attempting to change practice, sometimes in the face of strong opposition (Greenwood, 1994). It is important that any discussions of this kind are bound by the norms of confidentiality applying to all research.

Securing collaboration

Action researchers have reported difficulty in sustaining a project because, as work develops, it becomes clear that not all participants are truly committed. For example, Webb (1989) found that the sister on her action research ward had a different and personal agenda from that agreed at the start, and as a result the project did not develop beyond the early stages of problem identification. Meyer (1993b) and Webb (1990a) both ran into difficulties when doctors did not collaborate as they had agreed in relation to changed medication practices and Hunt (1987) could not change pre-operative fasting times because of lack of agreement by anaesthetists.

In an attempt to overcome such difficulties, Whyte (1989) did not begin his three action research projects until collaboration had been extensively negotiated: 'In all three cases, the projects began only after extended periods of vigorous discussion during which the professional researchers felt free to express their ideas and opinions and encouraged the practitioners to do likewise' (1989: 374). Nolan and Grant (1993) identify the requirements for action research as:

- a shared and explicit set of values acting as a guide for practice;
- recognition that a problem area exists;

- a common understanding of the problem;
- a perceived need for change;
- the situation is amenable to change;
- there is a focus of involvement and team building.

These are termed 'pre-conditions' by Gibbon and Little (1995), who decided that their stroke care setting was appropriate for an action research project because these conditions were already in existence.

However, it could be argued that the need for an action research project may arise precisely because there are problems in a particular setting where there is an unrecognised need for change or everyone involved does not agree on how to proceed. It is then part of the action research process to discuss and attempt to resolve these kinds of issues and to write about the process so that others can learn and benefit from them. In practice these kinds of problems have been encountered and tackled within action research projects, and have been discussed by researchers as questions of power and control.

Power and control

In the examples of lack of collaboration by doctors discussed earlier, issues of power and control were operating. In other cases, it appeared that managers – who may or may not have been nurses – had their own agendas. In Webb's self-medication project, for example, managers supported the scheme and provided a small quantity of resources. This legitimated the work and made it difficult for others to sustain their opposition (Webb, 1990a). However in Webb's previous attempt with action research, managers were aware of problems created by the ward sister's management style but had not dealt with them and hoped that the researcher would do so instead (Webb, 1989). Meyer had backing from managers which meant that, although she encountered opposition, the project did carry on when the first ward sister lost her motivation and changed to another job: a second sister, who was committed, was brought in to replace her (Meyer, 1995a).

East and Robinson (1994) talk about questions of power in the action research setting in terms of 'inner' and 'outer' context. They point out that: 'Much of nursing research is inward looking and acontextual, as if nothing important happens beyond the ward door or even the individual patient's bedside. Yet, in equal measure, most management research ignores nursing' (1994: 61).

In their action research, managers and ward sisters each blamed the other for lack of progress in implementing changes, and East and Robinson (1994) agree that exploring 'both sides of the story, recognising the participative emphasis' is part of action research.

Another concern about power in action research concerns whether research is 'top down' or 'bottom up'. Some writers claim that it is a strength of action research that it adopts a 'bottom up' approach, giving participants a sense of 'ownership' in the project and the changes introduced, so that continuity is more likely to occur than with a 'top down' approach (Meyer, 1993a). However, the present state of affairs in nursing being what it is, with the lack of appreciation and application of research already identified earlier, the reality is that almost all the action research projects discussed in this chapter were initiated by researchers rather than by practising nurses. Exceptions to this are Webb's self-medication work, where she was approached by a group of enrolled nurses for help with implementing a proposal they had developed on a course, and Binnie's approach to the Institute of Nursing in Oxford to propose a collaborative project (Webb, 1990a; Titchen and Binnie, 1993b).

Evaluating action research

Those more used to traditional research approaches may criticise action research for a lack of validity, reliability and generalisability. Greenwood (1984) replies by stating that action research demonstrates face validity because the findings appear to fit reality. Another criterion for evaluating research that sets out to achieve a change is whether in fact that change was actually achieved (Greenwood, 1994). Reliability results from the fact that throughout the action research process, findings are fed back to participants, discussed, reflected upon, and used to further progress the research. Generalisability of action research, like that of all case studies, is not a claim made by researchers. Other researchers or practitioners wishing to relate the findings to their own situation bear the onus of convincing themselves that this is appropriate and then testing this judgement in their own projects (McTaggart, 1994). In order that they may do this, action researchers must document comprehensively how they went about the research, which methods were used and why, and whether these were successful. If they were not successful they must document why this was and what modifications were made. Difficulties encountered must be acknowledged as well as reporting strengths and achievements, in keeping with the fundamental requirement of action research for reflection (Carr and Kemmis, 1986).

Titchen (1995: 47) suggests a 'decision trail' of questions to be asked when evaluating an action research report, but believes that ultimately 'Valid action research is an ethical enterprise which rests on the researchers' honesty, trustworthiness and integrity'.

The ideas discussed in this section are summarised by Holter and Schwartz-Barcott (1993: 303) when they say:

> Knowledge developed through action research is grounded in actual practice . . . If the ultimate purpose in developing nursing knowledge is to improve nursing practice, then knowledge that is validated and revised through practical application is extremely important for knowledge in nursing.

Two examples of action research projects aiming to improve nursing practice, one in a hospital setting and one in the community, will be presented in the next two sections to illustrate and further develop the earlier discussion. In these two examples, confidentiality and anonymity are maintained by disguising all names except those of the researchers.

The Midvale demonstration wards project

At the time of the project, Midvale was a large health authority with two district general hospitals, both of which received nursing and medical students on placement from the local college of nursing and the university. The chief nurse was newly appointed, there having been no permanent occupant of this post for the past six years. As a result it was acknowledged that there had been a lack of nursing leadership and staff development in the district, together with an underresourcing of nursing services. The arrival of the new chief nurse coincided with publication of the Department of Health's Strategy for Nursing (Department of Health, 1989).

The chief nurse decided to implement the strategy in the district by, among other initiatives, setting up a demonstration wards project the main focus of which would be the introduction of primary nursing. The wards were to receive support and facilitation from a clinical nurse specialist (CNS) for practice development. Selection of four wards for the demonstration project was by competitive tendering, so that each ward in the two hospitals would have an equal chance of being selected. The criteria for selection were that the wards had to show that development initiatives were already taking place, a graduate or diplomate nurse had to be in a senior position, and nurse learners had to be allocated to the clinical area.

The chief nurse invited the professor of nursing at the local university to participate in the project and they put in a joint application for funding to the regional health authority for a nurse research assistant (RA) to evaluate the initiative. Because of the usual time taken up in securing funding, the project had been underway for several months before the RA, David Pontin, took up his appointment. During this period, however, support for the development wards had been limited because the CNS had gone on long-term sick leave.

The arrival of Pontin led to some ambiguity among project staff about the difference in roles between the CNS and himself. This was compounded by the CNS's absence. Staff seemed to feel that there was a void in support and that the RA would bridge the gap. This placed Pontin in a dilemma because he knew that, for the project to be a success, development work had to take place as soon as possible. He felt that he had the knowledge, skills and ability to do this work but not the managerial authority and insider knowledge to carry off the role. In addition his workload as evaluator of the project was a demanding one. The dilemma was resolved by deciding that he would include as much development work as he could while he was carrying out participant observation on the wards to collect initial baseline data. Thus he spent four days each week on the wards, one day per ward in rotation, in addition to formal meetings with ward staff. This period of joint activity lasted 12 weeks, after which the CNS returned from sick leave and Pontin reverted to a research role.

After this initial three months of intensive contact with the demonstration wards, he reduced his presence to one day per week plus attending any formal project meetings that took place. This allowed him to maintain the distinction in roles between himself and the CNS. However three months later the CNS left to take up a new post and the dilemma returned of how to maintain developments and ensure the success of the project. By this time the evaluation data collection work was building up and it was decided that the RA would spend two days each week on general ward contact and development work until a new development worker was appointed three months later. The new CNS maintained a high clinical profile from the start, in addition to performing an educative and consultative role, and this allowed the RA to return to his previous pattern of one-day-per-week of ward contact plus attending project-related meetings. The work pattern of the RA is summarised in Figure 14.2.

Months	April–August	August–October	October–January	January–March	March–June	June–End
CNS 1.	Development	Sick	Sick	Development	Left	
Researcher			Research and development	Research	Research and development	Research
CNS 2.						Development

Figure 14.2: Work patterns in the Midvale Project (Pontin, 1996).

Pontin wrote about these experiences in the following way:

> This is an example of the flexibility of researcher role that Patton (1990) talks about in his model of Dynamic Naturalistic Evaluation Inquiry. However, there can be problems with this wider degree of flexibility that is not found in other forms of research. I found the initial three months and the period from March to June when the CNS was absent very stressful. This was due in part to the increased responsibility I felt for the success of the project, as well as the volume of work inherent in my own role as 'researcher'. Also, I am not sure that ward staff ever really believed me when I said that I was not the replacement for the CNS. Even when there was a development worker in place, demonstration ward staff tried to involve me in activities that I considered to be the proper remit of the development worker. The price of flexibility in action research roles can be ambiguity in the minds of participants about who actually does what and what they are responsible for. This is despite participants' involvement in the project affairs from the outset. (Pontin, 1996: 194)

Pontin's involvement as an insider in the project obviously led demonstration ward staff to have confidence in him and to identify him as a trustworthy and credible facilitator of developments. The fact that he was an 'outsider' at the start of his involvement was overcome as he spent considerable periods of time on the wards and built up rapport both personally and professionally with participants. This occurred to such an extent that they came to view him as an 'insider' who was a co-participant with them in progressing the project. More information about this action research project can be found in articles written about the findings (Pontin and Webb, 1995, 1996; Webb and Pontin, 1996).

Titchen and Binnie (1993b) have written about the issues of being an insider and an outsider in action research. Their situation seemed in some ways clearer than that of Pontin, with Titchen being identified primarily as researcher and Binnie as 'actor'. Binnie occupied a managerial post in the hospital where primary nursing was being introduced and so had the authority to facilitate change. The benefits of the 'double act' they developed were that the continued presence of an insider was more likely to ensure continuity of change at the end of the project and that both researchers had support in the inevitably stressful development process. The stresses were different for the researcher and the actor, and there were times when each felt guilty about their relative contribution. Titchen realised that Binnie had more stress because of her direct involvement in the wards and hospital, while Binnie felt guilty that she was doing less 'writing' and often did not have time to read thoroughly the written material produced by Titchen. Although the 'double act' was extremely productive in terms of reflecting together on the action research process, dilemmas also arose over confidentiality when they 'told stories' to each other about events or conversations that had taken place in the research setting. In order to be aware of what was happening, they write that:

> Throughout the project, we collected data on the effects of our partnership within the study, and on how we influenced each other. We did this not only to address the issue of reflexivity, but also to explore the 'double-act' model for change in nursing. Through a process of description, hypothesis generation and testing, we plan to develop a set of guiding principles for such a partnership. (1993b: 863)

Reflection and documentation recorded in research logs or diaries are thus an essential aspect of the action research process and promote an analytical and self-critical stance on the part of the action researcher. Although the dilemmas and stresses were different, reflection with co-researchers and keeping a research diary were vital aspects, too, of the community nursing action research project carried out by Pat Turton which is discussed in the next section. This section gives detailed data about the actual dynamics involved in the project, in keeping with the reflexive nature of action research.

Living and dying with AIDS: action research in the community

Turton was an experienced district nurse who was seconded from her post as a university lecturer to a district health authority to develop a district nursing service for AIDS patients. However, on taking up the post she discovered that these patients, who were mostly gay men, were not in fact being cared for in the community. In addition, patient numbers were small in the region concerned. Patients were being nursed in two wards of a regional infectious diseases unit, were admitted there for terminal care, or were coming as out-patients for treatments which could be carried out at home (Turton, 1995).

Confidentiality was a major issue for patients, their carers and families and for nurses in the unit. Patients were reluctant to inform their GPs of their diagnosis for fear of the reaction and because of possible loss of confidentiality. The same worries were present in relation to district nurses, and men were concerned that a district nurse in uniform visiting their homes would allow neighbours to identify them as having HIV/AIDS. Many had been subject to harassment in the past, even having their homes vandalised and having to be re-housed, and their fears were thus realistic. Nursing staff at the hospital were very protective of their patients, having come to know them over a long period of time. They were also aware of the need for confidentiality and the fact that awareness of a diagnosis of HIV/AIDS could lead to family breakdown, loss of insurance benefits and to various forms of stigmatisation. Some nurses were gay or lesbian and worked in the HIV/AIDS field because of shared values and lifestyles, and patients were regarded as part of 'the family'.

Against this background, Turton (1995) chose to use action research to achieve the goal of setting up community nursing services so that patients could live and die at home if that was their wish.

HIV is predominantly viewed as a sexually transmitted disease. Qualitative methods such as ethnography are increasingly regarded – and promoted – as more fruitful than quantitative research methods in exploring HIV and sexuality (Chouinard and Albert, 1990). In North America and Western Europe it has been homosexual and bisexual men who have been most at risk. Little systematic research, however, had been done with gay men prior to the epidemic. This was largely because of legal, cultural and social attitudes as well as methodological problems. The result of this dearth of research is that: 'Individuals practising homosexual behaviour today still remain poorly understood as do the factors contributing to the persistence of particular high risk behaviours' (Carballo and Reeza, 1990: 277).

Ethnographic techniques are acknowledged to be ideally suited to studies aimed at gaining insight into the cultural aspects of and social relationships pertinent to practising homosexuals (Herdt, 1987; Bloor et al., 1992).

What has more commonly been termed 'action research' is also known as 'applied anthropology', and this approach provided guidance for setting up the project. Applied anthropologists have been employed as researchers and change agents in community health and mental health programmes, notably in the USA (Schensul and Schensul, 1978; Van Willigen, 1986). Turton's academic background was in anthropology and so her preference was towards using an ethnographic approach.

There is a recognition among British health-service researchers in particular that 'it has been extremely difficult to determine specific categories of need and match them with resources' and that 'the development of methodology to address this issue is crucially important for managers who have to deploy resources optimally and satisfy clients and carers' (Ong, 1991: 639). Hammersley suggests that:

> One aspect of the popularity of ethnography, which has been given increasing emphasis in the current cold economic climate, is the belief that this method offers a better source of information for social and educational policy making than does quantitative research. (Hammersley, 1992: 123)

Applied anthropology in relation to issues of health and illness aims, according to Helman, 'to demonstrate the clinical significance of cultural and social factors in both illness and health' (Helman, 1984:5). A consequence of this is that ethnography is 'being used with increasing frequency to examine selected concepts critical to the provision of nursing care' (Field, 1989: 91).

The usefulness of ethnography to both the practice and theory of nursing and as an action research approach is that ethnography provides 'an increasingly wide range of possibilities for understanding health behaviour and problem solving among providers and recipients of care' (Aamodt, 1989: 50). This is a particularly telling argument in relation to the needs of the terminally ill. Such patients' views of service provision are difficult to establish through questionnaires and/or interviews carried out by unknown researchers, although they are essential if services are to be responsive to their needs. Indeed, there is a danger that 'studies of palliative care which rely on data gained by patient interview may be biased to include patients with fewer problems' (Butters and Higginson, 1993: 105). Ethnographic fieldwork by a practitioner-researcher familiar to the patients and carers avoids this particular problem. The same argument applies to patients with HIV-related illness (Herdt, 1987).

Action researchers have two main roles, according to English (1991). First, they act as change agents, identifying and clarifying the need to change in a certain direction and then working and negotiating to bring about the change. Second, they are scientists and in this role they: 'record the events that occur, using whichever techniques are available and appropriate, reflect on them and draw conclusions about them' (English, 1991: 8).

Distinctions between applied anthropology and action research, therefore, lie more in the academic background of the researchers than in any fundamental difference in their approaches. In fact Hammersley suggests that action research, 'often referred to as case study, can be seen as a version of ethnography' (Hammersley, 1992: 362).

Thus, Turton decided to use her background and experience as an anthropologist and district nurse and to use a form of research and development that fitted with her commitment to consult and negotiate with those most affected, and to holistic care. However, at the start of the project she felt:

> . . . as if I was about to enter an exotic and foreign field, with a culture and language that was unfamiliar and would therefore have to be learnt before I could begin to understand what was determining the pattern of service provision and the means of developing community care for people with HIV/AIDS. (Turton, 1995: 136)

After some initial experience of visiting the infectious diseases unit and beginning to appreciate the enormity of the task in front of her, Turton decided that the best way to gain insight into patients' situations and needs, and to understand and respond to staff resistance, was to work as a nurse on the unit. She therefore adopted a staff nurse role, wearing the usual uniform and working the same shifts as regular staff. In this way she could begin to demonstrate her commitment, build up credibility, learn appropriate skills such as care of intravenous (IV) lines, and begin to collect ethnographic data by means of participant observation, interviews with patients and staff and by keeping a research diary. The following extracts from this diary record an early incident when ward staff were still extremely sensitive about confidentiality: 'One of the ward nurses a few months later commenting on the "secretive" atmosphere I encountered, said, "people were a bit reluctant, I know, to tell you anything or to welcome you really"' (Turton, 1995: 171).

An incident occurred with a patient in which:

> His partner had been injured in a car crash and would be hospitalised for some time. The (staff member) said 'the patient is at the top of the tree – in crisis'. Three factors made this a 'risky' referral and put me in a very difficult situation, first legally: the patient was on IV medication and needed help to administer the drug and I was not yet certified to give intravenous treatment; secondly with regard to timing: he was close to death and very anxious, as was his elderly mother who had unexpectedly had to take on the role of carer at this point because of his partner's road traffic accident. I had never met him or his carers. I therefore, decided to decline to go to the house to give the medication. I was aware that my lack of certification was known by the (staff member), whose background was in district nursing, and that entering a new situation and trying to build up a relationship with a family in crisis was likely to prove difficult. As a result of my decision the patient had to be brought to the ward. The third factor in the situation arose from the discrepancy in the IV procedure when carried out by the ward nurses as opposed to the junior doctor. I was instructed to carry out the procedure for the patient on his arrival, wearing gloves and apron. The doctor, however, knew the patient well and on entering the cubicle took over from me. She carried on without gloves or a sterile technique. The

patient assumed that my use of gloves was a sign of prejudice and he therefore lost confidence in both my attitudes and my expertise. The patient
remained on the ward and died there two weeks later. (Turton, 1995: 172)

Turton records that she felt that this was an 'initiation ceremony'
and that she had 'failed' in the eyes of ward staff (Alavi and Cattoni,
1995). However, as she continued to work on the ward, staff came
gradually to accept her and value her contribution, as the following
extract from an interview with a nurse shows:

It was important to be based here because you needed to be seen around a
lot especially in the initial phases to establish who you were and what you
were about. To gain acceptance, dare I say, you have to work at it. It was
important that you were seen as part of the team. Then we realised that . . .
you were having a hard time to get this thing going – to look after people in
the community. (Turton, 1995: 177)

Another field diary entry adds further evidence that, little by little,
Turton was becoming seen by ward staff as an 'insider':

The (staff member) had remarked in front of the ward nurses one coffee
time that a dying AIDS patient, a gay man, had appreciated my being with
him. She repeated that he had told her he felt better after the massage I had
given him and felt cared for when I was with him. The public nature of the
comments and the fact that they were repeated was significant. It was the
first acknowledgement that I might have something to offer 'the family'.
(Turton, 1995: 177–8)

Turton also noted in her diary that she was coming to see herself as
an insider too: 'But I note that I am already beginning to use the
term "we" when referring to (ward) staff' (Turton, 1995: 179).

At the start, then, the most influential actors in the project seemed
to be ward staff. As the project developed Turton began to collaborate
with two other AIDS CNSs working in neighbouring health districts.
They decided that, because none of them had many AIDS patients in
their own districts and patients came to the regional unit from a wide
geographical area, they would form a Community Liaison Team
(CLT) and work together to provide 24-hour cover for care in the
community. This would enable generic district nurses to give care and
be supported by the CLT. Setting up the team was crucial, not only for
service provision, but for providing Turton with professional and
personal support in a developing context in which the stresses were
multiple: gaining acceptance of the new service against hospital staff
resistance, winning over district nurses and their managers to the new
system, and coping with the often extremely distressing physical,
emotional and social aspects of caring for AIDS patients, many of
whom were in the terminal phase of illness.

District nurses were not accustomed to AIDS patients, nor were they trained in certain procedures such as male catheterisation (by female nurses), care of intravenous long lines and administration of intravenous medication. Turton, herself an experienced district nurse, believed that with one-to-one teaching and support they would be able to adapt. In fact they did this more rapidly than she and they anticipated, as an interview with a district nurse shows:

> Initially a lot of support is needed until skills and confidence are gained in HIV work. Later I needed to know that I could call someone anytime if I am worried or need support. But I want to care for my patient myself. I have found the CLT provide this. Compared with other specialist nurses they are much more willing to do joint visits and not to keep their specialist skills to themselves but to share them. I also think they provide a vital training role. (Turton, 1995: 238)

Patients' views of the DNs were summed up by a patient's partner, who wrote a 'consumer report' to the team which said:

> AIDS with all its horror and cruelty, cannot destroy the value of the human spirit. This spirit was reflected in the team of district nurses who took on board the demanding requirements of AIDS. They delivered an exacting daily service for nearly two years. My friend was only able to come home, which is what we both wanted, because of the high quality of the district nurses. They gave treatments that before were only provided in hospital and they did it with a high level of competence, kindness, compassion and friendliness. (Turton, 1995: 233)

Patients themselves also played a vital role as co-participants with Turton and the relationships she and the other two nurses in the CLT built up with them provided support in the form of positive feedback on their work, as this letter from a patient involved with Body Positive (BP) shows:

> Many of our members have greatly benefited from this existing service, without which we would not have known of the possibilities and choices available to us . . . the (CNS) post has been invaluable in forging links between the hospital, community services and people with HIV/AIDS . . . meeting the needs of the individual whether it be at home or in the hospital has greatly enhanced the quality of life for many people. (Turton, 1995: 225)

Describing the way the CLT worked and the process of reflection and self-criticism that took place as the three members struggled to find the most fruitful ways forward, one of the team members said:

> We called it action research because we didn't want to stop working to do research – we fit the theory to the practice and then the practice to the theory . . . We were learning what was needed while we were doing it and

then writing it up as if we knew what we were doing. We didn't know what we were doing – we made mistakes or we did not made mistakes. We talked to patients who identified a need – trying to meet it and getting it right or getting it wrong – thinking about it and trying again – that's what we called the action research cycle. (Turton, 1995: 377)

Turton's action research project links with some of the debates raised earlier in the chapter. In particular, she faced the problem of securing consent from participants and meeting resistance, but these dilemmas took different forms from those described by other authors. If she had not begun the project without securing full agreement and collaboration in advance, as suggested by Whyte (1989) and Nolan and Grant (1993), then almost certainly the project would not have got off the ground due to the degree of protectiveness shown by hospital staff over patients and their own roles in care. Furthermore, if Turton had agreed to withdraw if participants were not happy with her contribution, as discussed by Meyer (1993a), then again the work might well have not advanced very far. However, Turton and the other members of the CLT felt that they had a responsibility to patients to press on because they were convinced by patients that they wanted, and would benefit from, home care (Turton, 1995). To have not started the project or to have withdrawn part-way through would have been to allow professionals who were in a powerful position to veto developments that could have led to a quality service for less powerful actors, namely patients.

By pushing forward in the face of early difficulties and adopting a participant nursing role in the unit, Turton was able to set in motion the action research spirals of reflection, planning, action, evaluation and reflection which form the foundations of the approach (Kemmis and McTaggart, 1988).

Summary

Support for the action researcher in the inevitably stressful process of promoting and introducing change has already been identified as vital (Greenwood, 1994). For Turton (1995) this took the form of the CLT, whose other two members were carrying out a similar role to herself and were therefore in an ideal position to understand her stresses and the three team members acted as mutual supporters.

The 'insider/outsider' issue is raised in several of the reports discussed, and it seems as if there is no single ideal solution to this problem. Researchers have been in different starting positions in their projects, as shown in Figure 14.3.

	Starting position	Position reached within the action research project
Meyer 1993a	Former ward sister in same hospital	Insider
Pontin 1996	Outsider	Insider
Titchen and Binnie 1993b	Insider and outsider	Insider and outsider
Turton 1995	Outsider	Insider
Waterman 1994; Waterman et al.,1995	Former ward sister in same hospital	Insider
Webb 1989	Clinical teacher on same ward	Insider to some staff Outsider to ward sister
Webb 1990a	Clinical teacher in same hospital	Insider to some staff Outsider to reluctant participators (part-timers)
Webb 1990b	Clinical teacher in same hospital	Insider

Figure 14.3: Positions adopted by action researchers.

This illustrates that the role achieved within the action research project is not necessarily determined by the researcher's status beforehand. Action researchers known and not known to participants have achieved a high degree of acceptance, but this is not guaranteed even when a similar approach is used. Other factors already discussed, such as co-operation and power of those outside the immediate setting, such as managers and doctors, may influence the situation by their actions or inactions. Different groups of individuals within the project may have their own agendas and be powerful in promoting these. What is vital to the continuing development, criticism and evolution of action research in nursing is that these issues continue to be reported and discussed so that future work can build on experiences already gained.

Gaining informed consent continued to be a concern in the examples of Pontin (1996) and Turton (1995), just as it had been for earlier workers. Perhaps this is an inevitable feature of action research in a health-care setting where staff turnover can be rapid and the change process drawn-out. This is a feature that differentiates this work from action research by teachers, who are relatively autonomous in their own classrooms and whose work has relatively contained boundaries (Greenwood, 1994) in a way that they cannot exist in a multidisciplinary setting like health care.

Despite the difficulties experienced by nurse action researchers, the potential of action research to achieve the goal of narrowing the theory–practice gap continue to be enormous. The precise forms it takes should be in keeping with the demands and needs of each particular project, and rigid rules for carrying out action research would be at odds with its basic principles of democracy, participation and empowerment of participants to make things move in directions they wish. The examples quoted in this chapter have shown the degree of variety possible; it is for others who follow to work out solutions suited to their own particular contexts.

References

Aamodt AM (1989) Ethnography and Epistemology: Generating Nursing Knowledge. Qualitative Nursing Research: A Contemporary Dialogue. London: Sage.

Alavi C, Cattoni J (1995) Good nurse, bad nurse. Journal of Advanced Nursing 2: 344–9.

Bloor M, McKeganey NP, Finaly A, Barnard M (1992) The inappropriateness of psycho-social models of risk behaviour for understanding HIV-related risk practices among Glasgow male prostitutes. AIDS Care 4(2): 131–7.

Butters E, Higginson I (1993) Palliative care for people with HIV/AIDS: views of patients, carers and providers. AIDS Care 5(1): 105–10.

Carballo M, Reeza G (1990) AIDS, drug misuse and the global crisis. In Strang J, Stimson G (Eds) AIDS and Drug Misuse. London: Routledge.

Carr W, Kemmis S (1986) Becoming Critical. Brighton: Falmer.

Chouinard A, Albert J (1990) Human Sexuality: Research Perspectives in a World Facing AIDS. Ottawa: International Development Research Centre.

Department of Health (1989) A strategy for nursing – a report of the steering committee. London: HMSO.

East L, Robinson J (1994) Change in process: bringing about change in health care through action research. Journal of Clinical Nursing 3: 57–61.

English P (1991) Action research and primary health care. Teamcare Valleys Discussion Paper (No. 5). Whitchurch: Teamcare Valleys.

Field PA (1989) Doing fieldwork in your own culture. In Morse J (Ed) Qualitative Nursing Research: A Contemporary Dialogue. London: Sage.

Gibbon B, Little V (1995) Improving stroke care through action research. Journal of Clinical Nursing 4: 93–100.

Greenwood J (1994) Action research: a few details, a caution and something new. Journal of Advanced Nursing 20: 13–18.

Hammersley M (1992) What's Wrong with Ethnography? Methodological Explorations. London: Routledge.

Hart E, Bond M (1995) Action Research for Health and Social Care. A Guide to Practice. Buckingham: Open University Press.

Helman C (1984) Culture, Health and Illness: An Introduction for Health Professionals. London: Wright.

Herdt G (1987) AIDS and anthropology. Anthropology Today 3(2): 1–3.

Holter L, Schwartz-Barcott D (1993) Action research: what is it? How can it be used and how can it be used in nursing? Journal of Advanced Nursing 18: 298–304.

Hunt M (1987) The process of translating research findings into nursing practice. Journal of Advanced Nursing 12: 101–10.

Kemmis S, McTaggart R (Eds) (1988) The Action Research Planner. 3rd edn. Geelong: Deakin University Press.

Lauri S (1982) Development of the nursing process through action research. Journal of Advanced Nursing 7: 301–7.

Lewin K (1946) Action research and minority problems. Journal of Social Issues 2: 34–46.

McNiff J (1988) Action Research: Principles and Practice. London: Macmillan Education.

McTaggart R (1994) Participatory action research: issues in theory and practice. Educational Action Research 2(3): 313–37.

Meyer J (1993a) New paradigm research in practice: the trials and tribulations of action research. Journal of Advanced Nursing 18: 1066–72.

Meyer J (1993b) Lay participation in care: a challenge for multidisciplinary team-work. Journal of Interprofessional Care 7(1): 57–66.

Meyer J (1995a) Lay participation in care in a hospital setting: an action research study. Unpublished PhD thesis, University of London.

Meyer J (1995b) Action research. Stages in the process: a personal account. Nurse Researcher 2(3): 24–37.

Nolan M, Grant G (1993) Action research and quality of care: a mechanism for agreeing basic values as a precursor to change. Journal of Advanced Nursing 18: 305–11.

Ong BN (1991) Researching needs in district nursing. Journal of Advanced Nursing 16: 638–47.

Patton M (1990) Qualitative Evaluation and Research Methods. 2nd edn, London: Sage.

Pontin D (1996) The effect of primary nursing on the quality of nursing care: an action research study of nursing development work. Unpublished PhD thesis, University of Manchester.

Pontin D, Webb C (1995) Assessing patient satisfaction. Part 1. The research process. Journal of Clinical Nursing 4: 383–9.

Pontin D, Webb C (1996) Assessing patient satisfaction. Part 2. Findings: nursing, the hospital and patients' concerns. Journal of Clinical Nursing 5: 33–40.

Schensul SL, Schensul JJ (1978) Advocacy and applied anthropology. In Weber G, McCall G (Eds). Social Scientists as Advocates. London: Sage.

Susman G, Evered R (1978) An assessment of the scientific merits of action research. Administrative Science Quarterly 23: 582–603.

Titchen A (1995) Issues of validity in action research. Nurse Researcher 2(3): 38–48.

Titchen A, Binnie A (1992) Research partnerships: collaborative action research in nursing. Journal of Advanced Nursing 18: 858–965.

Titchen A, Binnie A (1993a) What am I meant to be doing? Putting practice into theory and back again. Journal of Advanced Nursing 18:1054–65.

Titchen A, Binnie A (1993b) Research partnerships: collaborative action research in nursing. Journal of Advanced Nursing 18: 858–65.

Turton AJP (1995) Developing a community nursing service for people with HIV disease: an action research project incorporating ethnographic methods. Unpublished PhD thesis, University of Manchester.

Van Willigen J (1986) Applied Anthropology: An Introduction. Boston, MA: Bergin & Garvey.

Waterman H (1994) The meaning of visual impairment: developing ophthalmic nursing practice. Unpublished PhD thesis, University of Manchester.

Waterman H, Webb C, Williams A (1995) Changing nursing and nursing change: a dialectical analysis of an action research project. Educational Action Research 3(1): 55–70.

Webb C (1989) Action research: philosophy, methods and personal experiences. Journal of Advanced Nursing. 14:403–10.

Webb C (1990a) Self-medication for elderly patients. Nursing Times Occasional Papers 86(16):46–9.

Webb C (1990b) Partners in research. Nursing Times 86(32): 40–4.

Webb C, Mackenzie J (1993) Where are we now? Research-mindedness in the 1990s. Journal of Clinical Nursing 2: 129–33.

Webb C, Pontin D (1996) Introducing primary nursing: nurses' opinions. Journal of Clinical Nursing. 3(6) 351–8

Whyte WF (1989) Advancing scientific knowledge through participatory action research. Sociological Forum 4(3): 367–85.

Chapter 15
Evaluation research for the development of health care and health services

Brenda Roe

Introduction

Evaluation, as opposed to evaluation research, has been undertaken within nursing for some years, in particular in nurse education (Marsland and Gissane, 1992: 233) and in relation to nursing development units (NDU) (Pearson, 1983, 1991). This chapter describes the difference between evaluation and evaluation research, along with discussion of the relevant literature. Two examples of the application of evaluation research in health and social care are briefly presented by way of illustration, and how it relates to clinical nursing practice and its outcomes is explored. The strengths and limitations of evaluation research are considered and its appropriateness for the development of health care and health services is also discussed with reference to nursing. Specific examples of published research that has evaluated health care and health services are presented.

Evaluation research

Evaluation research is recognised as important for evaluating the impact of health promotion, health care and health services (Marsland and Gissane, 1992; Tones and Tilford, 1995). Evaluation research is generally considered to be research, as it adopts a systematic approach using a wide variety of research designs and methods, ranging from single case studies to randomised controlled trials (Bond and Tierney, 1992) in order to provide objective empirical information that is then measured against specified goals, objectives and outcomes (Suchman, 1967; Luker, 1981; Tones and Tilford, 1995). The origins of evaluation research are generally considered to be in the social sciences (Suchman, 1967; Luker, 1981) and the modern revival and interest that has arisen since the 1960s is due to large-scale government-funded education and public health programmes, particularly those in the United States, undertaken to help inform public and fiscal policy (Scriven, 1991; Rossi and Freeman, 1993: 5 and 9). Evaluation is a subjective process of assessment or appraisal which does not systematically use research methods or logic (Suchman, 1967; Luker, 1981) and is generally used within nursing education (Marsland and Gissane, 1992) although early mention has been made in relation to nursing care in North America (Derryberry, 1939).

Evaluation and clinical nursing practice

The nursing process, with its roots in the United States, has evaluation as its last stage and is used to review whether assessed needs, planned goals and implemented nursing care have been achieved (Yura and Walsh, 1978; Roper et al., 1980). Evaluation and evaluation research have been compared and contrasted with elements of the nursing process, where it was observed that evaluation is often secondary to the main focus of assessing patients' needs, identifying goals and the delivery of nursing care (Luker, 1981). Luker (1981) also concluded that the disproportionate emphasis on assessment was to the detriment of evaluation and argued that a greater emphasis on the evaluation stage within a process–outcome approach could be a way forward for evaluation research in nursing. The nursing process lends itself to the evaluation format of structure, process and outcome, as suggested by Donabedian (1969), and is an approach that continues to be used in research evaluating health care and health services today (St Leger et al., 1993; Button et al., 1996).

Evaluation research for health care and health services

Since the introduction of the NHS Research and Development strategy within the UK (Department of Health, 1991, 1993a) evaluation of health care and health services has been an important aspect of health services research and contributes to ensuring that health care and the delivery of health services are based upon sound evidence, and where possible effectiveness (NHSE, 1996). The word evaluation when used on its own in the context of health services research ascribes it the traditional evaluation research label or meaning, that it is based upon systematic and empirical enquiry. Nurses comprise the largest workforce within the NHS (Department of Health, 1995: 6) and are major contributors to health care delivery and services in both hospitals and the community, 24 hours a day and seven days a week. Evaluation research into clinical nursing practice and nursing care systems is therefore important and it is generally agreed that innovations or developments in nursing should not be widely adopted until they have been evaluated (Bond and Tierney, 1992).

Dissemination and utilisation of research evidence to inform clinical nursing practice has already been recognised as an important research and development endeavour (Funk et al., 1989, 1991; Closs and Cheater, 1994; Dunn et al., 1997) (see Chapter 1). Dissemination and development have been defined as generic processes, with dissemination relating to the presentation of information, in particular research evidence, to improve practice and development being a planned and systematic process of implementation to promote, change or improve skills, competencies or nursing care systems. Dissemination could just relate to one single project outcome whereas development relates to the synthesis and interpretation of all available information, data or evidence and its implementation (Department of Health, 1993b: Appendix 2). Development and dissemination are now key features of health services research policy (Department of Health, 1993b) with the Second International Conference on the Scientific Basis of Health Services held in Amsterdam, the Netherlands, having 'Using the Evidence' as its primary theme. Evidence has been categorised into three groupings: the dissemination of evidence, its implementation, and the evaluation of evidence in practice. Using evidence can focus on dissemination and directing results to those who need them. Implementation of evidence or development includes overcoming obstacles to change, matching guidelines to patients and settings and health care or health services. The evaluation of evidence in practice includes monitoring the use and resulting effects of evidence, dissemination and development in relation to specified goals and outcomes. Establishing or measuring the impact of dissemination or development initiatives in this context constitutes evaluation research and reaffirms its importance for health care and health services.

Specified goals and outcomes

A further distinguishing feature of evaluation research, as opposed to evaluation, is that it is also undertaken with pre-specified goals or objectives that are used to measure the effects or success of the activity, intervention or service that is being evaluated (Luker, 1981; St Leger et al., 1993). Identifying the goals or objectives, more latterly known as outcomes, is therefore an essential step when undertaking evaluation research to determine the effectiveness of developments in health care or health services. Outcomes are, traditionally speaking, the independent variables that are measured to determine the success or effectiveness of an intervention, with the initial research design adopted, sample size recruited and statistical analysis undertaken allowing the confidence we can attribute to there being a direct causal relationship between the intervention and its outcome (see Chapters 7, 8, 9 and 10).

Outcome measurements are recognised as an important aspect of the evaluation of health services and health care (Coulter, 1992; Wilkin et al., 1993; UK Clearing House on Health Outcomes Briefing, 1993). They can include objective and subjective measures of clinical information such as diagnoses or physiological readings (see Chapter 8), standardised quality of life measures such as health status, psychological well being or life satisfaction (see Chapter 9 and Bowling, 1991, 1995) or consumers' views on their satisfaction with health care or services (Fitzpatrick, 1991, 1993). When dealing with health services, the intervention or process of health care itself can also be considered to be an outcome.

Outcomes and nursing

Evaluating the outcomes of nursing care has been attempted to identify the unique nature and contribution that nursing makes to patient care (Bond, 1992; Higgins et al.,1992). This also supports the notion of nursing being therapeutic and producing effects that can be measured or described (Kitson, 1991; McMahon and Pearson, 1991). Outcome measures need to be valid, reliable and sensitive (see Chapter 9). It is generally acknowledged that developing outcomes which meet such criteria is difficult. As with health services and health care in general, the actual intervention or process of nursing care itself can be considered as an outcome and needs to be examined. Bloch (1975) and Pearson (1987) have both contended that just looking at outcomes alone is too simplistic and that the process of care itself needs to be examined to see how it has contributed to a favourable or unfavourable outcome of nursing care.

Higgins et al. (1992) obtained data on outcome measures as part of a larger study evaluating skill mix and effectiveness of nursing care. They developed a number of patient-focused standards that related to the outcome of nursing care on 15 surgical and medical wards in seven acute hospitals. Initial testing reported that these outcome measures showed promise as being valid and reliable for evaluating nursing care and were easy to use in the clinical setting. Researchers in Newcastle have also looked at outcome measures for nursing and have developed a specific instrument that measures patients' experiences of and satisfaction with their nursing care, known as the Newcastle Satisfaction with Nursing Scales (NSNS) (Priest et al., 1995). This scale is now being more widely used in research projects throughout the UK. Measuring goals, objectives and outcomes of nursing care is in keeping with evaluation research that measures the outcomes of developments in health care and health services.

Two examples of evaluation research in health and social care

Kazi (1996) described the use of single case designs with both quantitative and qualitative methods as part of an evaluation research project undertaken in education social work. The practitioners found that by using a single case design they could continuously assess the outcome data along with their clients, and this provided an opportunity for collaboration and accountability. Three case studies were presented, one involving a primary school girl aged 8 years who was referred to a social worker at the request of her mother to help with aggressive and destructive behaviour at home. The conventional single case approach was used, where A denotes the baseline when measurement has started before the intervention, or when the intervention has stopped and the measurement is continued, B is when the same measure is used during an intervention phase and C when an intervention phase is changed to another. In the case of the primary school girl, the social worker asked her parents to keep a record of all notable episodes of behaviour along with a log of any antecedents or consequences. An intervention programme, which consisted of advice and support for both parents, was started to enhance their management of their daughter's behaviour. This was essentially a B design as no previous baseline data were available.

The qualitative data provided by the parents were then quantified to the number of days per week when bad behaviour did not occur, which was then represented on a graph. Over a six-week period, the girl's behaviour improved from one day per week when bad behaviour did not take place to six days per week when bad behaviour did not take place. Kazi (1996) notes that this is a weak research design and that the only inference that could be drawn was that the behaviour improved, and that it could not be concluded that this was due to the intervention. However he appreciates that this design can provide useful information on progress for both the social worker and the client.

A second case reported by Kazi (1996) involving a 7-year-old girl, also referred by her mother, used an AB design providing before and after data. Baseline recordings were obtained for the three problem behaviours of swearing, temper tantrums and night-time enuresis. The behaviours were recorded by the mother and a star was awarded for those days when the behaviours were absent. As with the previous case, qualitative recordings were then converted to quantitative data and represented graphically so that they could be reviewed by the social worker and the clients. The social worker aimed to develop the mother's parenting skills, improve the relationship between the parent and the child and subsequently improve the child's behaviour. The intervention comprised behaviour modification for each of these three behaviours. Evaluation of the quantitative data showed that immediate improvement and benefit occurred in all three behaviours once the intervention had commenced. Kazi (1996) concluded that single case designs for evaluation research are useful for practising social workers and that they could also be used by other public sector professionals, such as those in health, social services or education, as part of their work.

An example of evaluation research in health care is provided by Oakley and colleagues (1990) who undertook a randomised controlled trial to evaluate the impact of social support on outcomes of pregnancy. Pregnant women with a history of low birth weight babies were recruited from antenatal clinics at four hospitals ($n =$ 509). The women were then randomly assigned to either the intervention group, which received social support in addition to standard antenatal care, or the control group, which received standard antenatal care only. Social support was provided by four midwives in the form of home visits, where they listened to mothers' concerns, provided advice and information, collected medical and social information and initiated referral to other health professionals. Midwives also provided 24-hour telephone contact. Information on the outcomes of pregnancy were obtained from obstetric notes and from a questionnaire sent six weeks after delivery.

Babies of mothers in the intervention group had higher mean birth weights than those in the control group and there were also fewer very low birth-weight babies born to mothers in the intervention group. More women in the control group were admitted to hospital during their pregnancy than in the intervention group. Spontaneous labour and vaginal delivery were more common in women in the intervention group. Fewer epidurals were also used by women who had received the social support. Mothers and babies who received the social support were also significantly healthier (including physical and psychosocial health and use of health services) in the early weeks than those in the control group who had received standard antenatal care. Oakley et al. (1990) concluded that the policy implications of their findings were that less impersonal and more sensitive antenatal care, which has continuity, is important. A more comprehensive presentation of this project on social support and motherhood is available and provides a detailed example of evaluation research that took the form of a large randomised controlled trial with important findings for health care and health services (Oakley, 1992).

Strengths and limitations of evaluation research

Evaluation research is mainly concerned with establishing whether desirable goals have been achieved and can include both process and outcomes. General research, on the other hand, has a much wider range of purposes (Tones and Tilford, 1995: 50–1). General research or 'blue sky research' is often for the pursuit of new knowledge to enhance understanding or to develop new technologies. Its findings are generally published within the academic press, whereas findings from evaluation research are generally there to inform or influence decision makers (Jamieson, 1984). The findings from evaluation research may be used to provide feedback on certain activities or projects, for the development of theory about activities and their contexts or for general dissemination, either locally or more widely. They may also be used to assess the value of activities in terms of their effectiveness, efficiency or equity (Tones and Tilford, 1995: 50).

As the questions for evaluation research are often set by a client wanting a service or project evaluated, the evaluation researcher may be constrained by this and limited in the direction he or she can take or the designs and methodologies incorporated. General researchers may have more scope to pursue certain lines of their own enquiry (Tones and Tilford, 1995: 50), although with the increased emphasis on the strategic and operational management of commissioned research and grants awarded this may no longer be the case. Where evaluation research is undertaken as an external activity by externally appointed researchers, participants may not see it as a threat. However, recognised limitations of evaluation research are where participants see the data collection as being disruptive to the service, or the evaluation activity may be perceived as worthless by the participants or even threatening, particularly if the end result of a project is the discontinuation of a service or programme. It behoves researchers to think this through at the beginning of a project and possibly to adopt a research design that establishes a more equal participation in evaluation activities by both researchers and participants (Tones and Tilford, 1995: 50) (see Chapter 14). Even when more equal participation is adopted there still may be different emphasis placed by participants and evaluators; for example, evaluators may be more interested in outcomes while participants may place more emphasis on the process itself. How a process empowers patients in relation to their health may be of greater importance to participants, although in the short term it may make no difference in terms of health outcomes (Tones and Tilford, 1995: 50).

Luker (1981) has argued that evaluation researchers are constrained by the need for strict methodological requirements that allow for causal inferences to be made from findings. She suggests that the randomised controlled trial provides the strongest case for internal validity and is strong on external validity where appropriate sampling techniques are used (see Chapter 7). She argues that the consequences of incorrect inferences or misleading generalisations are more serious in applied social research, to which evaluation research belongs, and that the randomised controlled trial is therefore the design of choice. However practical difficulties in the field can limit which experimental design is selected and having a control group, particularly in health care or health services, may pose a problem. A combined approach, using an experimental design in the context of structure, process and outcomes, as suggested by Donabedian (1966, 1969), may be a realistic way to proceed with evaluation research dealing with health care or health services.

Developments in health care settings and situations

Evaluation research is applied research that takes place in a real world setting and as such the features of the research are determined by the questions needing to be asked, the range of intervention strategies that can be implemented and the feasibility and moral considerations of whether or not a randomised controlled trial can be undertaken, particularly in relation to health care or health services. Evaluation of health care and health services is a concern for a variety of professionals, not least nurses who undertake clinical nursing practice in both hospital or community settings (Luker, 1981: 88; St Leger et al., 1993). Dissemination and development have been defined as generic processes, with developments being planned and systematic processes of implementation to promote, change, or improve skills, competencies or care systems (health care or health services).

Development relates to the synthesis and interpretation of all available information, data or evidence and their implementation (Department of Health, 1993b: Appendix 2) and, as such, it could be argued that some form of dissemination is implicit either as a precursor activity or within the developments themselves, as well as an end stage activity to disseminate any findings arising from an evaluation of the development initiative. Evaluation research is applied research that can be undertaken in the real-world settings of health care and health services and is essential to determine the impact or effects of dissemination and development activities. The stages would therefore be dissemination, implementation or development and then evaluation (research) within health care or health services. A number of key papers and research projects that have looked at evaluation of developments in health care and health services now follow, by way of example.

Evaluation of health care

Individualised outcome measures

Cook (1995) argues for the merits of individualised outcome measures within routine clinical practice, where the required outcomes of care may be defined differently for each individual client. This is in contrast to standardised outcome measures, such as health status measures, that are used for all clients. She maintains this is particularly useful for therapists, nurses and multidisciplinary teams who work with people who have complex and multiple disabilities and co-morbidities, where the treatment itself is not a standardised intervention. Spreadbury (1995) goes on to describe how outcomes for individualised care can be measured using the Binary

Individualised Outcome Measure (BIOM), a tool for use with clinical audit, care planning and patient documentation (Cook and Spreadbury, 1995) which was developed as part of a project undertaken in Trent Region, working with occupational therapists and nurses ($n = 50$). The intention was to design an individualised outcomes measure that could be incorporated into existing documentation and that would assist clinical staff in meeting a number of objectives. These objectives included clarifying the purpose of their service, improving patient care and the effectiveness and efficiency of services, providing evidence of effectiveness in order to be accountable and gaining personal job satisfaction through evidence of achievements (Spreadbury, 1995). One of the reasons for wanting to develop an outcome measure for individualised care was that care is client centred, with the goals and problems negotiated with both the client and/or carer. By involving the client in the therapy they are active participants and therefore more able to understand and measure changes that occur. The results or outcomes of the therapy can then be evaluated and the results aggregated for a number of patients. Spreadbury (1995) illustrates its application by presenting the case study of a 50-year-old client who had suffered a stroke. This approach, using goal identification, care planning and evaluation, is similar to the individualised outcomes of the nursing process (Roper et al., 1980) and lends itself to evaluation research of developments in health care by clinicians using case methodologies and aggregating their findings.

Dissemination of research evidence for continence care

A further example relevant to health care is a project undertaken by Williams et al. (1995) which evaluated nursing developments in continence care and looked at a method of disseminating research evidence to qualified nurses (registered and enrolled nurses) working in elderly care wards and community hospitals (15 sites throughout Oxfordshire, UK). A static group comparison research design involving an experimental group and control group with a pre-test, post-test and follow up was undertaken. The intervention comprised a clinical handbook of continence care (Roe and Williams, 1994) compiled from a systematic review of published literature on incontinence (Williams et al., 1995), issued in discussion groups once pre-test information had been collected. Individual nurses were invited by personal letter to attend a discussion group at their place of work, which provided an opportunity to share further information about the project as well as being a means for collecting data on their reported practice using self-completed questionnaires. Once data had been collected, the clinical handbook was distributed to nurses in the experimental groups and its contents presented and discussed. Nurses in the control group were informed that they would receive the handbook once the project was completed. Seven weeks later, a further discussion group was held at each site and nurses attending reflected on their practice and completed a further questionnaire. Data on the prevalence of urinary and faecal incontinence and documented practice were also collected from nursing staff and the medical and nursing notes by the researchers. A 54% response rate of qualified nurses was obtained at the pre-test ($n = 233$) and a 29% response rate at the post-test ($n = 124$). Significant improvements in reported practice on continence care were obtained between the pre- and post-test phase for 86% of variables ($n = 84$) for nurses in the experimental group compared to 59% of variables ($n = 54$) for nurses in the control group (McNemar's test, p <0.05). Limited documentation was found for continence care at each phase of the study, despite 41% of patients suffering from urinary incontinence ($n = 213$), 1% of patients suffering from faecal incontinence ($n = 8$) and 9% of patients suffering from a combination of urinary and faecal incontinence, within the study sites ($n = 45$). It was concluded that use of a clinical handbook and discussion groups was an effective method for disseminating information on continence care to practising nurses. For this knowledge to be translated into clinical practice it would require further work involving the collaboration of all members of the multidisciplinary team. This study illustrates how evaluation research can be used to assess development work in health care involving practising nurses.

Guidelines on health care can be used as an effective means of disseminating research evidence to health care practitioners and have been found to change clinical practice and benefit patient outcome (Effective Health Care Bulletin, 1994). They are now being widely used within health services as part of initiatives on clinical effectiveness and attempts to improve the efficiency and effectiveness of patient care and services (Eddy, 1990; McCormick and Fleming, 1992; Effective Health Care Bulletin, 1994; Klazinga, 1994; Deighan and Hitch, 1995; NHSE, 1996). Guidelines are effective if they take account of local circumstances and if they are actively disseminated within an educational intervention. Balanced incomplete block designs, randomised controlled trials that randomise the health professionals individually or in groups, and randomised crossover trials are recommended as providing the strongest evidence for effectiveness (Effective Health Care Bulletin, 1994) (see Chapter 13). Button and colleagues (1996,1998), as part of the NHS Executive Strategy for major Clinical Guidelines, developed a national Clinical Guideline for the Promotion and Management of Continence by Primary Health Care Teams (PHCT). The guidelines were developed through a process of managed consensus based upon scientific review and included a systematic review of published evidence for the health care of people with incontinence. The guidelines were implemented and evaluated within one healthcare setting, as part of the initial agreement for the commissioned work. The practice setting was an urban first-wave fundholding practice in the north-west of England with 12 000 registered patients. The evaluation research design adopted was acknowledged as being weak, as there was no control group due to the time and financial constraints of the project. The impact of the guideline was evaluated using a pre-and post-implementation survey of a random sample of 17% of patients aged 18 years and over ($n = 1503$ from 8908 records). Baseline information was collected concerning prevalence of urinary and faecal incontinence prior to implementation, along with related epidemiological data and the current management of incontinence. Patients were then invited to have their condition assessed and their care reviewed. A post-implementation survey of patients who had agreed to participate in a second round was undertaken to evaluate the impact of the guideline on patient care. It was also used to establish reasons why some sufferers chose not to seek help. Developments in the structure and process of health care included the production of a single assessment tool for incontinence which interfaced with the practice's computerised record keeping system, facilitating future clinical audit of patient records regarding incontinence, and screening for 'at risk' groups by including questions on incontinence within the over-75 screening programme and at cervical cytology clinics. The education and training needs of members of the PHCT were also identified and met. Due to a weaker research design, the fact that only one PHCT site could be included and the limited time available for implementation of the project, the impact of the guideline on clinical outcomes was not great and this clearly demonstrates the realities of working within the 'real world' with limited funding available. The guideline did not have any impact on the patients' perception of their incontinence as a problem nor its subjective severity, although there was some slight improvement in the approaches adopted by members of the PHCT in relation to assessment of incontinence and referral of patients to other health professionals. Further longitudinal evaluation of the impact of these guidelines was recommended.

Organisation and quality of health care

Evaluation research has also been used to look at the impact of different management styles on the impact of quality of health care (Whelan, 1988). The style of management of 16 oncology ward sisters was classified for three dimensions that included patterns of decision making, task orientation and socio-emotional orientation. This study did make allowances for the influence of confounding variables but could have been further strengthened by having a tight operational definition of 'management style'. Quality of care was assessed in terms of the nurses' confidential ratings, and variations in the ward sisters' task and socio-emotional orientations were found to be significantly correlated with differences in quality of care. This study serves to illustrate how developments in style of management can affect the quality of health care.

Maguire (1991) undertook evaluation research to study the impact of primary nursing on the quality of care of elderly people and specifically looked at the effectiveness of Senior Monitor in evaluating changes in nursing care over time. She concluded that irrespective of the organisation of care (primary nursing), the process of assessment itself was a powerful incentive for care to be improved in wards that had been matched in size, patient population, staffing level, skill mix and support services. This study demonstrates how evaluation research can be used to measure developments in health care and the author is realistic in the conclusion drawn, that the assessment itself can act as a powerful incentive to improve practice.

Donabedian (1966: 169) has addressed quality of health care and views outcomes as being the ultimate measures of its effectiveness and quality. He proposed that health care could be evaluated in relation to structure (resources, facilities and organisational settings), process (the activities between health professionals and patients) and outcome (change in health status as a result of health care) (Donabedian, 1980). This remains a very valuable approach to the evaluation of both health care and health services. Coulter (1992: 116), in a chapter that looks at evaluating the outcomes of health care, lists four levels of evaluation research within health services that relate to: outcomes of specific treatments, patterns of health care for particular patient groups e.g. antenatal care or care of people with chronic conditions, evaluation of organisations, such as hospitals or health centres and evaluation of health systems and services, that could relate to methods of payment for health care or approaches to purchasing or commissioning of health services.

Evaluation of health services

Systems of nursing care: nursing development units

Health services can be evaluated in terms of systems or organisation of services and their impact on health care and outcomes. The Nursing Development Unit (NDU) initiative is a system of nursing developments and innovations related to nursing roles, career structure and clinical practice (Turner Shaw and Bosanquet, 1993; Evans and Griffiths, 1994; Pearson, 1997). The NDU initiative arose in Burford, Tameside and then Oxford and was formally launched as a Nursing Developments Programme by the King's Fund in 1989 (Pearson, 1997). The King's Fund NDU programme was established as a focus for excellence in nursing and to improve patient care by developing nurses and nursing (Turner Shaw and Bosanquet, 1993). Four NDUs in Brighton, Camberwell, Southport and West Dorset were given pump-priming money by the King's Fund over a 3-year period. The Department of Health went on to fund the evaluation of these four units and provided funding for a further 30 demonstration sites (Moores, 1993). The evaluation of the four NDUs was undertaken by Turner Shaw and Bosanquet (1993), who described the process of setting up the units in order to gain knowledge to inform future policy and decisions on their effectiveness and benefits. They found the principle underlying the NDUs was that in order to develop clinical nursing practice it is necessary to develop nurses themselves. Improvement in the quality of patient care was taken as implicit and this would lead to an increased satisfaction for both nurses and patients. They were unable to find valid and reliable measures of these factors at the time the research was undertaken and so relied upon descriptions from the practitioners' perspective. The design of the study was a longitudinal case study approach, with data being collected at regular intervals, which allowed comparison with earlier findings.

In this way, the NDUs acted as their own 'control' over time, as Turner Shaw and Bosanquet (1993) felt it was not feasible or necessary to establish true control wards. Data were collected in two phases: the first to obtain baseline information on historical perspectives, which included how and why the NDU had been established and the specific ward chosen, and to record a profile of the structure and process of the early development of each NDU. The second phase repeated the data collection methods of phase one and examined the continuing development of the NDUs. Both quantitative and qualitative data were collected using techniques of participant observation, interview and staff questionnaires. All nursing staff who worked in the NDUs were surveyed and an 88% response rate was achieved ($n = 80$). Data were examined to provide information on the NDUs being agencies of change, costs and resources, and lessons for dissemination. Thirteen key recommendations arose from this study and it was concluded that NDUs do provide a way of developing nurses and clinical practice and they should be considered by health care organisations as providing high quality and effective care. Managers should champion NDUs and act as facilitators of developments, while the role of NDU leader was seen as discrete from that of ward manager and crucial as a change agent. Precise costings were not able to be obtained and systems need to be established so that value for money of innovations can be measured. A more recent evaluation of the King's Fund NDU programme has found that the most important features relate to development and change and the second most common feature related to carrying out research and evaluation. Where NDUs were not able to become established they had failed due to a lack of funding and managerial support (Pearson, 1997).

Continence services and primary health care teams

Another study has looked at the organisation of health services in relation to health interventions and patient outcomes on incontinence (Roe et al., 1996). An evaluation of health interventions by primary health care teams and continence advisory services on patient outcomes related to incontinence was undertaken in two health authorities, one with an established continence advisory service (CS) and one without, that opted to rely on members of its primary health care teams. The structure of both of these services was documented and compared with the recommended policy for continence services. The project comprised three stages. Stage I was a postal survey of random samples of adults in the community of the two health authorities (53% response rate, $n = 6139$). This provided a period and point prevalence of urinary incontinence (23%, 95% confidence intervals (CI) from 22.2% to 24.3% and 9%, 95% CI from 7.9% to 9.3% respectively). Information was also collected on demography and health status, using the Short Form 36 usually called the SF36 (Ware, 1993), contact with health professionals, use of formal contacts and services, health interventions and satisfaction with health care and services. Stage II went on to conduct more detailed telephone interviews with a convenience sample of incontinent people recruited from Stage I ($n = 376$) and provided further evaluation of health services and interventions on patient outcomes. Stage III was mainly a qualitative study that explored the impact of incontinence and effective and ineffective management.

The majority of people had spoken to their GP about their incontinence (71%, $n = 245$). Significantly more people with incontinence in the health authority with a continence service had completed a bladder chart to record their baseline micturition pattern and episodes of incontinence (21% $n = 49$ vs 10% $n = 25$, $x^2 = 9.9$, df = 1, p = 0.01), had seen a physiotherapist (14% $n = 25$ vs 6% $n = 10$, $x^2 = 5.6$, df = 1, p = 0.02), had received physiotherapy (8% $n = 17$ vs 2% $n = 5$, $x^2 = 6.3$, df = 1, p = 0.01) and undertook pelvic floor exercises (31% $n = 70$ vs 17% $n = 40$, $x^2 = 12.0$, df = 1, p = 0.0004) than those in the health authority without a service. This was the first study to evaluate continence advisory services and primary health care teams on patient outcomes related to incontinence. It would seem from these results that more people in the health authority with a continence service received appropriate health interventions aimed at restoration of continence, such as use of bladder charts, pelvic floor exercises and physiotherapy, although it should be noted that this health care activity was only undertaken for a minority of sufferers.

Where people had not contacted a health professional, significantly more people in the health authority without a service did not know to do so (58% $n = 34$) compared with people in the one with a continence service (33% $n = 15$) ($x^2 = 5.1$, df = 1, p = 0.02). Significantly more people in the health authority with a service indicated that they did not want treatment or help, and so had not contacted a health professional, than those in the health authority without a service (81% $n = 50$ vs 47% $n = 33$, $x^2 = 14.4$, df = 1, p = 0.0002). This demonstrates the importance of health care providers making sure that the public knows what health services are available and where to go to access these services. These findings suggest that people in the health authority with a continence service had made an informed choice not to take up the health services that were available.

Significantly more people in the health authority with a continence service were satisfied with the health services or care they had received for their incontinence than people in the health authority without a service (72% $n = 88$ vs 60% $n = 73$; $x^2 = 6.2$, df $= 2$, p $= 0.005$). This difference in satisfaction with health services was not mirrored in people's opinions of their continence status, with only a minority viewing their incontinence as cured, improved or better managed (44% $n = 192$) while the majority felt their incontinence was no different or worse (49% $n = 216$). A number of targets arose from this project related to prevalence of urinary incontinence, satisfaction with health care and continence status that could be used by purchasers and providers when evaluating their health services for people with incontinence.

Clinical audit

The drive to improve the quality of health care and health services has led to health professionals being involved with a variety of quality-assessment activities, namely clinical audit (see Chapter 16). The term 'audit' was originally limited to the examination of financial accounts but now also relates to the quality of, and change in, health care activities (Robinson, 1996). An evaluation of the progress of clinical audit in a variety of health professions, other than medicine and nursing, included professionals from clinical psychology, occupational therapy, physiotherapy and speech and language therapy (Kogan et al., 1994). The research element of the project looked at a sample of health professionals' experience of the progress of clinical audit and a development element created a framework that the professionals could use to evaluate the progress of their clinical audit work and guide the planning of future activities. Semi-structured interviews with the four sets of health professionals, and others who had an interest in the outcome of clinical audit, were undertaken in six sites. Qualitative data were collected for 135 audit activities within the six sites. Each project was categorised using the Donabedian framework (Donabedian, 1988), structure of care delivery, process of delivery and its outcomes, or a combination of these. Four main outcomes identified by the health professionals included a framework to guide analysis of their clinical audit, identification of factors that facilitated or constrained audit activity,and recognition of the potential impact of audit work along with recommendations for future progress. The researchers concluded that the development of audit by the therapy professions reflected the strengthening of health service management over the power or dominance of individual health professional groups. This was further evidenced by the topics chosen for audit being related to managerial concerns for measurable outcomes. Evidence from clinical audit was found to be useful for informing the contracting process between purchasers and providers and demonstrated the shift from solely a professional concern to one of management. This study used an evaluation approach and is a key research and development project that looked at clinical audit by health professionals in the context of health services and demonstrates the benefits of analysing empirical evidence to facilitate the development of a framework for good practice (Kogan et al., 1994; Robinson 1996).

Summary

This chapter has established that evaluation research is very much suited to investigating the impact and effect of dissemination and development work within health care and health services. Evaluation research is different from evaluation in that it utilises systematic empirical approaches, research designs and questions to measure the outcome of specific goals and objectives. Evaluation and evaluation research are not unfamiliar within clinical nursing practice. Individual outcome measures, for example the nursing process, could be collated and aggregated using case study approaches by practising nurses or other health professionals to evaluate their health care. Much larger evaluations of health services and systems can also be undertaken using standardised outcome measures. Evaluation research is particularly suitable for projects undertaking dissemination, implementation or development, and evaluation of health care or health services.

References

Bloch D (1975) Evaluation of nursing care in terms of process and outcome. Issues in research and quality assurance. Nursing Research 24: 256–63.
Bond S (1992) Outcomes of Nursing. Report no 57. Newcastle: Centre for Health Services Research, University of Newcastle.
Bond S, Tierney AJ (1992) Preface. International Journal of Nursing Studies 29(3): 229–30.
Bowling A (1991) Measuring Health. A Review of Quality of Life Measurement. Buckingham: Open University Press.
Bowling A (1995) Measuring Disease. Buckingham: Open University Press.
Button D, Roe B, Webb C, Frith T, Colin Thome D, Gardner L (1998) Consensus Guidelines for the Promotion and Management of Continence by the Primary Health Care Team. London: Whurr Publishers.
Button D, Roe B, Webb C, Frith T, Colin Thome D, Gardner L (1996) The

Development, Implementation and Evaluation of Consensus Guidelines for the Promotion and Management of Continence by Primary Health Care Teams. Unpublished Report. Runcorn: Castlefields Health Centre.

Closs SJ, Cheater FM (1994) Utilization of nursing research: culture, interest and support. Journal of Advanced Nursing 19: 762–73.

Cook S (1995) The merits of individualised outcome measures within routine clinical practice. Outcomes Briefing 6: 15–18.

Cook S, Spreadbury P (1995) Trent Occupational Therapy Clinical Audit and Outcomes Project. Sheffield: Trent Regional Health Authority.

Coulter A (1992) Evaluating the Outcomes of Health Care. In Gabe J, Calnan M (Eds) The Sociology of the Health Service. London: Routledge.

Deighan M, Hitch S (1995) Clinical Effectiveness from Guidelines to Cost-Effective Practice. Brentwood: Earlybrave Publications Ltd.

Department of Health (1991) Research for Health. A Research and Development Strategy for the NHS. London: Department of Health.

Department of Health (1993a) Research for Health. London: Department of Health.

Department of Health (1993b) Report of the Taskforce on the Strategy for Research in Nursing, Midwifery and Health Visiting. London: Department of Health.

Department of Health (1995) Making it Happen. Public health – the contribution, role and development of nurses, midwives and health visitors. Report to the Standing Nursing and Midwifery Advisory Committee. London: Department of Health.

Derryberry M (1939) Nursing accomplishments as revealed by case records. Public Health Records 54: 20-35.

Donabedian A (1966) Evaluating the quality of medical care. Millbank Memorial Fund Quarterly 44: 166–206.

Donabedian A (1969) Some issues in evaluating the quality of nursing care. American Journal of Public Health 59: 1833–6.

Donabedian A (1980) Explorations and Quality Assessment and Meaning, Vol I: The Definition of Quality and Approaches to its Assessment. Ann Arbor, MI: Health Administration Press.

Donabedian A (1988) Quality assessment and assurance: unity of purpose, diversity of means. Inquiry 25: 173–92.

Dunn G, Crichton N, Williams K, Roe B, Seers K (1997) Using research for practice: a UK experience of the Barriers Scale. Journal of Advanced Nursing. 26(6): 1203-10

Eddy DM (1990) Guidelines for policy statements: the explicit approach. Journal of the American Medical Association 263(16): 2239–43.

Effective Health Care Bulletin (1994) Implementing Clinical Practice Guidelines. December 1994, Number 8. Leeds: Nuffield Institute for Health, University of Leeds.

Evans A, Griffiths P (1994) The Development of a Nursing-Led In-Patient Service. London: King's Fund.

Fitzpatrick R (1991) Surveys of patient satisfaction. I: designing a questionnaire and conducting a survey. British Medical Journal 302: 1129–32.

Fitzpatrick R (1993) Scope and measurement of patient satisfaction. In Fitzpatrick R, Hopkins A (Eds) Measurement of Patients' Satisfaction with their Care. London: The Royal College of Surgeons.

Funk SG, Tornquist EM, Champagne MT (1989) A model for improving the dissemination of research. Western Journal of Nursing Research 11(3): 361–7.

Funk SG, Champagne MT, Wiese RA, Tornquist EM (1991) Barriers: The barriers to research utilization scale. Applied Nursing Research 4(1): 39–45.

Higgins M, McCaughan D, Griffiths M, Carr-Hill R (1992) Assessing the outcomes of nursing care. Journal of Advanced Nursing 17: 561–8.

Jamieson I (1984) Evaluation: a case of research in chains? In Adelman C (Ed) The Politics of Evaluation. London: Croom Helm.

Kazi MAF (1996) Single case evaluation in the public sector using a combination of approaches. Evaluation 2(1): 85–97.

Kitson AL (1991) Therapeutic Nursing and the Hospitalised Elderly. London: Scutari.

Klazinga N (1994) Compliance with practice guidelines: clinical autonomy revisited. Health Policy 28: 51–66.

Kogan M, Redfern S, Kober A, Norman I, Packwood T, Robinson S (1994) Clinical Audit in Four Health Professions: Report to the Department of Health. London: Nursing Research Unit, London University.

Luker K (1981) An overview of evaluation research in nursing. Journal of Advanced Nursing. 6: 87–93.

McCormick KA, Fleming B (1992) Clinical Practice Guidelines. Health Progress. December: 30–4.

McMahon R, Pearson A (1991) Nursing as Therapy. London: Chapman & Hall.

Maguire J (1991) Quality of care assessed: using senior monitor index in 3 wards for the elderly before and after change to primary nursing. Journal of Advanced Nursing 16: 511–20.

Marsland D, Gissane C (1992) Nursing evaluation: purposes, achievements and opportunities. International Journal of Nursing Studies 29(3): 231–6.

Moores Y (1993) Foreword. In Turner Shaw J, Bosanquet N (1993) A Way to Develop Nurses and Nursing. London: King's Fund.

NHSE (1996) Promoting Clinical Effectiveness. A framework for action in and through the NHS. London: Department of Health.

Oakley A (1992) Social Support and Motherhood. Oxford: Blackwell.

Oakley A, Rajan L, Grant A (1990) Social support and pregnancy outcome. British Journal of Obstetrics and Gynaecology 97: 155–62.

Pearson A (1983) The Clinical Nursing Unit. London: Heinemann.

Pearson A (1987) Outcome Measures. In Pearson A (Ed) Nursing Quality Measurement Quality Assurance Methods for Peer Review. Chichester: Wiley.

Pearson A (1991) Primary Nursing. Nursing in the Burford and Oxford Nursing Units. London: Chapman & Hall.

Pearson A (1997) An evaluation of the King's Fund Centre Nursing Development Network 1989–1991. Journal of Clinical Nursing 6(1): 25–34.

Priest J, McColl E, Thomas L, Bond S (1995) Developing and refining a new measurement tool. Nurse Researcher 2(4): 69–81.

Robinson S (1996) Evaluating the progress of clinical audit: a research and development project. Evaluation 2(4): 373–92.

Roe B, Williams K (1994) Clinical Handbook for Continence Care. London: Scutari.

Roe B, Wilson K, Doll H, Brooks P (1996) An Evaluation of Health Interventions by Primary Health Care Teams and Continence Advisory Services on Patient Outcomes Related to Incontinence. Vol I: Main Report. Oxford: Health Services Research Unit, University of Oxford.

Roper N, Logan WW, Tierney AJ (1980) The Elements of Nursing. Edinburgh: Churchill Livingstone.

Rossi PH, Freeman HE (1993) Evaluation. A Systematic Approach. London: Sage.

Scriven M (1991) The Evaluation Thesaurus. London: Sage.

Spreadbury P (1995) Measuring the outcome of individualised care. Outcomes Briefing 6: 19–21.

St Leger AS, Schneiden H, Walsworth Bell JP (1993) Evaluating Health Services' Effectiveness. Buckingham: Open University Press.

Suchman EA (1967) Evaluation Research. New York: Russell Sage Foundation.

Tones K, Tilford S (1995) Health Education. Effectiveness, Efficiency and Equity. London: Chapman & Hall.

Turner Shaw J, Bosanquet N (1993) A Way to Develop Nurses and Nursing. London: King's Fund.

UK Clearing House for Information on Health Outcomes (1993) Outcomes Briefing. Issue 1. Leeds: Nuffield Institutes for Health, University of Leeds.

Ware JE (1993) Measuring patients' views: the optimum outcome measure. SF36: a valid, reliable assessment of health from the patient's point of view. British Medical Journal 306: 1429–30.

Whelan J (1988) Ward sisters' management styles and their effects on nurses' perceptions of quality of care. Journal of Advanced Nursing 13: 125–38.

Wilkin D, Hallam L, Doggett M (1993) Measures of Need and Outcome for Primary Health Care. Oxford: Oxford Medical Publications.

Williams K, Roe B, Sindhu F (1995) An Evaluation of Nursing Developments in Continence Care. Report No 10. Oxford: National Institute for Nursing.

Yura H, Walsh MB (1978) The Nursing Process. Assessing, Planning, Implementing, Evaluating. New York: Appleton Century Crofts.

Chapter 16
The relationship between clinical audit and research

Francine M. Cheater and S. José Closs

Introduction

Audit has become an expected part of the working life of health care professionals since its formal introduction into the NHS in 1989 in an attempt to improve clinical performance (NHS Executive, 1996a). Audit programmes involving nurses, doctors, therapists and other health care practitioners have been established in most acute and community trusts and the same is true of general practice (Robinson 1996; Baker et al., 1995; Willmott et al., 1995; Stern and Brennan, 1994; Buttery et al., 1994). In addition to unidisciplinary audit, multi-disciplinary and cross-sectoral involvement in audit are increasingly encouraged (Department of Health, 1993a). Although audit was initially promoted as a professionally led activity, more recently there has been a requirement to incorporate the involvement of purchasers (Department of Health, 1993a) and patients in the process as well (Kelson, 1996; Duff et al., 1996; Department of Health, 1993a). Policy for the development of audit has subsequently evolved beyond clinical audit to a wider quality management programme (Clinical Outcomes Group, 1994; NHS Management Executive, 1994; Department of Health, 1993a). The Total Quality Management philosophy (TQM), or Continuous Quality Improvement (CQI), successfully adopted in industrial settings, has been viewed as a possible solution to promoting quality and managing change within health care settings in the UK and elsewhere (Oakland, 1993).

Alongside these developments, the drive towards evidence-based health care (clinical effectiveness) to improve patients' outcomes and value for the use of resources has gathered increased momentum.

Clinical effectiveness is one of the six priority areas identified within the Priorities and Planning Guidance for the NHS 1997/1998 (NHS Executive, 1995). Supported by a broad coalition of practitioners – researchers, educators, managers, policy makers and others – the so-called 'evidence-based health care movement' aims to accelerate and improve the application of evidence from sound research to clinical practice (Haynes et al., 1996). Clinical audit is viewed as a key component of clinical effectiveness, a tool that can be used by practitioners and purchasers to determine the extent to which effective methods of care are being implemented (NHS Executive, 1996b). There is, therefore, a clear relationship between audit and research. Research informs the development of criteria and standards for monitoring the quality of care, through the systematic process of clinical audit. Audit is a method to improve the quality of patient care through which research can be introduced into routine clinical practice.

This chapter begins by defining the purpose and nature of audit and research. The similarities and differences between the two processes are then examined according to the defined stages of the audit process. This is followed by a discussion of the purchaser's role in audit as a means of ensuring clinically effective services. Finally, the need to integrate audit within the wider context of health care quality management is addressed.

Definition of terms

Audit

Audit was formally introduced into the NHS in the late 1980s, although quality assurance within nursing has a long, established history (Kitson and Harvey, 1991; Royal College of Nursing, 1990). Among many health care practitioners, however, there still exists considerable conceptual confusion about the true purpose and nature of audit (Idall et al., 1997; Harvey, 1996). Although there are a number of similarities, the distinctions between audit and research activities are not always made clear (Closs and Cheater, 1996; Barton and Thomson, 1993). Indeed, some medical practitioners have suggested that audit is a form of research (Nixon, 1992; Russell and Wilson, 1992). The attitude that audit represents poor quality research also exists, particularly among some medical staff (Barton and Thomson, 1993). The bewildering array and inconsistent use of jargon in much of the quality management literature are also unhelpful. Professional differences in approaches and perspectives to quality assessment have also led to misunderstanding (Morrell et al., 1995; Kitson, 1994), particularly when multidisciplinary or interface audits are undertaken. The Department of Health's definition of audit has evolved since 1989. Unlike earlier versions, the most recent definition explicitly identified the need for change in response to evaluation. Audit is defined as a: 'clinically-led initiative which seeks to improve the outcomes of patient care through structured peer review whereby clinicians examine their practices and the results against agreed standards and modify their practice when indicated' (NHSE, 1996a: 2).

Audit is most often conceptualised as a systematic, cyclical or spiral process, consisting of a series of steps to monitor and improve practice. This is consistent with the concept of TQM or CQI, in which small cumulative changes contribute to significant improvement over time. Audit includes three key elements: agreed criteria for 'good' practice; methods of measuring against these criteria; and mechanisms for implementing appropriate change (Taylor, 1996; Harvey, 1996; Shaw 1990).

Research

There are numerous descriptions of research in the literature. One definition is 'an attempt to increase the available knowledge by the discovery of new facts or relationships through systematic enquiry' (Macleod Clark and Hockey, 1989: 4)

The adoption of a broad definition of research, such as the one above, befits a clinical discipline like nursing that requires a range of approaches to research, both quantitative and qualitative, in the pursuit of scientific enquiry. Narrower interpretations of research focus specifically on hypothesis testing and the generation of inference based on controlled experimental designs (explanatory research) and the application of such inferences in randomised controlled trials in a range of clinical settings (pragmatic research) (Balogh, 1996; Schwartz and Lellouch, 1967). The pragmatic randomised controlled trial (RCT) is considered to be the best method of assessing the effectiveness of clinical interventions and is the focus of evidence-based medicine (Haynes et al., 1996).

The aim of research is to generate or extend a body of scientific knowledge. Although the main purpose of clinical research is to produce new knowledge about what is best practice, evidence from descriptive, exploratory and qualitative studies often provides the essential groundwork from which problems in practice are identified and understood and hypotheses are generated and tested.

Audit is easily distinguished from research if defined according to its narrower, positivist definition, but the differences become less clear when a broader definition of research is used (Closs and Cheater, 1996; Waterman, 1996). For example, there is an abundance of descriptive, exploratory research that has identified large variations between observed and desired levels of clinical practice in nursing and other areas of health care. In the UK, for example, the pioneering research project, The Study of Nursing Care, produced a series of mainly descriptive studies about the practice of nursing that aimed to stimulate improvements in the quality of nursing care (McFarlane, 1970). The focus of this work is clearly related to audit as it provided a basis from which standards of care could subsequently be developed. However, the studies themselves did not include the formulation of standards, the measuring of performance against these standards, the implementation of change nor the measurement of improvements in practice that are the essential characteristics of audit.

However, there is one research approach, action research, that appears to be very similar to audit (Closs and Cheater, 1996; Balogh, 1996; Waterman, 1996). Superficially, the processes of action research and audit look identical. Action research is a cyclical, locally initiated problem-solving process that enables practitioners to reflect on their practice, identify areas for improvement, identify solutions and implement and monitor changes to practice (Webb, 1989). However, the aim of action research is not only to implement change but also to generate theory (Waterman, 1996; Greenwood, 1994). The generation and/or testing of theory are essential characteristics of research that differentiate it from activities such as audit. Audit may use theory but does not generate or test it (Closs and Cheater, 1996).

Purpose

Research and audit are often defined in terms of their differences in purpose (Balogh 1996; Barton and Thomson, 1993; Smith, 1992). 'Research is concerned with discovering the right thing to do; audit with ensuring that it is done right' (Smith, 1992: 905). Barton and Thomson suggested that the fundamental difference between audit and research is determined by two questions: research asks 'what should we be doing?' and audit asks 'are we doing what we should be?'

The main aim of clinical research is to establish what is effective practice, adding to a scientific body of knowledge that is generalisable. In contrast, audit is initiated by practitioners (and others) to monitor and evaluate the quality of care in local situations. The findings of audit are usually specific to the setting in which it was undertaken (Bull, 1993). Audit can be used to assess the extent to which current best evidence, determined by research, is being implemented (NHS Executive, 1996b). Doing the 'right thing', however, is not the only factor likely to influence quality. There may be differences in skills, experience, facilities and support within health care settings that also have an impact on quality (Sheldon, 1994) and may also need auditing. Similarly, access, equity, relevance, acceptability and efficiency (Maxwell, 1984) are dimensions of health care quality, in addition to effectiveness, that may also require systematic evaluation. Whereas the primary purpose of research is to contribute to a generalisable body of knowledge from which best practice can be determined, the purpose of audit is to enable practitioners to assess and improve practice in specific, local circumstances. Although audit and research are distinct as to their purpose, the two activities are similar in a number of ways and each process informs and supports the other (Closs and Cheater, 1996; Harvey, 1996; Barton and Thomson, 1993).

Links between audit and research

Research is usually motivated by existing scientific knowledge, theory and/or the interests of the researcher. Audit is usually specific to a particular setting and initiated through local needs, problems or interests (Closs and Cheater, 1996). Research is a systematic process which begins by defining a specific question or hypothesis, collecting, analysing and interpreting data and disseminating findings to the wider scientific and clinical community (Figure 16.1). The ultimate aim of research may be the improvement of health care but, with the exception of action research, the end point of the process for researchers is usually dissemination of findings, rather than the implementation and monitoring of changes per se.

Audit is also a systematic process that requires a clearly defined question, the identification of measurable criteria and target standards, the collection and analysis of data, the measurement of performance against standards, the implementation of appropriate change and re-audit to establish the extent to which local improvements have been made (Figure 16.1).

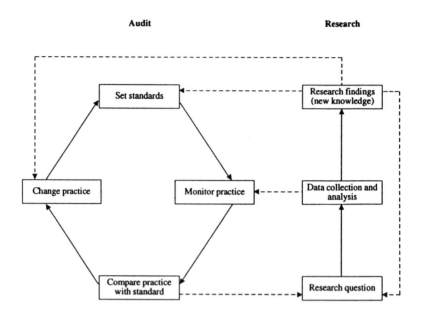

Figure 16.1: Relationship between audit and research. Reproduced with permission from Closs SJ, Cheater FM (1996) Audit or research – what is the difference? Journal of Clinical Nursing 5: 249–56.

There are clearly similarities between some of the stages of audit and research and the activities interrelate in a number of ways. The similarities, differences and links between audit and research are now discussed according to key stages of the audit process namely: identification of criteria and standards, monitoring of practice, comparison of practice with standards and implementing change.

Criteria and standards

Numerous definitions of 'criteria' and 'standards' exist in the litera-ture and the terms frequently are used interchangeably or collec-tively to mean indicators of quality. The definitions identified in Figure 16.2 are useful in clarifying the distinction between the two terms. In undertaking audit it is necessary to define precisely the element of care that denotes 'good' practice (a criterion) and to agree a quantitative level of performance (a standard) that indicates compliance with the criterion. Only if quantitative measures are used can current practice be reliably compared with best practice.

Where sound research evidence exists, it should be used to inform the development of audit criteria and standards. Thus research supports audit by determining current best practice from which evidence-based criteria can be developed. Current initiatives to promote clinical effectiveness such as evidence-based guidelines (Grimshaw et al., 1995), systematic reviews and meta-analyses produced by agencies such as the Cochrane Collaboration (Cullum, 1997; Chalmers, 1993) and the NHS Centre for Reviews and Dissemination (Sheldon and Chalmers, 1994) and publications such as effective health care bulletins (Torgerson et al., 1995), *Evidence-Based Medicine* and *Evidence-Based Nursing* can inform the development of audit criteria and standards. Important, ongoing work being undertaken to develop a nursing contribution to the Cochrane Collaboration is identifying randomised controlled trials and systematic reviews of effectiveness that specifically evaluate nursing practice (Cullum, 1997).

An audit protocol is a comprehensive set of criteria for a specific clinical condition (e.g. asthma management) or aspects of organisation (e.g hospital discharge procedure) that can be used to assess quality of care (Baker and Fraser, 1995). The Eli Lilly National Clinical Audit Centre has an established audit protocol programme that uses a systematic process for the identification of audit criteria, based on the strength of the research evidence and impact on patient outcome (Baker and Fraser, 1995). Evidence-based audit protocols are being developed in collaboration with nurses working in NHS trusts locally, in areas of care in which they have a leading role (e.g. the management of adults with urinary incontinence in the community; the management of intravenous peripheral lines). Externally developed protocols, therefore, can provide nurses and other practitioners with criteria sets derived from systematic evaluation of the available research, which they can use to undertake audit.

Criterion*

Clearly definable and precisely measurable element of care that is relevant to the definition of good quality. It must be so clearly defined that it can be said with confidence whether it is present or absent.

Standard**

The percentage of events that should comply with the criterion.

Figure 16.2: Definitions of criteria and standards.
*Royal College of General Practitioners (1994)
**Baker R, Fraser R (1995)

Where evidence is lacking, sound judgements need to be made about what constitutes best practice. This may be particularly true for disciplines such as nursing or primary care, where there are considerable gaps in the information base about effective practice. For many clinical conditions, therefore, systematically developed guidelines are likely to consist of evidence-linked and consensus-based recommendations (Grimshaw and Russell, 1993). In the UK, for example, national guidelines on topics such as the management of lymphoedema, acute pain and continence commissioned by the Department of Health (Von Degenberg and Deighan, 1995) provide nurses with a mixture of evidence-based recommendations and recommendations derived from consensus, from which audit criteria may be developed.

Although audit is predominantly concerned with the quantitative assessment of processes and outcomes of care, qualitative methods are increasingly being used to inform the development of valid criteria. Precipitated in part by the need to incorporate users' perspectives on quality of care (Kelson, 1996) a range of qualitative approaches are now being used. For example, the College of Health uses a qualitative technique called a 'consumer audit' to identify what patients, their carers and potential users think of services and want from them (Kelson, 1995). The critical incident technique (Flanigan, 1954) has been used with patients, enabling them to recall the details of a particular experience, focusing on incidents that they judged to be important to them (Kelson, 1996). Similarly, Norman et al. (1992) found the use of the critical incident technique an effective method of eliciting indicators of high and low quality of nursing care from patients and their nurses. Significant event auditing (critical event auditing) is a similar technique that has been used by members of the primary health care team to identify and define quality issues of relevance to the practice (Pringle and Bradley, 1994; Berlin et al., 1992; Bradley, 1992).

Increasingly, qualitative data, derived from focus groups and in-depth interviews, are also being used to identify issues of importance to patients in the development of patient opinion questionnaires and to highlight problems that may require evaluation (Kelson, 1996; Baker, 1993). Thus, qualitative approaches are increasingly being used in the earlier stages of audit to identify problems and to define indicators of quality, prior to the evaluative stage of the process (Closs and Cheater, 1996).

Local standards may be set according to nationally determined targets, where such information is available. For example, the *Health of the Nation* document set standards for a reduction in the prevalence of pressure sores by 5–10% per annum (Department of Health, 1991). However, the usefulness of prevalence data as an indicator of quality care is doubtful (Moffatt and Franks, 1997). Provided adjustment is made for differences in the risk of developing a sore, incidence data are preferable to prevalence data, as they produce information on pressure-sore incidence developing over time and show whether or not preventive strategies are effective (Moffatt and Franks, 1997).

The setting of standards may be determined locally to take account of variability of patients, clinical settings and resources (Baker and Fraser, 1995). Thus realistic, rather than absolute, standards may be agreed (e.g. 80% rather than 100% compliance), with the intention that new standards might be set at a higher level when the initial standards are reached and the cyclical or spiral process continued.

Monitoring practice

Asking, observing and reviewing records are the three main ways to monitor practice (Poulton, 1994). Many of the methods used to collect audit data (e.g. questionnaires, interviews, observation and record review) are therefore the same as those used in research. Also, validated instruments developed for the purpose of research, for example, symptom scales such as the Beck Depression Inventory (Beck et al., 1961), health related quality of life measures such as the Nottingham Health Profile (Hunt et al., 1986) and patient satisfaction questionnaires such as the Newcastle Satisfaction with Nursing Scales (Thomas et al., 1996) are borrowed for use in audit. Practitioners undertaking audit, like researchers carrying out research, are concerned with ensuring that data are complete and accurate. Drawing on the knowledge of research methods ensures the process of data collection is rigorous (Harvey, 1996). All practitioners are now expected to undertake audit as part of their clinical role. For the most part, therefore, audit involves collecting existing data that are readily available as part of routine clinical practice (Closs and Cheater, 1996). Researchers may also use existing data but more often the need for complex information requires the use or development of advanced data-collection methods, yielding detailed information that would not normally be required for audit (Closs and Cheater, 1996).

Sample size is another issue around which confusion between

audit and research frequently arises. In order to draw sound inferences about a population, research samples need to be of adequate
size to be representative so that the results are generalisable. The use
of unbiased sampling methods, therefore, is essential to this process.
For the purpose of a valid audit, however, sample sizes need not
necessarily be large (Barton and Thomson, 1993). Audit is applied to
local situations, and therefore the population of concern may be
small. For example, a local mental health trust audit of the management of deliberate self-harm during the previous 12 months may
identify a total of 20 patients. Thus 20 patients would comprise the
total population eligible for inclusion in this audit. In this case it is
valid to audit 20 patients and to judge whether a given standard of
care was met. Sometimes, audit of a single patient may be justified,
particularly when adverse events (such as unexpected death) occur
(Balogh, 1996; Closs and Cheater, 1996).

However, the characteristics of the population and the frequency
of the condition/problem being audited will determine the
approach needed. For example, a district-wide audit of leg ulcer
management is likely to require an unmanageably large number of
patients to be audited so sampling would be considered. A sampling
method would be chosen to ensure that the information gathered
was representative of the total population of patients with leg ulcers
in the district. Limited resources, therefore, require decisions to be
made about which areas of care should be audited. Decisions need to
take account of factors such as impact on health, number of patients
affected, willingness to change and resource implications.

Comparison of practice with standards

Where practice falls short of pre-set standards, the reasons are identified and possible solutions are agreed. Ultimately, the aim of audit
is to make appropriate changes to improve practice. More than one
change is frequently introduced concurrently and comparisons are
made from similar samples in successive cycles (re-audit) (Closs and
Cheater, 1996). It is therefore difficult, if not impossible, to show
conclusively that the interventions implemented are responsible for
any demonstrated change (Barton and Thomson, 1993). This is not
the purpose of audit, however, but rather the aim of research where
causal attributions are of fundamental concern (Balogh, 1996).
Research establishes the effectiveness of interventions in leading to
improvements in outcomes. Audit applies the evidence from
research, where appropriate, for the purpose of improving practice.

In quantitative research, statistically significant differences must be reached to determine that findings were not due to chance alone. Audit aims to produce small, incremental improvements at each cycle, not necessarily reaching statistical significance but producing clinically significant improvement over time (Closs and Cheater, 1996; Barton and Thomson, 1993). As Barton and Thomson (1993: 53) stated:

> Dismissing audit because it does not fit into the parameters of research is denying the important differences between audit and research. Equally, ignoring the methods and analytical approaches of research in the setting of audit will deny audit the access to valuable techniques and approaches.

Implementing change

As already discussed, the prime purpose of audit is to create change, where indicated. The expanding body of research concerned with effective methods of implementing change, therefore, is directly relevant to audit. Research thus not only informs the development of audit criteria and standards but also contributes to our understanding of how to effect changes in clinical practice through audit. Implementation strategies are drawn from four main theoretical bases: the social influences model; the diffusion of innovations theory; adult learning theory; and marketing approaches (Lomas, 1994). Implementation strategies include: educational materials; academic detailing/educational outreach (one-to-one and small group education); audit and feedback; reminders; opinion leaders (individuals identified as influential by their peers) (Cheater and Closs, 1997). Research involving primarily doctors suggests that active implementation strategies, rather than passive dissemination of information, are more likely to be successful in changing clinical performance (Grimshaw et al., 1995; Lomas, 1994). For example, the introduction of guidelines, through multidisciplinary academic detailing (educational outreach) targeted at general practitioners and members of the practice team, led to improvements in the recording of key data associated with effective care of diabetic patients (Feder et al., 1995).

The Framework for Appropriate Care Throughout Sheffield (FACTS) project aims to create a reproducible, effective framework for changing doctors' clinical behaviour (Hodgkin et al., 1996). The researchers concluded that there is no single way to promote change successfully. Instead, multifaceted interventions, tailored to address the barriers that are preventing change and promoted by a credible source, were found to have an appreciable effect in generating change (Hodgkin et al., 1996). However, while much can be learned from the medical literature, the transferability of these research findings to nurses and other health care practitioners is largely unknown. Research is therefore needed to identify optimally effective methods of implementing change that are targeted at nurses and other health care practitioners (Cheater and Closs, 1997).

In addition to the literature on change, a considerable body of research has evaluated the impact of audit from which valuable lessons can be learned (Baker et al., 1995; Kogan and Redfern 1995; Willmott et al., 1995; Buttery et al., 1994; Kerrison et al., 1993). For example, Walshe (1995) identified seven key characteristics of successful audit programmes based on extensive research commissioned by the Department of Health. These factors included the need for clinical leadership, a clear audit strategy, the availability of audit support staff, effective structures and systems to support audit, training and education of practitioners, and practitioners' and managers' involvement in the audit process. Similar factors for achieving effective nursing audit were identified by Kitson et al. (1994) and included: teamwork; facilitation; leadership; organisational commitment to quality improvement, and communication. Research of this nature, therefore, has the potential to improve audit activity at a strategic and organisational level by identifying the ingredients that are essential to its success.

Use of findings

Quantitative research methods that use unbiased sampling techniques produce conclusions that may be generalisable. In contrast, the results of local audit are usually specific to the population/ sample and the setting in which it was undertaken. Audit findings, therefore, should not be generalised, although the supporting methods and standards may be of value in audits elsewhere. There is an expectation that research findings will be disseminated to the wider scientific and clinical community. Audit findings, however, may be restricted to local dissemination where practice has been shown to be deficient. Audit, like research, is subject to ethical scrutiny and the rules of confidentiality apply equally (Rix and Cutting, 1996). In many instances, however, audit findings are published for dissemination to the wider clinical community. For example, it is common practice for primary care audit groups to disseminate anonymous findings from multi-practice audits so that individual practice teams can compare their level of performance with that of their peers elsewhere (Baker et al., 1995). The findings can provide a basis for constructive dialogue between peers at different practices. Audit findings from different centres, however, need to be interpreted with caution. Local resources, skill mix and patient characteristics may vary significantly, so that direct comparisons are not necessarily meaningful (Closs and Cheater, 1996). Similar criticisms have been raised in connection with the publication of outcomes data in national league tables (McKee and Hunter, 1995).

It can be seen that research supports the process of audit at a number of levels. Research also frequently generates more questions, for which other studies need to be carried out. Audit, in turn, can inform the research agenda by identifying gaps in the existing knowledge base and raising further questions for future research (Harvey, 1996). The similarities and differences between audit and research are summarised in Table 16.1.

So far, discussion has focused predominantly on the relationship between audit and research from the perspectives of providers of health services. Although the principles distinguishing audit and research are the same regardless of stakeholder (e.g. provider, purchaser or patient) it is important to consider purchasers' involvement in audit and how it links with the provision and delivery of evidence-based health services.

Purchasers' involvement in audit

Initially, audit was promoted as a professionally led activity recognising only a peripheral role for management (Lord and Littlejohns, 1995). More recently, there has been a requirement to incorporate purchasers' (including GP fundholders') interests into the process and audit has become part of contracting and service development (Department of Health, 1993a; NHS Management Executive, 1994). For example, quality specifications related to acceptability of services to patients (e.g. provision of user/carer information) or to patient access (e.g. waiting times for inpatient and outpatient appointments) derived from the Patients' Charter and the Health of the Nation standards, have become part of contract negotiations (Lord and Littlejohns, 1995). In April 1996, the new funding arrangements for audit, which were included in the overall allocation to purchasers, gave them greater influence on the content and development of audit in primary and secondary care (NHS

Table 16.1: Characteristics of clinical audit and research

	Clinical audit	Research
Purpose	To monitor and improve local clinical practice, by providing data that show what actually happens, and how it compares with a predetermined standard of best possible practice.	To extend the body of generalisable scientific knowledge in order to provide a sound basis for clinical practice.
	The ultimate aim is to improve the delivery of patient care.	The ultimate aim is to add to scientific knowledge. (The knowledge should then be used as a basis for best possible patient care.)
Type of process	Clinical audit is a systematic and critical analysis of the quality of patient care leading to improvements in practice.	Research is a process of systematic scientific enquiry which aims to discover new facts or relationships that can be generalised to populations.
	It is most commonly conceptualised as a *cyclical* process of setting desirable standards, monitoring local practice, comparing practice with the agreed standard, and changing practice if it does not reach that standard. This process should be repeated in order to reach and then maintain the required standard.	The research process is usually conceptualised as linear, beginning with the research question, reviewing the relevant literature, identifying the best methods for obtaining the required data, identifying an appropriate sample, collecting data, analysing results and publishing findings. New research questions usually arise, stimulating further research, but these are not usually a straightforward repetition of the original study.

Table 16.1: (contd)

	Clinical audit	Research
Theoretical basis	Audit is usually driven by local interests/needs/problems. It should use research findings to set standards for practice. If none is available, the results of a consensus meeting or expert local opinion are used.	Research is usually driven by existing scientific knowledge theory and/or the interests of the researcher. The underlying theory may be new or established, and is usually derived from earlier research.
Methods	Audit uses mainly data which exist by virtue of practice.	Research often involves the collection of detailed data, which require additional and sometimes sophisticated methods of data collection.
		Action research is a similar activity to audit, but in addition it tests and generates theory.
	Similar methods of data collection may be used for each, including questionnaires, interviews, record review and others.	
Sample	Clinical significance is required. It is possible to audit one patient or 1000 patients and see whether an agreed standard has been reached.	Rigorous criteria must be met in quantative sampling techniques if statistical significance is to be obtained, thereby producing results which can be generalised.
	Where unmanageably large numbers of cases are to be audited, sampling may be used to ensure a valid indication of the quality of care is obtained.	Some qualitative research employs theoretical sampling, but this does not allow generalisability.
Use of findings	Primarily by those who have been audited, allowing them to use the findings as a basis for improving their own practice.	Should be widely disseminated, so that findings are accessible to all those who may have an interest.

Table 16.1: (contd)

	Clinical audit	Research
	Multicentre audits may stimulate debate and exchange of ideas between centres.	Provide a base for best possible practice as well as for audit standards.
		Stimulate new research questions.
	Where large audit data sets have been obtained via careful sampling techniques, data may sometimes be used for research purposes.	
Confidentiality	Important for clinical staff. Confidentiality allows practitioners to be more honest about clinical problems and their attempts to solve them.	Confidentiality for research subjects is accepted ethical practice.
Time frame	Changes in practice should be made as an integral part of the audit process.	It may take years for research findings to change practice, if they are used at all.

Reproduced with permission from Closs SJ, Cheater FM (1996) Audit or researcher – what is ther difference? Journal of Clinical Nursing 5: 249–560.

Executive, 1996c). Purchasers were expected to have a more active role in audit, including negotiation over the choice of audit topics, to reflect local, regional and national priorities. Indeed, NHS Executive guidance suggested that purchasers' concerns may constitute 40% of their local providers' audit programmes (NHS Management Executive, 1994). Quality specifications in contracts are now commonly used by purchasing authorities, although they are often rudimentary, open to different interpretations and inconsistently applied (Gray and Donaldson, 1996; Rumsey et al., 1994). Additionally, there is increasing pressure on purchasers to negotiate contracts with providers on agreed patterns of care that are clinically effective (NHS Executive, 1995). The expectation is that purchasers should 'spend as much time successfully challenging ineffective or inappropriately accessed practices as trying to contract within budget' (Gill, 1993: 18).

Linked to this, purchasers have been encouraged to use contracts to introduce systematically developed guidelines to their providers, in order to increase clinical effectiveness (NHS Executive, 1995). Guidelines are expected to be linked to purchasers' and providers' audit programmes and to promote dialogue on the effectiveness of underlying clinical practice. Consequently, purchasing authorities require robust, external mechanisms for monitoring adherence to clinical standards and guidelines that complement, and are compatible with, their providers' internal audit monitoring activities (Miles et al., 1996). As yet, few purchasing authorities appear to have adequate monitoring mechanisms in place (Miles et al., 1996; Rumsey et al., 1994).

The use of audit for contract monitoring has predictably led to tensions between purchasers and providers (Cheater and Keane, 1996; Thomson et al., 1996; Rumsey et al., 1994).

Purchasers may place greater emphasis on the potential of audit to influence purchasing decisions. Providers are interested in achieving improvements in patient care, whereas purchasers may emphasise a need to identify where good and poor practice occurs (Thomson et al., 1996). Purchasers and providers often hold generalised assumptions about each other that may prevent effective dialogue between the two professional groups (Littlejohns et al., 1996; Thomson et al., 1996). Differences partly reflect the contrasting organisational aims of purchasers and providers.

Until recently, many purchasers have not chosen to, or have been unable to, use audit as a stimulus for change or as a source of information on clinical effectiveness (Cheater and Keane, 1996; Lord and

Littlejohns, 1995; Rumsey et al., 1994). This situation may be slowly changing and purchaser–provider interaction may be beginning to make some impact on clinical audit (Thomson et al., 1996) as part of a wider framework to promote clinical effectiveness (Department of Health, 1993). However, to date, there is little evidence to suggest that service contracts themselves are effective in achieving the desired quality improvements in health services, although there has been little rigorous evaluation of the process (Miles et al., 1996). Gray and Donaldson (1996) suggest that rather than continuintg to rely on quality specifications in contracting, greater efforts should be directed towards creating effective management of quality improvement through enhanced collaboration between purchasers and their providers. Indeed, good professional relationships between purchasers and providers have been identified as the key to successful audit programmes (Walshe, 1995).

Purchasers clearly have a central role in promoting and monitoring the use of clinically effective practices in their providers, and audit provides one mechanism through which this may be achieved. However, what strongly emerges from the literature is the need for this to take place within a mutually supportive and collaborative relationship, if genuine improvements in patient care are to result (Thomson et al., 1996; Walshe, 1995; Thomson and Barton, 1994).

Integration of audit into wider quality initiatives

Since audit was first introduced into the NHS, national policy has promoted its integration into wider quality programmes (Clinical Outcomes Group, 1994; Department of Health, 1993a). There was a growing recognition that any approach to improving quality of health care has to be integrated to have any chance of success. As funding and responsibility for monitoring audit came under the control of local purchasers, the organisation of audit by many providers has come under review. Increasingly, audit was viewed as one aspect of quality that should link explicitly with other systems for quality improvement as part of a provider's overall organisational strategy (Department of Health, 1993b). Hence, the expectation that audit would inter-relate with organisations' existing systems for patients' complaints and risk management, continuing education and research and development. For example, issues emerging from patients' complaints or risk management may generate priorities for clinical audit. Evidence of the clinical effectiveness of interventions provides the basis for standards that are monitored in audit programmes (as discussed earlier) and where shortfalls in the quality of care are identified, educational interventions may be required. Where evidence is lacking, the need for research and development is identified.

Evaluation of the audit programmes suggested that, initially, few providers succeeded in linking these different but related activities (Buttery et al., 1994), although subsequently developments towards greater integration have occurred (Cheater and Keane, 1996). However, the historical division between clinical and managerial aspects of quality has produced artificial professional and departmental boundaries that have, in some cases, been difficult to break down (Cheater and Keane, 1996; Moss and Garside, 1995).

Numerous national and local developments are under way that are testing and evaluating integrative approaches to quality improvement. For example, the Assisting Clinical Effectiveness (ACE) Project is a joint venture between providers and purchasers, with patient involvement, to implement evidence-based guidelines linked to clinical audit and continuing professional development (Humphris and Littlejohns, 1996). The lessons that are emerging from such projects will be useful to providers and purchasers who are grappling with the complexities of establishing coherent approaches to quality improvement.

Total Quality Management

The total quality management (TQM) (or continuous quality improvement (CQI)) approach has been viewed as a possible way of organising and involving the whole organisation in improving the efficiency and quality of services in the NHS. One definition of TQM is: 'a participative, systematic approach to planning and implementing a continuous organisational improvement process' (Kaluzny et al., 1992: 257).

This approach focuses on establishing procedures that ensure consistent quality rather than controlling problems after they have arisen (Potter et al., 1994). Joss and Kogan (1995) suggested that TQM provides the umbrella under which a great number of quality initiatives, including audit, could be managed within an organisation. Imported from the setting of industry, TQM has primarily been a management-led initiative, the principles of which have been adapted and implemented in a number of acute and primary care settings with varying degrees of success.

An evaluation of the effectiveness of TQM programmes in 17 departments of NHS organisations indicated that none of them fully met all the criteria for success (Pollitt, 1996; Joss and Kogan, 1995). A number of conceptual and organisational difficulties in applying the principles of TQM were identifed. Applying a corporate approach to quality, as in TQM, within the culture of the NHS, in which strong, professional groups and systems and approaches to quality already exist, was one of the main difficulties encountered (Joss and Kogan 1995; Potter et al., 1994). However, a recent study of the application of TQM principles in 18 general practices indicated that beneficial changes were achieved in most practices (Lawrence and Packwood, 1996). It may be easier to implement TQM in smaller, more contained organisations like general practices rather than in larger, more complex health care environments such as acute hospitals. Nevertheless, what clearly emerges from the literature is that wholesale adoption of quality improvement approaches originating in the private sector is unlikely to be successful in the NHS without considerable adaptation. The implementation process itself demands considerable time and resources. Pollitt (1996: 108) provides a very useful analysis of the use of business approaches to quality improvement in the NHS and concludes: 'There remains, therefore, a middle way. The aim would be to combine the strengths of professionalism with the insights and dynamism of commercial consumerism, while discarding the weaknesses of both.' Whether or not TQM programmes in health care settings are sustainable and cost-effective approaches to quality management has still to be determined. On logical grounds alone it is clearly desirable to ensure that quality approaches in health organisations, including audit, are coordinated and integrated and not, as is still frequently the case, discrete, episodic 'bolt-on extras'.

Summary

It is clear that there are many similarities between the processes of conducting audit and undertaking research. Each has a complementary but distinct purpose: research generates the evidence that determines what is best practice, while audit is a method through which sound research evidence can be applied to routine clinical practice. Audit was introduced into the NHS at a time of great change in the organisation and delivery of health services. In the hurly-burly, the essential purpose of audit and its relationship to research has sometimes become muddled. Effective audit is the key to promoting clinical effectiveness and nurses have an enormous role to play in this endeavour. Without a clear understanding of the differences as well as the linkages between audit and research, however, there is a real danger that neither activity will fully achieve its ultimate objective of improving the quality of patient care. The formal implementation of audit in the NHS has identified many valuable lessons from which to learn for the future. The need for audit to be a two-way, collaborative interaction between health professionals and purchasers, if decision making is to become genuinely evidence based, is one of the key messages that has emerged. Similarly audit, to be fully effective, needs to be firmly integrated into a wider quality management approach, which transcends professional, managerial and organisational boundaries. This is a complex task and one that is fraught with difficulties. However, innovative work at both national and local level is being undertaken to try to establish how this can be achieved most effectively. The aim of the NHS is: 'to secure, through the resources available, the greatest possible improvement in the physical and mental health of the population' (NHS Executive, 1996b). Used appropriately and effectively, audit and research are fundamental to achieving this aim.

References

Baker R (1993) Focus groups. Audit Trends 1: 106–7.

Baker R, Fraser R (1995) Development of review criteria: linking guidelines and assessment of quality. British Medical Journal 311: 370–3.

Baker R, Hearnshaw H, Copper A, Cheater F, Robertson N (1995) Assessing the work of the medical audit advisory groups promoting audit in general practice. Quality in Health Care 4 (4): 234–9.

Balogh R (1996) Exploring the links between audit and the nursing process. Nurse Researcher 3(3): 5–16.

Barton A, Thomson R (1993) Is audit bad research? Audit Trends 1: 51–3.

Beck A, Ward C, Mendelson M (1961) An inventory for measuring depression. Archives of General Psychiatry 4: 561–71.

Berlin A, Spencer J, Bhopal R, Van Zvanenberg T (1992) Audit of deaths in general practice: pilot study of the critical incident technique. Quality in Health Care 2(1): 231–5.

Bradley C (1992) Turning anecdotes into data: the critical incident technique. Family Practice 9: 98–103.

Bull A (1993) Audit and research: complementary but distinct. Annals of the Royal College of Surgeons of England 75: 308–11.

Buttery Y, Walshe K, Coles J, Bennet J (1994) The development of audit. Findings of a national survey of health care providers units in England. London: CASPE Research.

Chalmers I (1993) The Cochrane Collaboration: preparing, maintaining and disseminating systematic reviews of the effects of health care. Annals New York Academy of Science 703: 156–63.

Cheater F, Closs S (1997) The effectiveness of methods of dissemination and implementation of clinical guidelines for nursing practice. A selective review. Journal of Clinical Effectiveness in Nursing 1(1): 4–15.

Cheater F, Keane M (1995) An evaluation of the development of clinical audit in the North West Region. Research Report No. 6. Leicester: Eli Lilly National Clinical Audit Centre, Department of General Practice and Primary Health Care, University of Leicester.

Clinical Outcomes Group (1994) Clinical Audit in Primary Care. Report of the Primary Health Care Clinical Audit Working Group. London: Department of Health.

Closs SJ, Cheater FM (1996) Audit or research – what is the difference? Journal of Clinical Nursing 5: 249–56.

Cullum N (1997) Identification and analysis of randomised controlled trials in nursing: a preliminary study. Quality in Health Care 6(1): 2–6.

Department of Health (1991) Health of the Nation. London: HMSO.

Department of Health (1993a) Clinical Audit. Meeting and Improving Standards of Care. London: HMSO.

Department of Health (1993b) Health Circular 93/553. Press Release, 11 February. London: HMSO.

Duff L, Kelson M, Marriot S, McIntosh A, Brown S, Cape J, Marcus N, Traynor M (1996) Clinical guidelines: involving patients and users of services. Journal of Clinical Effectiveness 1(3): 104–11.

Feder G, Griffiths C, Highton C, Elridge S, Spence S, Southgate L (1995) Do clinical guidelines introduced with a practice based education improve the care of asthmatic and diabetic patients ? A randomised controlled trial in general practices in East London. British Medical Journal 311: 1473–8.

Flanigan W (1954) The critical incident technique. Psychological Bulletin 51: 327–58.

Gill M (1993) Purchasing for quality: still in the starting blocks? Quality in Health Care 2: 1117–18.

Gray J, Donaldson L (1996) Improving the quality of health care through contracting: a study of health authority practice. Quality in Health Care 5 (4): 201–5.

Greenwood J (1994) Action research: a few details, a caution and something new. Journal of Advanced Nursing. 20: 13–18.

Grimshaw J, Russell I (1993) Achieving health care through clinical guidelines, 1: Developing scientifically valid guidelines. Quality in Health Care 2: 243–8.

Grimshaw J, Freemantle N, Wallace S, Russell I, Hurwitz B, Watt I, Long A, Sheldon T (1995) Developing and implementing clinical practice guidelines. Quality in Health Care 4: 55–64.

Harvey G (1996) Relating quality assessment and audit to the research process in nursing. Nurse Researcher 3(3): 35–46.

Haynes R, Sackett D, Muir Gray J, Cook D, Guyatt G (1996) Transferring evidence from research into practice: 1. The role of clinical care research evidence in clinical decisions. Evidence-Based Medicine 1(7): 196–7.

Hodgkin P, Eve R, Golton I, Munro J, Musson G (1996) Changing clinical behaviour on a city-wide scale: lessons from the FACTS project. Journal of Clinical Effectiveness 1(1): 8–10.

Humphris D, Littlejohns P (1996) Implementing clinical guidelines: linking learning and clinical audit. Audit Trends 4 (2): 59–62.

Hunt S (1984) The Nottingham health profile. In Wenger N, Mattson M, Furberg C, Elinson J (Eds) Assessment of Quality of Life in Clinical Trials of Cardiovascular Therapies. New York: Le Jacq.

Hunt SM, McEwan J, McKenna SP (1986) Measuring Health Status. London: Croom Helm.

Idall E, Rooke L, Hamrin E (1997) Quality indicators in clinical nursing: a review of the literature. Journal of Advanced Nursing 25: 6–17.

Joss R, Kogan M (1995) Advancing Quality: Total Quality Management in the National Health Service. Buckingham: Open University Press.

Kaluzny A, McLaughlin C, Simpson K (1992) Applying Total Quality Management concepts to Public Health Organisations. Public Health Reports – Hyattsville 107(3): 257–64.

Kelson M (1995) Consumer involvement in clinical audit and outcomes. London: College of Health.

Kelson M (1996) User involvement in clinical audit: a review of developments and issues of good practice. Journal of Evaluation in Clinical Practice 1 (2): 97–109.

Kerrison S, Packwood T, Buxton M (1993) Medical Audit: Taking Stock. London: King's Fund Centre.

Kitson A (1994) Achievements with quality improvement in the NHS. Quality in Health Care 3 (Suppl.): S25–30.

Kitson A, Harvey G (1991) Bibliography of Nursing: Quality Assurance and Standards of Care 1932–1987. London: Scutari Press.

Kitson A, Harvey G, Hyndman S, Sindhu F, Yerrell P (1994) The impact of a nursing quality assurance approach, the Dynamic Standard Setting System (DySSSy) on nursing practice and patient outcomes (the ODyDDDy project). Report No. 4, Vols 1, 2, 3. Oxford: National Institute for Nursing.

Kogan M, Redfern S (1995) Making Use of Clinical Audit. A Guide to Practice in the Health Professions. Buckingham: Open University Press.

Lawrence M, Packwood T (1996) Adapting total quality management for general practice; evaluation of a programme. Quality in Health Care 5(3): 151–8.

Littlejohns P, Dumelow C, Griffiths S (1996) Implementing a national clinical effectiveness policy: developing relationships between purchasers and clinicians. Journal of Clinical Effectiveness 1(4): 124–8.

Lomas J (1994) Teaching old (and not so old) docs new tricks: effective ways to implement research findings. In Dunn E (Ed) Disseminating Research Findings /Changing Behaviour. Research Methods for Primary Care. Volume 6. Newbury Park, CA: Sage Publications. pp. 1–18.

Lord J, Littlejohns P (1995) Are purchasers ready for clinical audit? In Walshe K (Ed) Evaluating clinical audit: past lessons, future directions. Proceedings of a conference organised by the Royal Society of Medicine and CASPE Research with the support of the Department of Health. pp. 55–70.

McFarlane J (1970) The Proper Study of the Nurse. London: Royal College of Nursing.

McKee M, Hunter D (1995) Mortality league tables; do they inform or mislead? Quality in Health Care 4: 5–12.

Macleod Clark J, Hockey L (1989) Further Research for Nursing. London: Scutari Press.

Maxwell R (1984) Quality assessment in health. British Medical Journal 12: 1470–2.

Miles A, Bentley P, Price N, Polychronis A (1996) Purchasing quality in clinical practice: Precedents and problems. In Miles A, Lugon M (Eds) Effective Clinical Practice. Oxford: Blackwell Science. pp. 183–204.

Moffatt C, Franks P (1997) Pressure sore risk: a challenge in the community. British Journal of Community Health Nursing 2(2): 96–105.

Morrell C, Harvey G, Kitson A (1995) The reality of practitioner-based quality improvement. A review of the use of the Dynamic Standard Setting System in the NHS of the 1990s. National Institute of Nursing. Report No. 14. Oxford: National Institute of Nursing.

Moss F, Garside P (1995) The importance of quality: sharing the responsibility for improving patient care. British Medical Journal 310: 996–9.

NHS Executive (1995) Improving the effectiveness of clinical services. EL(95) 105. Leeds: NHS Executive.

NHS Executive (1996a) Clinical Audit in the NHS. Using Clinical Audit in the NHS: a position statement. Leeds: NHS Executive.

NHS Executive (1996b) Promoting Clinical Effectiveness. A framework for action in and through the NHS. Leeds: Department of Health.

NHS Executive (1996c) EL (95) 103 NHS Executive letter. Leeds: NHS Executive.

NHS Management Executive (1994) Clinical audit : 1994/95 and beyond. EL (94) 20. National Health Service Management Executive. Leeds: Department of Health.

Nixon S (1992) Defining essential hospital data. In Smith R (Ed) Audit in Action. London: British Medical Journal.

Norman I, Redfern S, Tomalin D, Oliver S (1992) Developing Flanigan's Critical Incident Technique to elicit indicators of high and low quality nursing care from patients and their nurses. Journal of Advanced Nursing 17: 590–600.

Oakland J (1993) Total Quality Management. 2nd edn. Oxford: Butterworth-Heinemann.

Poulton B (1994) Setting standards of nursing care. Nursing Standard 14(51): 3–8.

Pringle M, Bradley C (1994) Significant event auditing: a users' guide. Audit Trends 2: 20–3.

Pollitt C (1996) Business approaches to quality improvement: why they are hard for the NHS to swallow. Quality in Health Care 5(2): 104–10.

Potter C, Morgan P, Thompson G (1994) CQI in an acute hospital. A report of an action research project in three hospital departments. International Journal of Health Care Quality Assurance 7(1): 4–29.

Rix G, Cutting K (1996) Clinical audit, the case for ethical scrutiny? International Journal of Quality in Health Care 9(6): 18–20.

Robinson S (1996) Audit in the therapy professions: some constraints on progress. Quality in Health Care 5(4): 206–14.

Royal College of General Practitioners (1994) Quality and Audit in General Practice: Meanings and Definitions. London: RCGP.

Royal College of Nursing (1990) Quality Patient Care: the Dynamic Standard Setting System. London: Scutari Press.

Rumsey M, Foster J, Walshe K, Coles J (1994) The Role of the Commissioner in Audit. London: CASPE Research.

Russell I, Wilson B (1992) Audit: the third clinical science? Quality in Health Care 1: 51–5.

Schwartz D, Lellouch J (1967) Explanatory and pragmatic attitudes in clinical trials. Journal of Chronic Diseases 20: 637–48.

Shaw C (1990) Criterion-based audit. British Medical Journal 300: 649.

Sheldon T (1994) Quality: link with effectiveness. Quality in Health Care. Raising Quality in the NHS: Progress 3 (suppl.): S41–5.

Sheldon T, Chalmers I (1994) The UK Cochrane Centre and the NHS Centre for Reviews and Dissemination: respective roles within the Information Systems Strategy of the NHS R&D Programme, co-ordination and principles underlying collaboration. Health Economics 3: 201–3.

Smith R (1992) Audit and research. British Medical Journal 305: 905–6.

Stern M, Brennan S (1994) Medical Audit in the Hospital and Community Health Service. London: Department of Health.

Taylor D (1996) Quality and professionalism in health care: a review of current initiatives in the NHS. British Medical Journal 312: 626–9.

Thomas L, McColl E, Priest J, Bond S, Boys R (1996) Newcastle satisfaction with nursing scales: an instrument for quality assessment of nursing care. Quality in Health Care 5(2): 67–72.

Thomson R, Barton A (1994) Is audit running out of stream? Quality in Health Care 3(4): 225–9.

Thomson R, Elcoat C, Pugh E (1996) Clinical audit and the purchaser–provider interaction: different attitudes and expectations in the United Kingdom. Quality in Health Care 5(2): 97–103.

Torgerson D, Ryan M, Donaldson C (1995) Effective Health Care Bulletins: are they efficient? Quality in Health Care 4(1): 48–51.

Von Degenberg K, Deighan M (1995) Guideline development: a model of multi-professional collaboration. In Clinical Effectiveness from Guidelines to Cost Effective Practice. London: Department of Health. pp. 93–109.

Walshe K (1995) The traits of success in clinical audit. Evaluating clinical audit: past lessons, future directions. Proceedings of a conference organised by the Royal Society of Medicine and CASPE Research with the support of the Department of Health, 27 April 1995. pp. 13–21.

Waterman H (1996) A comparison between quality assurance and action research. Nurse Researcher 3(3) 58–68.

Webb C (1989) Action research: philosophy, methods and personal experience. Journal of Advanced Nursing 14: 403–10.

Willmott M, Forster J, Walshe K, Coles J (1995) A Review of Audit Activity in the Nursing and Therapy Professions. London: CASPE Research.

Chapter 17
Research and development in clinical nursing practice: the future

Brenda Roe and Christine Webb

Introduction

The purpose of this chapter is to summarise the main messages and lessons from preceding chapters on research methods and developments and provide suggestions for future directions for research and development initiatives related to clinical nursing practice.

Research in context

It is apparent that any research and development of clinical nursing practice is set in the wider context nationally and internationally of health care or health services research and the strengthening of research capacity for all health professionals. It forms part of the strategies for health services research and consequently faces competition for necessary resources. All of this is in the context of evidence-based health care and clinical effectiveness so that activities based upon custom and practice alone are eradicated in pursuit of cost-effective and efficient health services.

Nursing and nurses have had a long tradition of questioning the basis of clinical practice and endeavouring to improve patient care from the days of Florence Nightingale to the present (Abdellah and Levine, 1965). A variety of evolving research methods are available and it would appear that the nature of the research question asked determines the methods used rather than being fixed by or arguing for a naturalist versus positivist stance, which is anachronistic. This reflects the maturity of research and development within clinical nursing practice and the capabilities of those undertaking it. It is now generally accepted that a mix of methodological approaches has a lot to offer in answering questions, generating theory, providing evidence of cause or effect and elucidating context. There are strengths in qualitative and quantitative research and whether a study is large or small is no longer relevant. What is of more relevance is whether the research question is the right one and whether the research has been rigorously undertaken using the correct research design and methods involving an appropriate population and sample, sampling techniques and sample size. Data management and analysis should also be appropriate with particular attention to reliability, validity, health care processes and outcomes. Methods should be clearly documented so that it is clear how the work has been executed throughout every stage.

The chapters on qualitative and quantitative research methods provide clear guidance on how they may be used and considerations to be made. The importance of sampling techniques for all research, the rigorous analysis of data, their interpretation and the claims that can be made for the sample studied and wider populations is apparent. Literature searching, systematic reviews and meta-analyses are now acknowledged as research projects and methods in their own right. Rigorous searching and handling of published literature, unpublished research projects and their interpretations from pooled data are important irrespective of the research designs and methods chosen. Systematic reviews are not just limited to quantitative data but may also include qualitative research (Jensen and Allen, 1996; Rogers et al., 1996). Establishing the processes of nursing as well as their impact are essential outcomes. The economic impact of clinical nursing, in terms of direct and indirect costs as well as health outcomes, has been a neglected area (Drummond and Maynard, 1993) and should be strengthened in future studies. This may assist with providing evidence to establish the unique nature or value of nursing and its important contribution to health care and health services. There is some evidence that nurses working as clinical nurse specialists, such as community psychiatric nurses (Brooker and Butterworth, 1991), stoma nurse specialists (Wade, 1990), respiratory nurse specialists (Heslop and Bagnall, 1988), dermatology nurse specialists (Ersser et al., 1995), paediatric home care teams (While, 1991) or nurse practitioners (Brown and Grimes, 1993; Touche Ross, 1994; Richardson and Maynard, 1995), having clear clinical responsibilities, do improve patient outcomes. The incorporation of health economic data and cost effectiveness data in future studies investigating the role of nursing would be very beneficial.

Future research in clinical nursing practice requires the systematic reviewing of relevant evidence, well designed studies, their rigorous execution and interpretation along with comprehensive dissemination via publication and conference presentations. Continued efforts through research and development are required to obtain the evidence from which to inform the basis of clinical nursing practice and this remains an ongoing challenge.

Development of clinical nursing practice

The development component of research and development has only been a recent feature of health services research policy (Department of Health, 1993a, b; Roe, 1997) although development and innovation have been a feature of clinical nursing practice for some time. This has notably been in the form of nursing development units (NDUs), which have established initiatives related to nursing roles, career structures and clinical practice (Turner Shaw and Bosanquet, 1993; Evans and Griffiths, 1994; Pearson, 1997). Some of the early development initiatives (D) were not evaluated by empirical research (R), having the D component but not the R of R and D, although this was rectified in later studies (Turner Shaw and Bosanquet, 1993; Evans and Griffiths, 1994; Pearson, 1997).

Clinical nursing practice will continue to be developed by ensuring that rigorous research, based upon appropriate research questions and sound methodologies, continues to be undertaken. This can be achieved by ensuring that there are adequate opportunities and funding along with training scholarships for nurses to undertake research either as part of individual projects or as part of larger multidisciplinary research projects and teams. The research capability and capacity of nurses could also be further developed by ensuring they have knowledge and understanding of research methodologies and critical appraisal skills, so that evidence, as well as experience, is used to underpin their clinical practice. This would also assist them in raising questions about clinical practice they deemed no longer appropriate or that could be improved. Such initiatives for the development of research capacity within nursing have been clearly advocated in national policy (Department of Health, 1993b). This could be further assisted by the general development within health services of using evidence-based medicine (EBM) or health care (EBHC) along with evidence of clinical effectiveness (CE) to underpin all clinical practice (Kitson, 1997). The EBM language and terminology has been adapted for nursing (EBN) and it is envisaged that this evidence base will continue to be developed in the future (Cullum et al., 1997). The use of EBM, EBN and guidelines for health care practice based on clinical effectiveness is part of a larger national and international dissemination strategy, incorporating initiatives such as the Cochrane Library, so that health care is based upon evidence of effectiveness and that based upon unquestioned custom and practice is eradicated. It is anticipated that by adopting these approaches, clinical nursing practice and health care will be ultimately based on sound evidence of clinical and cost effectiveness ensuring efficient health services of determined quality. The incorporation of guidelines and EBM and EBN into general health services management for both purchasers and providers will also help to ensure their continued development within health care practice along with evaluation and incorporation into clinical audit. This would complete the research, development, evaluation and audit loop of managed quality health care systems.

Summary

Research and the development of clinical nursing practice continues to evolve as an academic and applied subject in its own right, as well as being part of the larger initiatives in health services and health care based upon strategies and policy for research, development, dissemination, utilisation, evaluation and audit. Continued opportunities and funding are required to increase the research capacity and capabilities of nurses and nursing so that the art and science of clinical nursing practice continues to be identified, understood and improved and the care given to patients is based upon sound empirical evidence.

References

Abdellah FG, Levine E (1965) Better Patient Care Through Nursing Research. London: Macmillian.
Brooker C, Butterworth T (1991) Working with families caring for a relative with schizophrenia: the evolving role of the community psychiatric nurse. International Journal of Nursing Studies 28(2): 189–200.
Brown S, Grimes D (1993) A Meta-Analysis of Care, Clinical Outcomes and Cost Effectiveness of Nurses in Primary Care Roles, Nurse Practitioners and Certified Nurse Midwives. Washington, DC: American Nurses Association.
Cullum N, DiCenso A, Ciliska D (1997) Evidence-based nursing: an introduction.

Nursing Standard 11(28): 32–3.

Department of Health (1993a) Research for Health. London: Department of Health.

Department of Health (1993b) Report of the Taskforce on the Strategy for Research in Nursing, Midwifery and Health Visiting. London: Department of Health.

Drummond MF, Maynard A (1993) Purchasing and Providing Cost-Effective Health Care. Edinburgh: Churchill Livingstone.

Ersser SJ, Venables J, Kaur V (1995) An Account of the Work and Role of a Clinical Lecturer Based in the Department of Dermatology Oxford 1990–1992. Unpublished Report. Oxford: National Institute for Nursing.

Evans A, Griffiths P (1994) The Development of a Nursing-Led In-Patient Service. London: King's Fund.

Heslop A, Bagnall P (1988) A study to evaluate the intervention of a nurse visiting patients with disabling chest disease in the community. Journal of Advanced Nursing 13: 71–7.

Jensen LA, Allen MN (1996) Meta-synthesis of qualitative findings. Qualitative Health Research 6(4), 553–60.

Kitson A (1997) Using evidence to demonstrate the value of nursing. Nursing Standard 11(28): 34–9.

Pearson A (1997) An evaluation of the King's Fund Centre Nursing Development Network 1989–1991. Journal of Clinical Nursing 6(1): 25–34.

Richardson G, Maynard A (1995) Fewer Doctors? More Nurses? A Review of the Knowledge Base of Doctor–Nurse Substitution. Discussion Paper 135. York: University of York.

Roe B (1997) Some observations on policy for research and development in the NHS. Journal of Clinical Nursing 6(3): 171.

Rogers A, Williams G, Popay J (1996) Rationale and standards for systematic review of qualitative literature in health services research. Conference proceedings. Qualitative Health Research Conference, Bournemouth: 50.

Touche Ross (1994) Evaluation of Nurse Practitioner Pilot Projects. London: Touche Ross/South Thames RHA/NHSE.

Turner Shaw J, Bosanquet N (1993) A Way to Develop Nurses and Nursing. London: King's Fund.

Wade BE (1990) Colostomy patients: psychological adjustment at 10 weeks and one year after surgery in districts which employed stoma care nurses and districts which did not. Journal of Advanced Nursing 15: 1297–304.

While AE (1991) An evaluation of a paediatric home care scheme. Journal of Advanced Nursing 16: 1413–21.

Index